Hematology

Hematology
Pathophysiologic Basis for Clinical Practice
Third Edition

Edited by

Stephen H. Robinson, M.D.

George C. Reisman Professor of Medicine, Harvard Medical
School; Chief of Hematology and Associate Chief of
Medicine, Beth Israel Hospital, Boston

Paul R. Reich, M.D.

Lecturer in Medicine, Harvard Medical School, Boston;
Vice President for Medical Affairs, Pilgrim Health Care, Inc.,
Norwell, Massachusetts

Little, Brown and Company
Boston/Toronto/London

Library of Congress Cataloging-in-Publication Data

Hematology : pathophysiologic basis for clinical practice / edited by Stephen H. Robinson and Paul R. Reich.—3rd ed.
   p. cm.
   Rev. ed. of: Hematology / Paul R. Reich. 2nd ed. c1984.
   Includes bibliographical references and index.
   ISBN 0-316-73864-6
   1. Hematology. 2. Anemia. 3. Myeloproliferative disorders.
I. Robinson, Stephen H. II. Reich, Paul Richard. Hematology.
   [DNLM: 1. Hematologic Diseases—physiopathology. WH 100
H4874533]
   RB145.R44 1993
   616.1′5′071–dc20
   DNLM/DLC   92-48886
   for Library of Congress   CIP

Printed in the United States of America

MV-NY

Contents

Contributing Authors

Kenneth A. Bauer, M.D.
Associate Professor of Medicine, Harvard Medical School;
Chief, Hematology-Oncology Section, Brockton/West
Roxbury Veterans Administration Medical Center and
Associate Physician, Beth Israel Hospital, Boston

Glenn J. Bubley, M.D.
Assistant Professor of Medicine, Harvard Medical School;
Attending Physician, Department of Medicine, Beth Israel
Hospital, Boston

Justine Meehan Carr, M.D.
Instructor in Pathology, Harvard Medical School; Medical
Director, Hematology Laboratory, Beth Israel Hospital,
Boston

Steven E. Come, M.D.
Associate Professor of Medicine, Harvard Medical School;
Director, Hematology-Oncology Division, Beth Israel
Hospital, Boston

Joseph Paul Eder, Jr., M.D.
Assistant Professor of Medicine, Harvard Medical School;
Associate Physician, Department of Medicine, Beth Israel
Hospital, Boston

Stacey M. Gore, M.D.
Instructor in Medicine, Harvard Medical School; Associate
Physician in Medicine, Hematology-Oncology Department,
Harvard Community Health Plan, Boston

Marshall E. Kadin, M.D.
Associate Professor of Pathology, Harvard Medical School;
Director of Hematopathology and Senior Pathologist, Beth
Israel Hospital, Boston

Margot S. Kruskall, M.D.
Associate Professor of Pathology and Assistant Professor of Medicine, Harvard Medical School; Medical Director of Blood Bank, Beth Israel Hospital, Boston

Roger F. Lange, M.D.
Assistant Clinical Professor of Medicine, Harvard Medical School; Associate Physician, Department of Medicine, Beth Israel Hospital, Boston

David M. Mastrianni, M.D.
Instructor in Medicine, Harvard Medical School; Associate Physician, Department of Medicine, Beth Israel Hospital, Boston

Paul R. Reich, M.D.
Lecturer in Medicine, Harvard Medical School, Boston; Vice President for Medical Affairs, Pilgrim Health Care, Inc., Norwell, Massachusetts

Stephen H. Robinson, M.D.
George C. Reisman Professor of Medicine, Harvard Medical School; Chief of Hematology and Associate Chief of Medicine, Beth Israel Hospital, Boston

Lowell E. Schnipper, M.D.
Theodore and Evelyn Berenson Associate Professor of Medicine, Harvard Medical School; Chief of Oncology and Associate Chief of Medicine, Beth Israel Hospital, Boston

Lawrence N. Shulman, M.D.
Assistant Professor of Medicine, Harvard Medical School; Clinical Director, Hematology-Oncology Division, Brigham and Women's Hospital, Boston

Peter F. Weller, M.D.
Associate Professor of Medicine, Harvard Medical School; Associate Physician, Department of Medicine, Beth Israel Hospital, Boston

Catherine Wheeler, M.D.
Instructor in Medicine, Harvard Medical School; Associate Physician, Department of Medicine, Beth Israel Hospital, Boston

Preface

The preceding two editions of this book were authored by Dr. Paul R. Reich. However, since the publication of the second edition in 1984, there has been a revolution in biology that has affected all fields in medicine, with hematology in the forefront. Because "pathologic material," consisting of blood, bone marrow, and lymph node specimens, is so readily available from patients with hematologic disorders, new discoveries concerning the roles of oncogenes, chromosomal abnormalities, and alterations in molecular biology in the pathogenesis of disease are being made at an especially rapid rate in this field. Some of these discoveries have already found application in the treatment of hematologic disorders. Thus, recombinant growth factors such as erythropoietin and GM-CSF are being used routinely to increase red blood cell and white blood cell production in several hematologic contexts, and all trans-retinoic acid has been found to be effective in inducing hematologic remissions in patients with acute promyelocytic leukemia by inducing the leukemic cells to differentiate into mature non-proliferating neutrophils.

These many changes led us to believe that multiple authors would be best able to describe the different areas of hematology, and we decided that this should be a project for the members of the Hematology-Oncology Division at the Beth Israel Hospital and Harvard Medical School. The Hematology-Oncology Division comprises a large number of physicians with different areas of expertise, covering the entire spectrum of hematology. Several of the chapters in this third edition are entirely new, but others are similar to those in the previous editions, although they have been revised and updated. The new authors were asked to present comprehensive, readable accounts of the different areas of hematology, including significant new findings; however, they have avoided undue detail and complexity in order to provide a readily comprehensible picture.

This book provides a fine introduction to hematology for medical students studying pathophysiology. At the same time, the text is comprehensive enough to be useful for senior medical students, house officers, and general physicians dealing with hematologic problems in hospital and office settings.

We have retained in this book a series of helpful guides for the student and physician. There is a series of photomicrographs illustrating the major morphologic abnormalities encountered in hematologic disorders, as well as tables describing the approaches to major clinical problems in hematology and case development problems that should help the reader to solidify his or her understanding of the major issues in this broad and interesting field.

S.H.R.
P.R.R.

Hematology

1 Physiology of Hematopoiesis

Stephen H. Robinson

All of the cells in the peripheral blood have finite life spans and thus must be renewed continuously. The mechanisms responsible for regulating steady-state hematopoiesis and the capacity to modulate blood cell production in response to stresses such as anemia or infection consist of a series of progenitor cells in the bone marrow and a complex array of regulatory factors. There has been an explosion of information about hematopoiesis, based on the development of assays for different progenitor cells and the new techniques of molecular biology that have made an increasing number of pure growth factors available for study. This information is still growing rapidly. Understanding this field is made more complex by the fact that both the cells and the factors that are involved in hematopoiesis have been named according to biologic assay systems, and these names have little apparent relevance to clinical medicine.

Hematopoietic Stem Cells

The primitive cells ultimately responsible for hematopoiesis are referred to as stem cells. These cells look like immature lymphocytes and are present in very small numbers in the bone marrow so that they cannot be identified morphologically. When a stem cell divides, it must have the capacity both to self-replicate and to give rise to differentiated progeny. Self-replication is necessary to maintain the stem cell pool; otherwise the marrow would become aplastic. Thus, division of a stem cell may give rise to two new stem cells, two cells destined to differentiate into one of the several pathways of bone marrow development, or one new stem cell and one cell programmed to differentiate. The most immature stem cells are multi- or pluripotential and thus capable of giving rise to differentiated progeny along multiple cell lines. More mature stem cells are committed to a single pathway of development. Thus, as shown in Figure 1-1, a multipotential stem cell gives rise to pluripotential stem cells of either the lymphoid or myeloid pathway. (The term *myeloid* refers to marrow.) The myeloid pluripotential stem cell gives rise to third-order progenitor cells, each of which is committed to

1

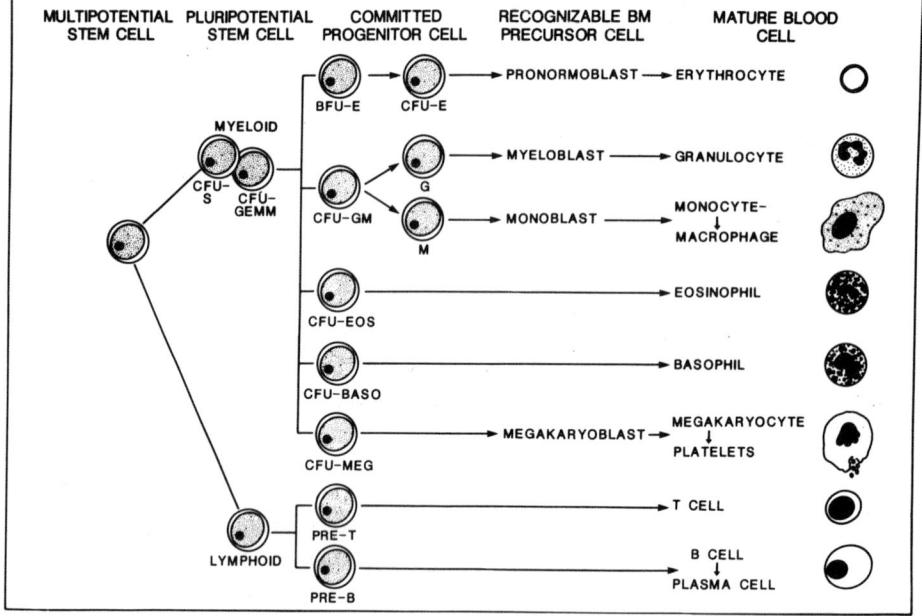

Fig. 1-1. A model of hematopoietic stem cell differentiation. Illustrated are progenitor cells of increasingly restricted potentiality, which give rise to the maturing cells recognizable in bone marrow preparations as the immediate precursors of peripheral blood elements. BM, bone marrow; CFU, colony-forming unit; S, spleen; GEMM, granulocyte-erythrocyte-monocyte (or macrophage)-megakaryocyte; BFU, burst-forming unit; E, erythroid; GM, granulocyte-monocyte (or macrophage); EOS, eosinophil; BASO, basophil; Meg, megakaryocyte. (From S. H. Robinson, Hematopoiesis. In J. H. Stein (ed), *Stein's Internal Medicine* (3rd ed.). Boston: Little, Brown, 1990. Reproduced by permission.)

one of the major pathways of bone marrow cell differentiation into erythrocytes, neutrophils, monocytes, eosinophils, basophils, or megakaryocytes.

Several generalizations apply to this hierarchical scheme of stem cell development. The most primitive stem cells are pluripotential, have a large amplification potential in regard to the number of mature cells produced after a long series of cell divisions, and are generally in a resting state under normal conditions but readily enter into active cell division when the need for new blood cell formation arises. The more mature, committed progenitor cells have a smaller capacity for self-replication and a smaller amplification potential. They are normally in a state of active cell division and are primarily responsible for the ongoing production of blood cells under normal steady-state conditions. As these committed stem cells divide and become more mature, they lose their capacity for self-replication, and they become progressively more responsive to lineage-specific growth factors such as erythropoietin or granulocyte colony-stimulating factor (G-CSF). The term *stem cell* is often used to connote very immature cells with a large capacity for self-replication. The term *progenitor cell* usually refers to a more mature cell that has lost some or all of its self-replicative capacity and is committed to a single pathway of differentiation. The term *precursor cell* is used for the recognizable cells in the bone marrow that are derived from committed progenitor cells and give rise to the mature cells that enter the peripheral blood.

Stem Cell Assays

Total body irradiation ablates marrow stem cells, leading to the disappearance of hematopoiesis from the bone marrow. Transfusion of a lethally irradiated animal with bone marrow or even peripheral blood cells from a normal, unirradiated animal can lead to restoration of bone marrow cellularity and prevent death of the animal. Such experiments were successful because of the presence of stem cells in the marrow and in the peripheral blood, and represented the first instances of experimental bone marrow transplantation. In 1961, Till and McCulloch found macroscopic colonies of cells in the spleens of irradiated mice that had then been rescued by intravenous injection of marrow cells from normal donor mice. These investigators demonstrated that each spleen colony was derived from a single pluripotential stem cell in the donor bone marrow; the colonies consisted of various combinations of erythroid, granulocytic, and megakaryocytic cells. Similar colonies were found in the bone marrows of the recipient mice, but these were difficult to assay because they were contained within a bony vault. Enumeration of spleen colonies was the first means of quantitating stem cells in a mammalian system and heralded the modern era of research in hematopoiesis. Till and McCulloch referred to the myeloid pluripotential stem cells that gave rise to spleen colonies as colony-forming units–spleen, or CFU-S, and this form of nomenclature became the standard when other stem cells and regulatory factors were subsequently identified.

Soon thereafter, it was found that in vitro culture of marrow cells in a semisolid matrix such as soft agar enriched with what were then crude growth factors gave rise to colonies consisting of granulocytes, macrophages, or both granulocytes and macrophages. The cells responsible for forming these colonies are now called CFU-G, CFU-M, and CFU-GM, respectively (see Fig. 1-1). The growth factors that support growth of these colonies are referred to as G-CSF, M-CSF (or CSF-1), and GM-CSF; CSF stands for colony-stimulating factor. Thereafter, in vitro assays were developed for a large number of the progenitor cells depicted in Figure 1-1. The myeloid pluripotential stem cell in humans, equivalent to the CFU-S in mice, cannot yet be assayed. Derived from this pluripotential cell is the CFU-GEMM, a less self-replicative stem cell that can be assayed in vitro, where it gives rise to colonies composed of multiple cell types, including granulocytes, erythroid cells, macrophages, and megakaryocytes. The CFU-GEMM in turn gives rise to progenitor cells committed to the different cell lineages of the bone marrow.

Erythropoiesis

Descending from CFU-GEMM are burst-forming units–erythroid (BFU-E), early progenitor cells committed to erythroid cell differentiation. In culture BFU-E give rise to "bursts" of several smaller colonies. During this process each BFU-E goes through a few cell divisions, leading to the development of several more mature erythroid progenitor cells known as CFU-E, each CFU-E giving rise to the individual small colonies of maturing erythroid cells that constitute the erythroid burst. BFU-E development is supported primarily by a factor or factors known as burst-enhancing factor derived from T lymphocytes, whereas growth of CFU-E is dependent on erythropoietin. GM-CSF turns out to be at least one form of burst-enhancing factor, as is described later in this chapter.

The CFU-E gives rise to a series of cells that are recognizable microscopically in bone marrow preparations as the precursors of mature erythrocytes. Approximately four cell divisions take place during this relatively late portion of the erythroid maturation sequence. The first recognizable erythroid cell in the bone marrow is the proerythroblast or pronormoblast, which on Wright or Giemsa stain is a large cell with basophilic cytoplasm and an immature nuclear chromatin pattern (Plate 1). Subsequent cell divisions give rise to basophilic, polychromatophilic, and finally orthochromatophilic normoblasts, which are no longer capable of mitosis (Plates 2–4). During this maturation process a progressive loss of cytoplasmic RNA occurs as the product of protein synthesis, hemoglobin, accumulates within the cell; as a result the color of the cytoplasm evolves from blue to gray to pink. At the same time the nuclear chromatin pattern becomes more compact and clumped until, at the level of the orthochromatophilic normoblast, there remains only a small dense nucleus, which is finally ejected from the cell. The resulting anucleate erythrocyte still contains some RNA and is recognizable as a reticulocyte when the RNA is precipitated and stained with dyes such as new methylene blue (Plate 5). Normally, reticulocytes remain within the bone marrow for approximately 2 days as they continue to accumulate hemoglobin and lose some of their RNA. The reticulocyte then enters the peripheral blood, where, after about one more day, it loses its residual RNA and some of its excessive plasma membrane and becomes indistinguishable from adult erythrocytes.

Under normal conditions the transit time from the pronormoblast to the reticulocyte entering the peripheral blood is about 5 days. This interval can be decreased to 2 to 3 days in response to increased levels of erythropoietin, a hormone produced by the kidneys in response to tissue hypoxia. The actions of erythropoietin are described later in this chapter.

It is thought that under normal conditions a small number of erythroid precursor cells are defective and are destroyed in the bone marrow before giving rise to reticulocytes. This process is called ineffective erythropoiesis and is markedly exaggerated in hematologic disorders such as megaloblastic anemia and thalassemia.

Granulocytopoiesis and Monocytopoiesis

Neutrophils and monocytes, which evolve into macrophages when they enter the tissues, arise from a common committed progenitor, the CFU-GM. The CFU-GM is derived from the CFU-GEMM and it, in turn, gives rise to CFU-G and CFU-M, progenitor cells committed specifically to the granulocytic and monocytic pathways of development, respectively. As with erythroid cell development, there are primitive CFU-GM that give rise to large dispersed colonies, which are apparently analogous to erythroid bursts.

The myeloblast (Plate 6) is the earliest recognizable precursor in the granulocytic series that is found in the bone marrow. It is derived from the CFU-G. Like the pronormoblast the myeloblast is a large cell with a high ratio of nucleus to cytoplasm. This cell has abundant cytoplasmic RNA imparting a blue color on Wright stain and a nucleus with a delicate chromatin pattern and one or more nucleoli. A series of four to five cell divisions are associated with progressive loss of cytoplasmic RNA and basophilia as the products of the mature neutrophil, cytoplasmic granules, develop. At the same time the nuclear chromatin becomes compacted and inactive. On division the myeloblast gives rise to two promyelocytes, which contain abundant dark "azurophilic" primary granules that overlie both nucleus and cytoplasm (Plate 7). With subsequent cell divisions these primary granules become progressively diluted by the secondary, less conspicuous "neutrophilic" granules that are characteristic of the mature cells. This concomitant cell division and maturation sequence continues from promyelocytes to early myelocytes, late myelocytes, and then metamyelocytes, which are no longer capable of cell division (Plates 8 and 9). The nucleus of the metamyelocyte is indented or kidney-shaped and the cytoplasm is filled with neutrophilic granules. As the metamyelocyte matures the nucleus becomes more attenuated and the cell is then called a "band" or "stab" form (Plate 10). Subsequent segmentation of the nucleus gives rise to the mature neutrophil or polymorphonuclear leukocyte (Plate 11).

The bone marrow contains a large storage pool of band forms and mature neutrophils. On entering the peripheral blood, neutrophils are divided about equally into a circulating and a marginal pool. These two pools are in dynamic equilibrium and neutrophils from the axial circulation are constantly marginating to the luminal surface of blood vessels, while marginating cells are continually re-entering the active circulation. Thus, a large reserve capacity of phagocytes is available in the bone marrow, and a large fraction of the neutrophils present in the peripheral blood is always in the marginating pool, available for egress into the tissues in response to infection or inflammation.

The average interval from the initiation of granulopoiesis to the entry of the mature neutrophil into the circulation is 10 to 13 days. The mature neutrophil remains in the circulation for only about 10 to 14 hours before entering the tissues, where it soon dies after performing its phagocytic function.

Monocytes and Macrophages

There is no reserve pool of monocytes in the bone marrow as there is for neutrophils. Like neutrophils, on the other hand, monocytes spend only a short time in the peripheral blood before entering the tissues. However, they survive in the tissues for variably long periods. In the tissues monocytes eventually become transformed into macrophages, long-lived phagocytic cells that retain some capacity for continuing cell division. Cells of the so-called reticuloendothelial system, now called the mononuclear phagocyte system, including alveolar macrophages, Kupffer cells in the liver, and bone marrow osteoclasts, are derived from monocytes that were produced in the bone marrow.

Thrombocytopoiesis

The committed stem cell for megakaryocytic development is called the CFU-Meg. Thrombocytopoiesis proceeds from this cell through a series of progressively more mature progenitor cells that finally give rise to the megakaryoblast, a cell that is difficult to discern in the bone marrow morphologically but can be detected by special cytochemical stains. The megakaryoblast produces megakaryocytes, distinctive large cells that are the source of circulating platelets. Megakaryocyte development takes place in a unique manner. The nuclear DNA of megakaryoblasts and early megakaryocytes reduplicates without cell division, a process known as endomitosis or endoreduplication. As a result, a mature megakaryocyte has a polyploid nucleus, that is, multiple nuclei each containing a full complement of DNA and originating from the same locus within the cell. Mature megakaryocytes are 8 n to 36 n. The final stage of platelet production occurs when the mature megakaryocyte sends cytoplasmic projections into the marrow sinusoids and sheds platelets into the circulation.

It takes approximately 5 days for a megakaryoblast to become a mature megakaryocyte. Each megakaryocyte produces from 1,000 to 8,000 platelets. The platelet normally survives for 7 to 10 days in the peripheral blood. Approximately 30 percent of circulating platelets are normally present in the spleen, and this splenic pool is in active equilibrium with platelets in the circulation.

Hematopoietic Regulatory Factors

Until a few years ago, knowledge of hematopoietic regulatory factors was based on studies of biologic activities present in crude media that stimulated the growth of colonies of hematopoietic cells in in vitro cultures of marrow cells. Recently, many of these "colony-stimulating activities" have been cloned using recombinant techniques of molecular biology, permitting examination of the properties of purified growth factors both in vitro and in vivo. What emerges is a complex picture indicating that the growth and differentiation of progenitor cells in each pathway of bone marrow development are regulated by overlapping combinations of different growth factors and that the same growth factors are often operative in multiple pathways, particularly during early phases of hematopoietic cell differentiation (Table 1-1). Greater specificity of regulatory factors for a given lineage of cell development is achieved as differentiation proceeds.

The factors that determine when primitive pluripotential stem cells undergo cell division and either self-replicate or initiate differentiation into the multiple pathways of bone marrow cell development remain relatively unclear, whereas regulation of the later phases of cell development along specific cell lines is better understood. The "hematopoietic inductive microenvironment" and short-range regulatory factors seem to be most important for immature progenitor cells, whereas more circumscribed growth factors, such as erythropoietin, G-CSF, M-CSF, and thrombopoietin, are operative for more mature, committed progenitor cells. A tissue culture model of marrow cell growth, developed by Dexter and associates, has demonstrated that an adherent stromal layer, equivalent to the hematopoietic inductive microenvironment of the bone marrow, permits ongoing regeneration of stem cells and mature blood cells over several weeks to months. This microenvironment consists of

Table 1-1. The major hematopoietic growth factors

Growth factor*	Target cells
Stem cell factor	Early stem/progenitor cells
Interleukin-3	CFU-GEMM, BFU-E, CFU-GM, CFU-Meg, CFU-eos, CFU-G, CFU-M
GM-CSF	CFU-GM, BFU-E, CFU-GEMM, CFU-eos, CFU-Meg, CFU-G, CFU-M, maturing neutrophils, monocytes, and eosinophils
G-CSF	CFU-G, maturing neutrophils
M-CSF	CFU-M, maturing monocytes, macrophages
Erythropoietin	Late BFU-E, CFU-E, maturing erythroid cells, megakaryocytes (?)

*Meg-CSF and thrombopoietin are not included because they are not yet well characterized. Their target cells are thought to be the CFU-Meg and maturing megakaryocytes, respectively. Interleukin-6 stimulates growth of CFU-Meg and probably accounts for some or all of Meg-CSF activity; IL-6 also acts on B cells and plasma cells. There is equivocal evidence that erythropoietin may stimulate megakaryocyte production. Also omitted from this table are growth factors that act primarily on lymphoid cells, e.g., interleukin-2.
Reproduced from S. H. Robinson, Hematopoiesis. In J. H. Stein (ed.), *Steins's Internal Medicine* (3rd ed.). Boston: Little, Brown, 1990.

both cellular elements, including fibroblasts, fat cells, endothelial cells, macrophages, and T lymphocytes, and extracellular matrix, consisting of fibronectin, laminin, and complex mucopolysaccharides. The cells of the microenvironment elaborate growth factors such as interleukin-3 (IL-3) and GM-CSF, which operate over short range. These factors are also adsorbed to extracellular matrix material, which makes them available to nearby progenitor cells. Direct physical or chemical interactions between hematopoietic progenitor cells and microenvironmental cells and/or extracellular matrix constituents may also be necessary for the progenitor cells to undergo successful growth and differentiation.

Interleukin-3, otherwise known as multi-CSF, is produced by activated T lymphocytes and supports the growth of relatively immature hematopoietic cells, including CFU-GEMM, BFU-E, CFU-GM, and CFU-Meg. GM-CSF is produced by a variety of cells, including virtually all of the cellular components of the hematopoietic microenvironment alluded to previously. Although this growth factor was initially thought to be more or less specific for progenitor cells of the granulocytic and monocytic pathway, purified GM-CSF proved to enhance the growth of CFU-GEMM, BFU-E, and CFU-Meg, as well as CFU-GM, CFU-G, and CFU-M. Thus, the spectrum of activity of GM-CSF overlaps that of IL-3, although IL-3 appears to be more active on primitive progenitor cells and GM-CSF on more mature cells. G-CSF and M-CSF are more specific and act more distally in the differentiation pathway. G-CSF stimulates the differentiation of CFU-G into myeloblasts and M-CSF the differentiation of CFU-M into monoblasts, thus augmenting the rate of production of neutrophils and monocytes, respectively. GM-CSF, G-CSF, and M-CSF not only enhance the growth of the corresponding hematopoietic progenitor cells but also increase the rate of cell division of the precursor cells, for example, myeloblasts, promyelocytes, and myelocytes in the granulocytic series, that originate from these progenitor cells. Moreover, these factors affect the differentiated progeny of these cell lineages, activating the functional properties of neutrophils and monocytes and preparing them for their phagocytic function. There are other growth factors that influence the growth and differentiation of lymphoid cells and eosinophils, for example, IL-5 and IL-6. These, too, have effects on more than one cell lineage.

A recently discovered growth factor, known as stem cell factor or kit-ligand, acts on stem cells at an earlier level than is affected by any of the other growth factors yet characterized. Stem cell factor by itself does not increase hematopoietic colony formation, but in combination with other growth factors such as IL-3, GM-CSF, and erythropoietin causes a markedly synergistic effect in the growth of colonies derived from CFU-GEMM, BFU-E, and other progenitor cells.

The mechanisms that regulate the production of GM-CSF, G-CSF, and M-CSF and other growth factors are complex and incompletely understood. Activated macrophages and monocytes in areas of infection or inflammation release factors, such as interleukin-1 (endogenous pyrogen), tumor necrosis factor, and other "monokines." These intermediates in turn act on T lymphocytes, endothelial cells, and fibroblasts to engender the production of the various types of CSF that stimulate the increased production and the enhanced functional capacity of phagocytes necessary to do effective battle with the infectious or inflammatory lesion. Negative regulatory factors also come into play. Thus, lactoferrin produced by neutrophils in an inflammatory exudate acts as an inhibitor of CFU-GM development. Similarly, prostaglandin E produced by macrophages inhibits the production of monocytes, the precursors of macrophages, and to some extent neutrophils as well.

Regulatory systems also exist for erythropoiesis and thrombopoiesis. BFU-E growth is supported by stem cell factor, IL-3, and GM-CSF; indeed, GM-CSF represents at least one form of what was previously called burst-enhancing factor. Erythropoietin comes into play at the late BFU-E stage of development and becomes the primary regulator at the level of the CFU-E, causing these cells to undergo an increased rate of cell division and differentiation. This hormone also stimulates the rate of cell division and hemoglobin synthesis in the recognizable erythroid precursor cells of the bone marrow and causes bone marrow reticulocytes to "shift" prematurely into the peripheral blood.

Erythropoietin is a glycoprotein hormone that is produced primarily by the kidney, probably by tubule cells, in response to tissue hypoxia. The mechanism that senses low tissue oxygenation has not been elucidated but may involve hemoproteins. The liver is a secondary, usually minor source of erythropoietin production. By virtue of its action on late BFU-E, CFU-E, and maturing erythroid precursor cells, increased serum levels of erythropoietin produced in response to anemia or other causes of hypoxemia result in erythroid hyperplasia of the bone marrow and an associated reticulocytosis in the peripheral blood. In addition to stimulating an increase in the rate of reticulocyte production from the level of the progenitor cell, erythropoietin increases the number of reticulocytes entering the peripheral blood by creating increased permeability of the adventitial cells of the bone marrow through which reticulocytes pass to gain access to the circulation. This "shift" of bone marrow reticulocytes into the peripheral blood is an early effect of erythropoietin, occurring within 24 hours after administration of this hormone to an experimental animal. It leads to the presence of large polychromatophilic erythrocytes in Wright-stained preparations of peripheral blood. The fact that these immature reticulocytes are present in the circulation for 2 to 3 days before they lose their RNA and are no longer identifiable as reticulocytes, as compared to one day for reticulocytes released under normal conditions, must be taken into account when calculating the reticulocyte index, an estimate of the rate of effective red cell production by the bone marrow (see Chap. 2).

Now that erythropoietin has been purified and is available in recombinant form, a sensitive radioimmunoassay for serum levels of this hormone has become available. This is sometimes useful in evaluating patients with erythrocytosis (see Chap. 11).

Regulation of thrombopoiesis is less well understood. Early events, affecting the least mature progenitor cells, are stimulated by IL-3, GM-CSF, and the less well-defined factor, Meg-CSF, which is derived from activated T lymphocytes; Meg-CSF, in fact, may possibly be either IL-3 or GM-CSF. Later events, including endomitosis and the production of platelets by megakaryocytes, are stimulated by an as yet poorly defined humoral substance, thrombopoietin, which appears to have a role analogous to that of erythropoietin in the later phases of erythropoiesis.

Considerable progress has been made in regard to the properties of the hematopoietic growth factors. All are glycoproteins and most have internal disulfide bridges that are important to their structure and function. The genes for several of these factors have been localized to specific chromosomes, for example, that for erythropoietin to chromosome 7 and those for IL-3, GM-CSF, and M-CSF to chromosome 5; moreover, the c-fms proto-oncogene, which codes for the cell receptors for M-CSF, is also present on chromosome 5. Cell receptors for several hematopoietic growth factors have been identified and characterized. There are distinct receptors for each growth factor, but interaction of some growth factors with their receptors modulates the affinity of other growth factors to their receptors; for example, IL-3 inhibits binding of GM-, G-, and M-CSF and GM-CSF inhibits binding of G- and M-CSF to bone marrow cells. In general, the number of receptors per cell is quite low and the affinity of the receptor for the growth factor quite high. It appears that a low order of receptor occupancy by growth factor molecules is sufficient to initiate the physiologic effects of that factor on the cell.

Clinical Applicability of Hematopoietic Stem Cells

Stem Cell Disorders

Disorders of hematopoietic stem cells include aplastic anemia, paroxysmal nocturnal hemoglobinuria, the various forms of acute non-lymphocytic (myelogenous) leukemia, the myeloproliferative disorders, and the myelodysplastic syndromes. The fact that the myeloid pluripotential stem cell is the usual locus of disease in these disorders can be inferred from the fact that the three major cell lines derived from that cell, erythrocytes, granulocytes, and platelets, are all often affected. Moreover, in the myeloproliferative disorders there is frequently an increase in eosinophils and particularly basophils, two other cell lines derived from the myeloid pluripotential stem cell. Chronic myelogenous leukemia is now believed to arise at a still more primitive level, that of the multipotential stem cell; lymphoid as as well as myeloid cells appear to be involved in the neoplastic process, and some patients with this disease undergo transformation to acute lymphocytic leukemia. Direct evidence that these disorders originate at the level of the pluripotential stem cell has been obtained by chromosome analysis and by studies of black female patients who are heterozygotes for two isotypes of the enzyme glucose-6-phosphate dehydrogenase (G-6-PD). This is discussed in the chapter on the myeloproliferative disorders.

Bone Marrow Transplantation

Bone marrow transplantation is a means of replenishing an abnormal bone marrow with normal pluripotential stem cells. Allogeneic marrow transplantation is used for diseases due to abnormalities in stem cell function, such as aplastic anemia in which stem cells are deficient or defective, or acute leukemia in which stem cells have become malignant. Normal marrow cells from a histocompatible allogeneic donor are used to repopulate the diseased bone marrow. When the stem cells are malignant, the recipient receives massive chemotherapy, often combined with total body irradiation, in order to ablate residual malignant cells before normal marrow cells are transplanted. Even in aplastic anemia, irradiation and immunosuppressive therapy are given to the recipient to prevent rejection of the marrow graft and the development of graft-versus-host disease, in which donor lymphocytes produce a rejection reaction aimed at host tissues.

Autologous bone marrow transplantation is being used more and more widely to permit the administration of highly intensive regimens of chemotherapy in patients with malignant disorders. These cytotoxic regimens would normally produce prolonged periods of bone marrow aplasia, but the patient's bone marrow cells are harvested and cryopreserved before the administration of the chemotherapy and are then given back to the patient after the chemotherapy has been administered. Autologous bone marrow transplantation is used either when the bone marrow is uninvolved with the malignant process or when attempts can be made to "purge" small numbers of residual malignant cells from the prechemotherapy bone marrow harvest with specific monoclonal antibodies or drugs that are aimed at killing malignant cells while preserving normal hematopoietic stem cells. It is not yet clear, however, that such purging procedures are necessary to achieve successful control of the malignant disorder through the use of autologous marrow transplantation.

Growth Factors as Therapeutic Agents

Now that purified growth factors can be produced in large quantities, clinical trials are taking place to examine their ability to stimulate hematopoiesis in patients. Early trials have demonstrated that recombinant GM-CSF can partly offset the neutropenia that follows intensive chemotherapy for malignant disorders. This agent also hastens recovery of the peripheral blood counts after bone marrow transplantation. Recombinant erythropoietin reverses the anemia of chronic renal insufficiency. It is clear that we are entering an era in which these and other growth factors are assuming major therapeutic roles in clinical medicine.

Topics for Discussion: Physiology of Hematopoiesis

Topics suitable for term papers or seminars in hematology are listed in each chapter. They concern aspects of hematology that are undergoing change and development at the present time and that are not possible to summarize in a textbook. Students are expected to search primary resources, journal articles, and reviews in order to bring themselves and their classmates up to date in these important areas of hematologic investigation. The bibliographies for each chapter include review articles that should aid in researching these topics.

The hematopoietic inductive microenvironment as examined through bone marrow cultures

Clinical studies of recombinant hematopoietic growth factors

Implications of the fact that the genes for several hematopoietic growth factors are clustered on chromosome 5

Evidence that the CFU-S is a stem cell and has pluripotential properties

Clinical and physiologic relationships among GM-, G-, and M-CSF

Does thrombopoietin exist?

Selected Readings

Bradley, T. R., and Metcalf D. The growth of mouse bone marrow cells in vitro. *Aust. J. Exp. Med. Sci.* 44 : 287, 1966.

Brandt, S. J. et al. Effect of recombinant human granulocyte-macrophage colony-stimulating factor on hematopoietic reconstitution after high-dose chemotherapy and autologous bone marrow transplantation. *N. Engl. J. Med.* 318 : 869, 1988.

Clark, S. C., and Kamen, R. The human hematopoietic colony-stimulating factors. *Science* 236 : 1229, 1987.

Dexter, T. M., Allen, T. D., and Lajtha, L. J. Conditions controlling the proliferation of the hematopoietic stem cells in vitro. *J. Cell. Physiol.* 101 : 335, 1977.

Eschbach, J. W. et al. Correction of the anemia of end-stage renal disease with recombinant human erythropoietin: Results of a combined phase I and II clinical trial. *N. Engl. J. Med.* 316 : 73, 1987.

Groopman, J. E. et al. Effect of recombinant human granulocyte-macrophage colony-stimulating factor on myelopoiesis in the acquired immunodeficiency syndrome. *N. Engl. J. Med.* 317 : 593, 1987.

Pluznik, D. H., and Sachs, L. The cloning of mast cells in tissue culture. *J. Cell. Physiol.* 66 : 319, 1965.

Sieff, C. A. Hematopoietic growth factors. *J. Clin. Invest.* 79 : 1549, 1987.

Till, J. E., and McCulloch, E. A. A direct measurement of the radiation sensitivity of mouse bone marrow cells. *Radiat. Res.* 14 : 213, 1961.

Trentin, J. J. Determination of bone marrow stem cell differentiation by stromal hematopoietic inductive microenvironments (HIM). *Am. J. Pathol.* 65 : 621, 1971.

2 Anemia

Paul R. Reich
Stephen H. Robinson

Anemia is usually defined as a condition in which the amount of hemoglobin in a patient's circulatory system is reduced. A physiologic definition stresses the inability of an anemic individual to maintain normal tissue oxygenation. This may result from decreased hemoglobin content or reduced red cell number. If oxygen-carrying capacity is reduced, then compensatory mechanisms come into play, such as increased pulse rate, stroke volume, and, therefore, cardiac output; increased erythropoietin production; decreased affinity of hemoglobin for oxygen; and diversion of blood from less vital to more vital organs, such as the brain.

These compensatory changes and the inability of blood to meet tissue oxygen requirements lead to signs and symptoms of anemia. These are listed on page 22. The speed with which anemia develops determines which symptoms are prominent. In acute blood loss the decrease in blood volume leads to inability to maintain blood pressure. Shock, unconsciousness, and ultimately death follow. Once bleeding has stopped, plasma volume is replenished in 24 to 72 hours. However, red cell volume may not be replenished for days or weeks, depending on the magnitude of the bleeding. Thus patients recovering from blood loss may be free of the effects of low blood volume but may suffer the chronic symptoms of anemia until enough red cells are available for oxygen transport to meet tissue metabolic requirements.

Red Cell 2,3-Diphosphoglycerate (2,3-DPG)

Erythropoietin, by increasing the number of hemoglobin-containing erythrocytes in the peripheral blood, enhances blood oxygen-carrying capacity and thereby tissue oxygenation. Another mechanism by which tissue oxygenation is enhanced in the face of anemia involves the affinity of oxygen for hemoglobin. If oxygen is more easily released from hemoglobin, then less hemoglobin is required to maintain normal tissue oxygen supply. This is illustrated in

(MCV) and hemoglobin concentration; the hematocrit is computed from the MCV and RBC.

Other red cell indices (Wintrobe indices) can be calculated manually or by computer from the hemoglobin, hematocrit, and red blood cell count. The formulas for mean cell volume (MCV), mean cell hemoglobin content (MCH), and mean cell hemoglobin concentration (MCHC) are shown on page 19. Since these indices represent average values, their calculation does not replace a careful examination of the stained peripheral blood smear for abnormalities of red cell size, shape, or color.

Reticulocyte Count and Reticulocyte Production Index

Bone marrow erythroid activity is usually reflected in the peripheral blood reticulocyte count. To obtain this count, one drop of whole blood is mixed with two drops of new methylene blue and, after incubation for 15 minutes, a blood smear is made. One thousand red cells are scanned with an oil immersion lens (2,000 cells give better statistical accuracy with reticulocyte counts of less than 5 percent), and the number of cells with dark blue strands or particles, usually appearing as a reticular network, are counted (see Plate 5). Normal values are 0.5 to 1.5 percent or, in "absolute" numbers (reticulocyte count as a decimal multiplied by RBC), 20 to 100 $\times$ 10^9 per liter.

In the presence of anemia the reticulocyte percentage does not accurately reflect reticulocyte production, since each reticulocyte released is being diluted into fewer adult red cells. A better measure of erythroid production is the *reticulocyte production index* (RPI). The reticulocyte percentage is first corrected to a normal hematocrit of 0.45. For example, a reticulocyte percentage of 10 percent in a patient with a hematocrit of 0.23 would be equivalent to a percentage of 5 percent in a patient with a hematocrit of 0.45. This is equivalent to calculating the absolute reticulocyte count in terms of red cell number. Another correction is made because erythropoietin production in response to anemia leads to premature release of newly formed reticulocytes, and these stress reticulocytes take up to 2 days rather than 1 to mature into adult erythrocytes. If many polychromatophils are seen, then a correction factor of 2.0 is divided into the corrected reticulocyte percentage, for example

$$\text{RPI} = \frac{10 \times 23/45 \text{ (hematocrit correction)}}{2.0 \text{ (maturation time correction)}} = 2.5$$

Maturation factors from 1.0 to 2.0 are used, the higher numbers if there is a great deal of polychromatophilia in the peripheral blood smear, and the lower numbers if there is little. Polychromatophils are discussed further in Chapters 1 and 4.

The reticulocyte production index is an approximate measure of effective red cell production in the marrow. A normal marrow has an index of 1. In hemolytic anemia, with excessive destruction of red cells in the peripheral blood and a functionally normal marrow, this index may be three to seven times higher than normal. When there is marrow damage, erythropoietin suppression, or a deficiency of iron, vitamin B_{12}, or folic acid, the index is less than expected for the degree of anemia—that is, 2 or less. Ineffective erythropoiesis, with intramedullary (marrow) destruction of erythroid precursors, can be deduced if the marrow contains many normoblasts but the reticulocyte production index is low.

Red Cell Mass

Since PCV and hemoglobin concentration are affected by abnormalities in plasma volume, a patient with a normal mass of erythrocytes will have a low PCV if the plasma volume is abnormally large. Similarly a high hemoglobin concentration can be due to salt depletion and dehydration with a resulting low plasma volume. To avoid these sources of error, red cell mass can be directly measured by a radioisotope dilution assay. An aliquot of the patient's blood is incubated with radioactive chromium 51, which attaches to the β-chains of hemoglobin within the erythrocyte, and then unbound chromium 51 is washed free. A known number of counts per minute of radiochromium in a known volume of blood (e.g., 5 mL) is injected back into the patient. After allowing time for mixing, another 5-mL blood sample is drawn and the counts per minute of radioactivity determined. A simple calculation

$$\frac{\text{counts per minute injected}}{\text{counts per minute sampled}} = \frac{\text{red cell mass (mL)}}{5 \text{ mL}}$$

yields the red cell mass (in milliliters) independent of plasma volume. The only major source of error is the potential for damaging red cells during the labeling procedure. If this occurs, the damaged radioactive red cells are removed from the circulation by the spleen, and a falsely high red cell mass is obtained.

Normal values for red cell mass are *25* to *30* mL per kilogram of body weight in the male and *22* to *28* mL per kilogram in the female. Red cell mass determinations are not used often in the clinical practice of hematology, since the PCV and hemoglobin concentration usually accurately reflect red cell mass.

Approach to Patient with Anemia

Three steps are carried out in the diagnostic approach to an anemic patient (see pp. 22–23). First, the medical history is taken to ascertain

---

Approach to patient with anemia

I. History
  A. Symptoms of anemia
    1. Chest pain on exertion (angina)
    2. Dizziness and syncope (fainting)
    3. Fatigue and weakness
    4. Shortness of breath
    5. Rapidity of onset of symptoms
    6. Response of anemia to therapy in the past
  B. Blood loss
    1. Gastrointestinal—hematemesis (vomiting blood); melena (black stools); hemorrhoidal bleeding; hematochezia (red blood in stools)
    2. Bleeding at operation or delivery
    3. Respiratory—hemoptysis (coughing blood); epistaxis (nosebleed)
    4. Uterine—menorrhagia (excessive bleeding); metrorrhagia (irregular bleeding)
    5. Other—hematuria (blood in urine)
  C. Bleeding tendency
    1. Bleeding after trauma, operations, deliveries, and tooth extractions
    2. Bleeding into joints
    3. Menstrual bleeding (see above)
    4. Petechiae (capillary hemorrhages)
    5. Ecchymoses (bruises)
  D. Iron deficiency anemia
    1. Blood loss (see B.)
    2. Glossitis (sore or inflamed tongue)
    3. Pregnancies and iron supplementation
  E. Megaloblastic anemia
    1. Foul-smelling diarrhea with greasy stools
    2. Glossitis
    3. Paresthesias (tingling toes or fingers); difficulty with gait
  F. Drugs and toxins
    1. Alcohol
    2. Occupational exposures
    3. Therapeutic medications
  G. Miscellaneous
    1. Bone pain
    2. Jaundice (yellow skin), early development of (bilirubin) gallstones
    3. Weight loss
  H. Family history
    1. Anemia
    2. Racial and geographic derivation
    3. Jaundice, early development of gallstones
    4. Splenomegaly
II. Physical examination
  A. Vital signs
    1. Blood pressure, pulse
    2. Orthostatic hypotension (lowered blood pressure upon standing or sitting)
  B. Skin
    1. Leg ulcers
    2. Nail beds—koilonychia (spoon-shaped nails)
    3. Pallor (pale skin)
    4. Purpura, petechiae
    5. Spider angioma (spider-shaped capillaries) and other signs of chronic liver disease

C. Conjunctivae
1. Jaundice
2. Pallor
3. Petechiae
D. Fundi
1. Papilledema
2. Hemorrhages
E. Mouth
1. Lips—angular stomatitis (sores at angles of lips)
2. Mucus membranes—pallor, petechiae
3. Tongue—redness, atrophy of papillae
4. Uremic breath
F. Lymph nodes
1. Enlargement in cervical (neck), axillary, inguinal (groin), epitrochlear (near elbow), or other areas
G. Bones
1. Tenderness over sternum, ribs, or vertebrae
H. Cardiorespiratory system
1. Cardiac gallop
2. Heart murmurs
3. Peripheral edema
4. Pulmonary rales
I. Abdomen
1. Hepatomegaly
2. Splenomegaly
3. Masses
4. Ascites
J. Neurologic examination
1. Loss of vibratory or position sense
2. Positive Romberg sign (inability to stand upright with eyes closed)
3. Peripheral neuropathy
K. Pelvic and rectal examination
1. Bleeding
2. Tumors
III. Laboratory data
A. Hematocrit and hemoglobin
B. Red cell indices
C. Reticulocyte count
D. White cell count and differential
E. Platelet count
F. Peripheral blood smear
G. Bone marrow aspirate or biopsy
H. Special tests
1. Schilling test for vitamin B_{12} absorption
2. Serum iron and total iron-binding capacity
3. Serum ferritin
4. Vitamin B_{12} and folic acid serum levels
5. Others as determined by patient's problem

the patient's symptoms that provide clues to the cause of anemia (e.g., blood loss, drugs, and inherited diseases). Second, the physical examination is carried out to determine the effect of the anemia on vital functions and to help pinpoint its etiology (e.g., splenomegaly, tumors, bleeding). Important information obtainable from the history and physical examination is listed in the outline as are definitions of medical terms used for certain signs and symptoms. Finally, laboratory tests are performed to quantitate and characterize the

---

Suspected hematologic diagnoses for which bone marrow aspiration should be performed
Agranulocytosis Aplastic anemia Hypersplenism Idiopathic thrombocytopenic purpura Leukemia Lipid storage disease Lymphoma Megaloblastic anemia Metastatic tumor Multiple myeloma Waldenström's macroglobulinemia

anemia and the status of the other blood elements, white cells and platelets. Importantly, the peripheral blood smear is examined for clues to the etiology of the anemia. Often a bone marrow specimen must be examined before a definitive diagnosis can be made (pp. 26–27). Special tests (e.g., serum iron, ferritin, vitamin B_{12}, and folate levels) are often done to confirm the diagnosis made from the history physical examination, blood counts, blood smear, and bone marrow examination (if a marrow was indicated). The extent of the laboratory testing depends on the nature of the hematologic problem, and the list of special tests is by no means complete. Subsequent chapters will explain how all this information is used to diagnose and treat anemia.

Since examination of the peripheral blood and bone marrow is central to the diagnostic workup, an approach to the interpretation of these specimens is discussed here.

Peripheral Blood Smear

Blood obtained by venipuncture (anticoagulated with ethylene diaminetetraacetic acid [EDTA]) or by fingerstick is smeared on cover slips or glass slides and then stained with Wright stain. With the oil immersion objective (100×), the smear should first be examined for abnormalities in erythrocyte size or shape. Table 2-2 describes common morphologic abnormalities and the diseases associated with them. The white blood cells should be examined next, and a differential count performed. The platelet number can be estimated by counting how many of these small blue particles (Plate 12) are present in a high power field. Normally there is an average of 15 to 20 per high power field. The white cells and platelets are produced in the marrow, and many abnormalities that produce anemia may affect these blood elements as well. The diagnosis of anemia often is helped by study of all three blood elements, as is made clear in subsequent chapters.

Table 2-2. Common peripheral blood (red cell) abnormalities

Abnormality	Description	Associated diseases
Anisocytosis	Abnormal variation in size (normal diameter = 6–8 μm)	Any severe anemia, e.g., iron deficiency, megaloblastic
Microcytosis (Plate 18)	Small cells less than 6 μm (MCV < 80 fL)	Iron deficiency, sideroblastic anemia, thalassemia, chronic disease
Macrocytosis	Large cells, greater than 8 μm (MCV > 100 fL)	Megaloblastic anemia, liver disease, hypothyroidism, hemolytic anemia (reticulocytes), postsplenectomy
Macroovalocytosis (Plate 26)	Large (> 8 μm) oval cells	Megaloblastic anemia
Hypochromia	Pale cells with decreased concentration of hemoglobin (MCHC < 30 gm/dL)	Iron deficiency, sideroblastic anemia, thalassemia, anemia of chronic disease
Poikilocytosis	Abnormal variation in shape	Many severe anemias—e.g., megaloblastic, iron deficiency, hemolytic; certain shapes are diagnostically helpful (see following, Spherocytosis through Teardrop cells)
Spherocytosis (Plate 33)	Spherical cells without pale centers; often small, i.e., microspherocytosis	Hereditary spherocytosis, immunohemolytic anemia; small numbers are seen in many hemolytic anemias and after transfusion of stored blood
Ovalocytosis (Plate 34)	Oval cells	Hereditary elliptocytosis, iron deficiency
Stomatocytosis	Red cells with slit-like, instead of circular, areas of central pallor	Congenital hemolytic anemia, liver disease, artefact
Sickle cells (Plate 37)	Crescent-shaped cells	Sickle cell hemoglobinopathies
Target cells (Plate 19)	Cells with a dark center and periphery and a clear ring in between	Iron deficiency, thalassemia, hemoglobinopathies (S, C, SC, S-thalassemia), postsplenectomy, liver disease
Schistocytes, helmet cells (Plate 39)	Red cell fragments	Microangiopathic hemolytic anemia (disseminated intravascular coagulation, thrombotic thrombocytopenic purpura, etc.)
"Spur" cells	Cells with irregularly spaced projections, often with foot processes	Liver disease ("spur cell" anemia), disseminated intravascular coagulation, pyruvate kinase deficiency
Acanthocytosis	Small cells with thorny projections; similar to spur cells	Abetalipoproteinemia (hereditary acanthocytosis or Bassen-Kornzweig disease)

Table 2-2 (continued)

Abnormality	Description	Associated disease
"Burr" cells (Plate 36)	Cells with regular sharp projections	Uremia, burns, DIC
Teardrop cells (Plate 59)	Cells shaped like teardrops	Myelophthisic anemia (neoplastic, granulomatous, or fibrotic marrow infiltration), thalassemia
Nucleated red cells (Plates 4 and 58)	Erythrocytes with nuclei still present	Myelophthisic anemia (neoplastic, granulomatous, or fibrotic marrow infiltration), extramedullary hematopoiesis, severe blood loss or hemolytic anemia, hyposplenism
Howell-Jolly bodies (Plate 38)	Spherical blue bodies (Wright stain) within or on erythrocytes; nuclear remnants	Hyposplenism, severe blood loss or hemolysis
Heinz inclusion bodies	Small round inclusions seen under phase microscopy or with supravital staining	Congenital hemolytic anemias (e.g., glucose-6-phosphate dehydrogenase deficiency), hemolytic anemia secondary to oxidant drugs (dapsone, phenacetin), thalassemia (Hb H), certain hemoglobinopathies (Hb Zurich, Köln, Ube, I, etc.)
Pappenheimer bodies (siderocytes) (Plates 20 and 21)	Iron granules, staining blue with Wright or Prussian blue stains	Iron-loading anemias, hyposplenism, hemolytic anemias
Cabot rings	Purple, fine, ring-like, intraerythrocytic structures	Pernicious anemia, any severe anemia
Reticulocytosis (polychromatophilia) (Plates 5 and 25)	Blue, reticular (RNA) network in erythrocytes stained supravitally with new methylene blue; appear as macrocytes with diffuse basophilia (polychromasia or polychromatophilia) when Wright-stained	Hemolytic anemia, blood loss, following treatment of iron deficiency or megaloblastic anemias
Rouleaux (Plate 82)	Aggregated erythrocytes regularly stacked on one another	Multiple myeloma, Waldenström's macroglobulinemia, hypergammaglobulinemia

Bone Marrow Examination

A specimen of marrow can be obtained by *aspiration* of spicules through a hollow needle placed in the intramedullary cavity of the anterior or posterior iliac crest or the sternum. If aspiration fails (a so-called *dry tap*); if the marrow is thought to be infiltrated or replaced by granuloma, fibrosis, or tumor; or if aplasia of the marrow is suspected, then a bone marrow *biopsy* should be per-

Suspected hematologic diagnoses for which bone marrow biopsy should be performed
Amyloidosis
Aplastic anemia
Granulomatous diseases (tuberculosis)
Leukemia
Lymphoma
Metastatic tumor
Myeloproliferative syndrome (myelofibrosis)
Thrombotic thrombocytopenic purpura
Most conditions in which marrow aspirates are done

formed. A large-bore needle is inserted into the marrow and a core of intramedullary bone is cut and removed. The specimen (Plate 13) is decalcified, sectioned, and stained with hematoxylin and eosin (H&E), and if indicated, with special stains for fibrosis, amyloid, or tuberculosis. The suspected diagnoses for which bone marrow biopsy is often performed are listed above.

A bone marrow *examination* should include at least the procedures listed under Aspirate in the outline, page 28. The marrow spicules obtained by aspiration are smeared on either coverslips or glass slides. These preparations are then stained with either Wright or Giemsa stain and with Prussian blue for iron. The clot that remains after preparation of the smears is fixed, and sections are made and stained with H&E (Plate 14). Iron stains are done on the aspirated specimen and are examined for intracellular red cell iron, ringed sideroblasts (sideroblastic anemias), and iron stores (Plates 15–17). If a bone biopsy specimen is obtained, touch preparations should be made on glass slides at the time of the biopsy and stained with Wright or Giemsa stain. The marrow biopsy core is then submitted for sectioning and staining with H&E. The clot section and bone marrow biopsy sections are particularly useful for determining cellularity of the bone marrow. In current practice a biopsy is usually included as part of the bone marrow examination. Other special studies can be done as part of the bone marrow examination.

After all the relevant data are available, an attempt should be made to classify the anemia. Most often this is possible at the time of initial workup, but establishment of a definite and specific etiology may require special studies. In the next section a clinically useful classification scheme is described.

Classification of Anemias

Many different classifications of anemia have been proposed. In Table 2-3 two widely used classifications, morphologic and physiologic, are outlined. Used together, these offer a rational pathophysiologic approach to the laboratory diagnosis of anemia.

Bone marrow examination

  I. Aspirate
    A. Glass slide or coverslip smears of marrow particles
      1. Wright or Giemsa stain
      2. Iron (Prussian blue) stain
      3. Histochemical stains for enzymes to identify cell type
        (e.g., myeloblasts, monoblasts)
    B. Section of clot after fixation
      1. H&E stain
      2. Iron stain
  II. Biopsy obtained with Jemshidi or Westerman-Jensen needle
    A. Touch preparation or imprint stained with Wright or
      Giemsa stain
    B. H&E stain of section
    C. Special stains, if indicated, for tuberculosis, fungi, fibrosis,
      amyloid, and so forth
 III. Bacteriologic studies
 IV. Cytogenetic studies (e.g., Philadelphia chromosome)
  V. Phase microscopy (e.g., wet preparation for thalassemic inclusion
    bodies)
 VI. Cell markers (e.g., membrane immunoglobulins, antigens)

Table 2-3. Classification of anemias

I. Morphologic

Normocytic, normochromic (MCV and MCHC normal)	Microcytic, hypochromic (MCV low, MCHC low)	Macrocytic, normochromic (MCV high, MCHC normal)
Blood loss	Iron deficiency	Megaloblastic
Hemolytic anemia	Sideroblastic anemia	anemias
Aplastic anemia	Lead poisoning	Liver disease
Myelophthisic	Thalassemia	Postsplenectomy
anemia	Chronic disease	Hypothyroidism
Chronic disease,		Stress erythropoiesis
renal insufficiency		

II. Physiologic

Hypoproliferation	Excessive destruction or loss of red cells	Maturation abnormality
Aplastic anemia	Hemolytic anemia	Megaloblastic
Myelophthisic	Blood loss	anemias
anemia		Myelodysplasia,
Renal insufficiency		including
Chronic disease		sideroblastic
Endocrine deficiency		anemia
status		Thalassemia
		Iron deficiency

According to the morphologic classification, anemic patients with normal-sized cells and normal hemoglobinization have normocytic, normochromic anemia and usually are found to be suffering from either increased red cell loss (blood loss or hemolysis) or decreased red blood cell production (aplastic anemia, myelophthisic anemia, anemia secondary to chronic disease or renal failure). Hemolytic anemias are those due to increased red cell destruction. Aplastic anemias are those due to primary bone marrow failure. Myelophthisic anemias are caused by replacement of the bone marrow by malignant cells, granulomas, or fibrosis. The microcytic, hypochromic anemias are characterized by small, incompletely hemoglobinized red cells. These anemias have in common defective production of hemoglobin. An absence of iron stores, a defect in heme synthesis, as seen in the sideroblastic anemias, or defective globin synthesis, as seen in the thalassemia syndromes, accounts for most of the microcytic, hypochromic anemias. Macrocytic anemias with large erythrocytes are either megaloblastic, usually due to deficiencies in vitamin B_{12} or folic acid, or nonmegaloblastic, often caused by liver disease, stress erythropoiesis, the postsplenectomy state, or (rarely) hypothyroidism.

The physiologic classification of anemia stresses three pathophysiologic mechanisms. The first, failure of normal proliferation of bone marrow elements, may be due to toxins, replacement of the bone marrow by abnormal cells, or aplasia (hypocellularity). The second major category, excessive loss or destruction of red cells, covers hemolytic anemias and blood loss anemia. The third category, maturation abnormalities, includes the megaloblastic and sideroblastic anemias among others. Normally maturation of the erythrocyte proceeds in both the nucleus and the cytoplasm. In the nucleus the chromatin becomes more clumped and finally pyknotic, while cell size diminishes. In the cytoplasm the initial basophilia is gradually replaced by pink-staining hemoglobin, and finally, with maturity, the red cell cytoplasm becomes completely pink-staining. In the megaloblastic anemias nuclear maturation defects are prominent. The cell cytoplasm becomes normally hemoglobinized, but the nucleus remains large and reticulated rather than clumped and pyknotic. This nuclear-cytoplasmic dissociation is sometimes referred to as dyspoiesis. Defects in cytoplasmic maturation are characteristic of iron deficiency and thalassemia. Nuclear maturation proceeds normally, but cytoplasmic hemoglobinization is delayed and often incomplete. All of these maturation abnormalities result in ineffective erythropoiesis and premature destruction of erythroid precursor cells in the bone marrow and perhaps also at the reticulocyte level.

The reticulocyte count is very useful in discriminating among these three pathophysiologic mechanisms of anemia. The reticulocyte count is low in anemias due to underproduction of red blood cells in the marrow and with the ineffective erythropoiesis of the maturation disorders. It is high with the anemias due to increased red cell loss because of the effect of elevated levels of erythropoietin on the normal bone marrow.

Treatment of Blood Loss and Anemia

The effects of blood loss are twofold. First, there is a reduction in hemoglobin and therefore in oxygen-carrying capacity. Second, there is concomitant loss of plasma, decrease in blood volume, and inability to maintain normal blood pressure. In the past, whole blood was used to treat anemia without regard to whether the patient was suffering from decreased oxygen-carrying capacity or from decreased blood volume. Due to the scarcity of blood and the risk of transmitting viruses such as hepatitis B and C and human immunodeficiency virus (HIV), component transfusion has now become accepted and is a vital means of meeting the need for blood transfusion. If it can be determined that the patient's major problem is inability to supply oxygen to tissues, and not danger from decreased blood volume, then the appropriate component for therapy is packed red cells. These are prepared by centrifugation or sedimentation of whole blood and removal of plasma components. If the patient's major problem is loss of blood volume, then plasma or albumin prepared from plasma should be used as well. Albumin prepared from plasma is hepatitis and HIV virus–free.

Transfusion of blood as the sole means of treating anemia should be limited to patients who have hematologic diseases that are not presently amenable to treatment. In every case great effort should be expended to define and treat the underlying cause of the anemia. Transfusion can be used to tide the patient over while treatment is being undertaken. In no case should blood transfusion be used in place of an adequate diagnostic workup. In many patients, once the cause of the anemia has been defined, it may be possible to avoid transfusion and its attendant dangers. Technical considerations in typing and crossmatching blood are considered in Chapter 9.

Case Development Problem: Anemia

A 24-year-old Nigerian foreign exchange student comes to the emergency ward after having passed out twice on the street. He reports having had diarrheal stools that were black and possibly bloody. A nurse orders an emergency hematocrit and it is reported as 0.30 (30%). A peripheral blood smear is ready.

1. How would you proceed with this patient?

The history, physical examination, blood counts, and peripheral blood smear form the basis for the initial workup of any patient with a suspected hematologic abnormality. In this case, however, the order in which these examinations are carried out is most important. Since the history suggests that the syncope is secondary to gastrointestinal bleeding and decreased blood volume, the first step is to obtain his vital signs, particularly blood pressure and pulse. Once these have been established as satisfactory, a brief history and a test for blood in stomach and rectum should follow. In this urgent situation the examination of the blood smear comes last. The nurse reports that she has obtained a blood pressure of 120/80 mm Hg with the patient in a lying position and 90/60 with him in the sitting position.

2. How do you account for this discrepancy?

These findings indicate that the patient has *orthostatic hypotension.* This means that his blood volume has been reduced to the point that his vascular tree is unable to compensate by vasoconstriction for the decreased blood volume. This leads to a marked drop in both systolic and diastolic blood pressures when he assumes the sitting or standing position. It is an important clinical sign of decreased blood volume.

3. What other physical findings are most likely present?

This patient very likely has a rapid pulse; pallor of the skin, mucus membranes, conjunctivae, and nail beds; and a "hemic" heart murmur.

4. The laboratory reports his hemoglobin as 10 gm per deciliter and his red cell count as 3.0×10^{12} per liter. Calculate and interpret his Wintrobe indices.

Mean corpuscular volume is 100 femtoliters, mean corpuscular hemoglobin is 33 picograms, and mean corpuscular hemoglobin concentration is 33 gm per deciliter. This indicates that he has a normocytic, normochromic anemia.

He gives a further history of having had a duodenal ulcer; his gastric aspirate and stool when tested for occult blood are both strongly positive. A repeat hematocrit is 0.29 (29%).

5. Does this stabilization of his hematocrit indicate that he has stopped bleeding?

No, because it may take upwards of 1 to 2 days for extravascular fluid to enter the *intra*vascular space and dilute the remaining red cells. This dilution will ultimately lead to a further decrease in his hematocrit. The important point to remember is that the hematocrit may not indicate the degree of blood loss until many hours or days have passed. Signs of orthostatic hypotension and tachycardia are therefore very important in assessing the magnitude of acute blood loss.

6. What blood products would you advise for transfusion should his condition fail to stabilize? Why?

This patient obviously has two deficits. First, he has lost red cells that are necessary for carrying oxygen to tissues. He has also lost plasma proteins that are necessary to maintain intravascular volume. The components that he needs—namely, red cells and plasma—should therefore be replaced. They can be given as packed red cells and either albumin or plasma, or as whole blood. (Whole blood is rarely used in current transfusion practice.)

His bleeding suddenly stops before surgical measures can be undertaken. Eight hours after admission to the hospital, his hematocrit is stable at 0.30 (30%) and his reticulocyte count has risen to 9 percent. Macrocytes with bluish or polychromatophilic cytoplasm are present in great numbers in his peripheral blood smear.

7. Calculate and interpret his reticulocyte production index.

$$RPI = \frac{\dfrac{9 \times 30}{45}}{2} = 3$$

His reticulocyte production index is calculated to be 3. This means that his bone marrow production is approximately three times normal. This has come about in response to his anemia and inadequate tissue oxygenation. Since there are large numbers of polychromatophils, a correction factor of 2 is used. These macrocytes account for a high normal mean corpuscular volume.

8. If you assume a normal red cell mass of 2,000 mL for this patient, how many milliliters of red cells will he produce per day with a reticulocyte production index of 3?

Normal individuals with a reticulocyte count of 1 percent replace about 1 percent of their red cells each day. In his case this would be 20 mL. Since his reticulocyte index is 3, he is able to produce 3 × 20, or 60 mL per day.

Topics for Discussion: Anemia

Oxygenation and deoxygenation of hemoglobin
Intracellular phosphate compounds and regulation of hemoglobin
    oxygen affinity
Particle counters

Selected Readings

Bellingham, A. J., and Grimes, A. J. Red cell 2,3-diphosphoglycerate. *Br. J. Haematol.* 25 : 555, 1973.

Hillman, R. S., and Finch, C. A. *Red Cell Manual* (4th ed.). Philadelphia: Davis, 1974.

Jandl, J. H. Physiology of Red Cells, Section 2 and The Anemias, Section 3. In J. H. Jandl, *Blood: Textbook of Hematology.* Boston: Little, Brown, 1987.

Kapf, C. T., and Jandl, J. H. *Blood: Atlas and Sourcebook of Hematology.* Boston: Little, Brown, 1981.

McDonald, G. A., Dodds, T. C., and Cruickshank, B. *Atlas of Hematology (3rd ed.).* Baltimore: Williams & Wilkins, 1970.

Miale, J. B. *Laboratory Medicine in Hematology* (6th ed.). St. Louis, Mosby, 1982.

Reich, P. R. *Scope Manual of Hematology.* Kalamazoo, Mich.: Upjohn Company, 1972.

Surgenor, D. M. (ed.). *The Red Cell,* Vols. 1, 2. New York: Academic, 1975.

Thomas, H. M. et al. The oxyhemoglobin dissociation curve in health and disease: Role of 2,3-diphosphoglycerate. *Am. J. Med.* 57 : 331, 1974.

Westerman, M. P. The bone marrow: Structure, function, and pathology. I and II. *Semin. Hematol.* 18 : 177 : 241, 1981.

Wintrobe, M. M. et al. Basic Cytology: Section I. Origin and Development of the Blood and Blood-Forming Tissues. In M. M. Wintrobe et al. (eds.), *Clinical Hematology* (8th ed.). Philadelphia: Lea & Febiger, 1981.

Wintrobe, M. M. et al. The Diagnostic and Therapeutic Approach to Hematologic Problems: Principles of Hematologic Examination. In M. M. Wintrobe et al. (eds.), *Clinical Hematology* (8th ed.). Philadelphia: Lea & Febiger, 1981.

Wintrobe, M. M. et al. The Erythrocyte, Section 2: The Mature Erythrocyte; Erythropoiesis; Nutritional Factors in the Production and Function of Erythrocytes. In M. M. Wintrobe et al. (eds.), *Clinical Hematology* (8th ed.). Philadelphia: Lea & Febiger, 1981.

3 Microcytic Anemias

Glenn J. Bubley
Roger F. Lange

An important mechanism of anemia is defective hemoglobin synthesis, which results in small, poorly hemoglobinized erythrocytes. After Wright staining, instead of red cells with pink hemoglobin filling the cytoplasm, the cells are pale with only a rim of hemoglobin. Since hemoglobin is made up of two components, either of two pathophysiologic mechanisms can lead to decreased hemoglobin synthesis—defective heme or decreased globin production. *Heme* is made up of iron and porphyrins; deficiencies in either affect heme production. Deficiency of iron stores, failure to utilize iron properly, and defective heme or porphyrin synthesis are characteristic of iron deficiency anemia, anemia of chronic disease, and the sideroblastic anemias, respectively. In the thalassemia syndromes, *globin* production is decreased, thereby hindering hemoglobin synthesis and producing a microcytic anemia.

Iron Deficiency Anemia

Iron deficiency anemia is the commonest cause of anemia in the world. In order to understand the symptoms, etiology, and the treatment of this anemia, it is necessary to review normal iron and heme metabolism.

Iron Storage

HEMOGLOBIN

Iron exists in several compartments within the body (Table 3-1). The largest compartment is hemoglobin iron. Hemoglobin contains 0.34 percent elemental iron by weight. Therefore 500 mL of whole blood contains about 250 mg ($15 \, gm/dL \times 5 \, dL \times 0.0034$) of elemental iron. The iron is complexed to an organic compound, heme, a tetrapyrrole, which is discussed later. Iron in this compartment is preferentially used over and over again in the erythropoietic cycle. Iron released at the time of red cell destruction in reticuloendothelial cells is bound to transferrin and delivered to erythroid precursors in the marrow. There it is incorporated into new cells, thus completing the cycle.

Table 3-1. Important iron compartments in normal 70-kg man

Compartment	Iron content (mg)
Hemoglobin	2,300
Storage (ferritin, hemosiderin)	1,000
Myoglobin	130
Tissue	8
Transport	4

Adapted from V. F. Fairbanks and E. Beutler. Iron Metabolism. In W. J. Williams et al. (eds.), *Hematology*. New York: McGraw-Hill, 1972. p. 125.

STORAGE IRON

Storage iron exists in two forms: hemosiderin and ferritin. Hemosiderin is usually detected by its reaction with Prussian blue stain, with which it produces blue particles (Plate 15). In unstained marrow smears it appears as clumps of golden refractile pigment. The amount of hemosiderin in marrow storage sites reflects the state of iron balance; e.g., in patients with iron deficiency anemia, hemosiderin is absent from the bone marrow.

Ferritin, the other storage form of iron, is better characterized; it is a water-soluble complex of ferric hydroxide-phosphate and a protein, *apoferritin*. The ferric hydroxide-phosphate core and apoferritin shell form a semicrystalline structure visible with special stains (Prussian blue) or through the electron microscope. Apoferritin is a sphere with a diameter of 13 nanograms. It has a hollow central cavity, 6 nm in diameter, which communicates with the surface via six channels through which iron can enter. When iron is added to the molecule, it is deposited in the central core. Rather than being a smooth sphere, the iron core is partially divided into four "lobes" by protein indentation, and this may account for the characteristic tetrads seen in ultrastural studies of ferritin. When fully saturated, ferritin has a molecular weight near 900,000 and contains about 4,500 iron atoms per molecule. The iron is in a trivalent, polymerized form with the probable subunit structure of $(FeOOH_8) \cdot (FeO \cdot PO_3H_2)$. Tissues such as liver, spleen, kidney, and bone marrow all synthesize slightly different forms of ferritins, or isoferritins, which can be separated by gel electrophoresis. Apoferritin is bound to polyribosomes until it incorporates iron to form ferritin. The release of ferritin from the ribosome stimulates more apoferritin synthesis.

How iron is released from ferritin is unknown. Ferritin is thought to be a more readily usable storage form of iron than hemosiderin. Ferritin is also found in the intestinal mucosa, where it may help regulate iron absorption and excretion. Both forms of iron are stored primarily in the reticuloendothelial system (bone marrow and

Kupffer cells of liver and spleen). Ferritin granules have been found by electron microscopy in hemosiderin, and it is thought that hemosiderin may represent partially denatured, partially deproteinized ferritin.

Ferritin-containing iron can be measured in the serum by a radioimmunoassay procedure. Serum ferritin iron comes from the reticuloendothelial system, where it derives partly from senescent erythrocytes. It is transported to the hepatocyte, where iron is stored and where the ferritin may regulate transferrin synthesis. The latter possibility has not been verified experimentally, and a role for serum ferritin in signaling intestinal cells to absorb iron has not been demonstrated in humans. Serum ferritin levels do have a direct correlation with tissue iron stores, which are most conveniently assessed by examination of the bone marrow. However, inflammation, liver disease, malignancy, and increased red cell turnover may falsely elevate serum ferritin values in relation to iron stores. Values may also be falsely high after an oral dose of iron salts.

MYOGLOBIN

This heme-containing protein is found in muscle. Following severe muscle injury it may be detectable in urine.

TISSUE HEME IRON

This compartment is small, but very important, and consists of heme-containing proteins such as cytochromes, catalase, peroxidases, and flavoproteins. Defective synthesis of some of these proteins may be responsible for the skin, mucus membrane, and nail changes found in patients with iron deficiency anemia.

TRANSPORT IRON

The iron-binding protein in serum, *transferrin,* migrates in the β-globulin region when serum is electrophoresed on cellulose acetate. Normally in serum there is 120 to 200 mg per deciliter of transferrin protein, or 250 to 400 μg per deciliter of iron-binding capacity. One third of transferrin normally contains bound iron, which is carried from the sites of red cell senescence and intestinal mucosal cells to the hematopoietic cells of the bone marrow. The total iron-binding capacity (TIBC) consists of the transferrin that has iron bound to it (i.e., the serum iron level) plus the unbound or unsaturated iron-binding capacity (UIBC) of transferrin.

Iron Absorption

The average daily American diet contains 10 to 15 mg of elemental iron, and a normal individual absorbs 5 to 10 percent of ingested iron, or 0.5 to 1.5 mg per day. The absorption of iron depends on many factors. Food and heme iron may be better absorbed than inorganic iron salts. Foods vary in the availability of iron for absorption, meat protein being a particularly good source because its iron is primarily heme iron; in other foods iron exists in its aggregated ferric form. Flour in the United States is fortified with 3 mg of iron per 100 gm of flour (20 percent of the recommended daily allowance per cup of flour). However, the form of iron used, primarily phosphates, is poorly absorbed. Low iron stores and increased iron requirements often increase the percentage of iron absorbed to 20 percent or more. It may be absorbed from almost any level of the small intestine, but the upper levels, particularly the duodenum, are the most efficient sites. In iron-deficient individuals absorption may occur at lower levels as well.

Iron complexed in organic compounds, such as the heme in hemoglobin or myoglobin from animal meat, is absorbed by a mechanism different from that of the absorption of inorganic iron salts. Heme from hemoglobin or myoglobin is absorbed intact in the upper-intestinal mucosal cells with the iron in the ferric or trivalent state, after which the iron is split by the enzyme heme oxygenase and released for entry into the bloodstream. Iron salts are absorbed in the mucosal cell in the ferrous or divalent state and then converted to the trivalent ferric form. Absorption of inorganic iron salts is increased by reducing agents such as vitamin C and hydrochloric acid, which convert ferrous to ferric iron. Absorption is decreased by phosphates and phytates (hexaphosphoinositol) that form insoluble complexes with the iron.

Iron absorption is primarily regulated by the amount of storage iron and the red cell production rate. Increased red cell production and decreased stores lead to greater absorption, and decreased production and normal or increased stores lower absorption. How production rate and storage iron influence mucosal cell absorption is controversial. It is clear that iron in the mucosal cell is carried across the cell by an active transport mechanism. Regulation of iron transport across the cell is linked to the iron content of the mucosal cell. When body iron stores are high, iron is diverted into ferritin and stored in the intestine, and if stores are low or red cell production high, iron passes directly through the mucosal cell into the plasma. Iron stored as ferritin in the mucosal cell is ultimately lost into the intestinal lumen when the epithelial cell is sloughed. This serves as a mechanism for iron excretion. However, only small quantities of iron, about 1 milligram per day, are normally excreted in this manner.

These physiologic control mechanisms can be overcome by ingestion of toxic quantities of iron tablets—e.g., taken accidentally by a child. Some types of clay and the antibiotic tetracycline depress iron absorption. Various factors that influence iron absorption are shown on page 39.

Factors influencing iron absorption
Causing increased absorption
Anemia
Ascorbic acid
Depletion of iron stores
Hydrochloric acid
Hypoxia
Increased erythropoiesis (especially ineffective erythropoiesis)
Liver disease
Causing decreased absorption
Certain clays
Magnesium trisilicate
Malabsorption syndromes
Phytates
Tetracycline
Phosphates

Iron Transport

Ferrous iron must be oxidized to ferric iron before binding to transferrin. Transferrin moves ferric iron from wherever it enters the plasma (intestinal mucosal or reticuloendothelial cells) to transferric receptors on the membranes of normoblasts in the bone marrow. From there iron enters the cytoplasm by *micropinocytosis,* a process consisting of normoblast membrane invagination of transferrin-bound iron and then cytoplasmic vacuole formation. The iron is released and transferrin returns to the plasma and is reutilized. A similar process has been proposed for transport of iron from intestinal lumen into mucosal cells. In the normoblasts, iron is complexed into heme in the mitochondria and then incorporated into hemoglobin. Before its incorporation into heme in the mitochondria, excess iron is packaged in the cytoplasm in ferritin micelles. These siderotic or iron-containing granules of normoblasts are seen in Prussian blue stains. Normoblasts containing siderotic granules are called sideroblasts (Plate 16).

The process, from initial binding to the normoblast to incorporation into hemoglobin, takes 6 to 8 minutes. It appears that the intracellular free heme level regulates the normoblast's uptake of iron. If mitochondrial heme synthesis is impaired, as may occur in sideroblastic anemias, iron uptake is enhanced and mitochondria become large and filled with iron. These structures surround the normoblast's nucleus, forming a *ringed sideroblast* (Plate 17). There is also an increase in the number and size of the siderotic (ferritin) granules in the cytoplasm of these cells.

Reticuloendothelial cell regulation of iron metabolism is important to the pathogenesis of the anemia of chronic disease. In iron deficiency, iron derived from hemoglobin in senescent red cells is promptly released by reticuloendothelial cells and reutilized. In chronic diseases, such as infections and malignancies, the reticuloendothelial cells fail to release iron to transferrin, and this leads to iron deficiency within the developing normoblasts and often a hypochromic anemia, despite adequate or even increased iron stores in the reticuloendothelial cells.

CONGENITAL ATRANSFERRINEMIA

Rare individuals congenitally lack transferrin and suffer from a severe, refractory, hypochromic anemia despite excess iron stores. Studies indicate that their iron is not delivered selectively to early normoblasts and cannot be efficiently utilized for hemoglobin production.

Iron Requirement

Table 3-2 shows the iron requirements for different types of individuals. Iron is lost in the feces in blood, bile, and exfoliated mucosal cells. Normal adult men and nonmenstruating women lose only about 1.0 mg per day (range 0.6-1.6/day). Small amounts are also eliminated in the urine and in sweat. Humans have a very limited ability to increase excretion of iron, and regulation of iron balance is achieved by changing gut absorption depending on the body's requirement for iron. Patients with excessive iron stores usually cannot correct their imbalance without the help of therapeutic blood removal by phlebotomy.

Iron Kinetics

A dynamic picture of iron metabolism can be obtained by use of trace amounts of radioactive iron. These studies have increased our understanding of iron metabolism, but now are rarely used in clinical practice.

Radiolabeled iron bound to transferrin is injected into a patient. Curves based on hourly sampling of the peripheral blood and counts of the radioactivity in the plasma are shown in Figure 3-1. In the normal person 50 percent of the injected radioactivity disappears from the circulation in approximately 90 minutes. This iron is taken up by the bone marrow and in 7 to 10 days is found in hemoglobin

Table 3-2. Normal human iron requirements

Individual	Iron requirement (mg/day)
Normal adult man	0.5–1.0
Normal menstruating woman	1.2–2.0
Pregnant woman	2.4–4.0
Lactating woman (with amenorrhea)	0.5–1.0
Postmenopausal woman	0.5–1.0
Infant	1.0

Fig. 3-1. Radioiron clearance from plasma. (Adapted from T. H. Bothwell et al. The study of erythropoiesis using tracer quantities of radioactive iron. *Br. J. Haematol.* 2 : 1, 1956.)

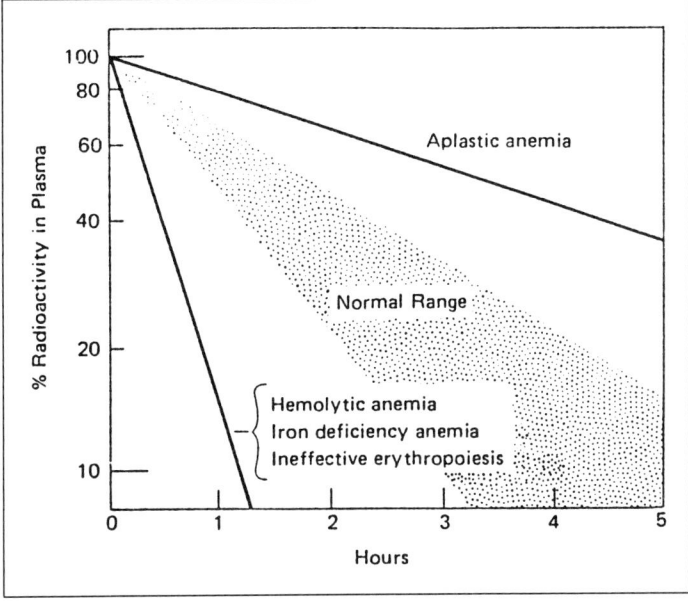

in circulating erythrocytes. Usually the clearance of iron from the plasma is expressed as *plasma iron turnover* (PIT).

$$PIT = \frac{\text{plasma iron} \times \text{plasmacrit}}{T\ 1/2 \times 100}$$

where PIT = mg iron/dL whole blood/day

      plasma iron is in μg/dL plasma

plasmacrit = 100 − hematocrit (%)

    T 1/2 = time (min) to clear 50% of injected radioiron

    Normal people clear 0.65 mg of iron from every deciliter of whole blood each day, or about 26 mg of iron leaves the plasma daily. Increased turnover has a correlation with increased erythropoiesis, either effective (as in hemolytic anemia) or ineffective (intra-marrow red cell destruction), and with deficient iron stores. Decreased turnover is seen with anemias due to reduced erythropoiesis (as in aplastic anemia).

    Another measurement of clinical importance is the percentage of injected labeled iron that appears in circulating red cells in 7 to 10 days. In normal people and iron-deficient patients at least 80 percent of injected radioiron may be counted in circulating red cells. In patients with marrow aplasia or ineffective erythropoiesis considerably less radioiron is incorporated into circulating erythrocytes.

    Finally, red cell life span can be determined by following red cell radioactivity over a period of weeks or months. In normal individuals radioactivity declines rapidly at about 120 days, the usual life span of red cells. In patients with hemolytic anemia, erythrocyte life span is foreshortened, and a sharp decline in radioactivity occurs considerably sooner. As we will see in Chapter 6, determination of red cell life span by labeling hemoglobin iron in a cohort of erythroid precursors requires more time than by "random" labeling of cells of various ages with radiochromium. For this reason radioiron is seldom used clinically to assess erythrocyte life span.

Etiology

From a knowledge of normal iron metabolism, it is easy to predict the derangements likely to produce a deficiency of normoblast iron. Excessive iron loss, greater than absorption, is the most common cause of iron deficiency anemia. Chronic intestinal or uterine bleeding accounts for most adult cases. Gastric or duodenal ulcers, esophageal varices, hiatal hernia, colonic diverticula, and tumors often account for bleeding in men and women. Menstrual losses and losses related to pregnancy and delivery are common in young adult women. Bleeding from otherwise silent colon cancers must be considered in all cases of iron deficiency in adults. In tropical areas bleeding secondary to intestinal parasites, particularly hookworms, is a common cause of iron loss.

Intravascular hemolysis, for example, the hemolysis associated with dysfunctioning prosthetic heart valves, may also result in excessive iron loss. This occurs when the hemoglobin released from the red cells exceeds the capacity of the serum protein haptoglobin to bind free hemoglobin, and the iron is excreted by the kidney as free hemoglobin or is shed in renal tubular cells as hemosiderin.

Hereditary hemorrhagic telangiectasia is a rare autosomal dominant disorder that manifests itself, usually in later life, as red or purple nodular, vascular lesions of the skin and mucus membranes. The mucosal lesions in the nose and gastrointestinal tract may chronically rupture and bleed, resulting in blood loss and iron deficiency anemia. This disease is rarely suspected unless the characteristic lesions are seen on the face, lips, tongue, palms, or soles. They blanch when pressure is applied with a glass slide. No effective treatment, except possibly estrogens, is available.

Excessive demand, exceeding iron absorption, is a problem for the 1- to 2-year-old infant, young adolescent, and pregnant woman. In the infant, inadequate iron in a predominantly cow-milk diet accounts for lowered iron stores. This, coupled with an increased demand for iron for erythropoiesis (the full-term infant requires 160 mg, and the premature, 240 mg of iron during the first

---

Important normal values relevant to iron metabolism

  I. Iron balance
    Iron requirement: 1.0–1.5 mg/day
    Absorption of elemental iron: 10% (can increase to 20% or more)
    Dietary iron: 15 mg/day
    Ferrous sulfate tablets (300 mg): 60 mg elemental iron
    Total storage iron: 1,000 mg in males; 400 mg in females
    Whole blood elemental iron content: 50 mg/dL
  II. Serum levels
    Iron: 80–160 μg/dL (new SI units: 14–29 μmol/L = μg/dL × 0.179)
    Total iron-binding capacity (TIBC): 250–400 μg/dL (SI units: 45–72 μmol/L)
    Percent saturation of TIBC: 15–45
    Ferritin: 12–250 μg/L
 III. Ferrokinetic values (radioiron)
    Plasma iron turnover: 0.65 mg/dL whole blood/day
    Percent of injected radioiron in circulating erythrocytes: ≥80% (8–10 days after injection)
    Red cell life span: 120 days
  IV. Marrow
    Sideroblasts: ≥30% of normoblasts
    Ringed sideroblasts: none

year of life) often leads to iron deficiency anemia at about age 1 or 2. Although 50 mg of iron is supplied by physiologic destruction of fetal red cells, more is required from the diet. For this reason iron supplementation is recommended for infants, especially when premature.

The young adolescent is faced with increased demands for iron because of rapid growth. On top of that requirement, the female adolescent begins to menstruate, losing approximately 45 mL of blood per menstrual period. Since 100 mL of blood contains 50 mg of elemental iron, there is an increased requirement of about 25 mg of iron per month or 1 mg per day in menstruating females. For this reason, unless iron is present in sufficient quantities in the diet or iron supplements are taken, iron deficiency anemia occurs in young females.

Pregnancy also increases demand for iron. There is a saving of about 200 mg of iron due to cessation of menses. However, expansion of the mother's red cell mass requires 400 mg of iron, and the fetus and placenta require another 400 mg. Blood loss at delivery, including blood in the placenta, accounts for another 300 mg. The total requirement for a single pregnancy, therefore, is about 1,100 mg. This is more than the average mother's total iron storage compartment. If iron supplementation is not provided, decreased maternal or fetal iron stores result, thereby increasing the chances of iron deficiency in mother or infant.

Malabsorption of iron is an uncommon cause of iron lack. Diseases of the intestinal mucosa, such as celiac disease in children and tropical and nontropical sprue, are associated with an inability to absorb normal quantities of iron from the diet. It is often possible to increase iron stores in such patients by giving large amounts of iron orally, or parenterally if oral administration is not feasible.

Subtotal gastrectomy often leads to iron deficiency many years after the operation. Multiple mechanisms probably account for the patient's decreased iron stores. Rapid transit through the duodenum, achlorhydria, perioperative blood loss, and occult bleeding secondary to recurrent ulceration have all been suggested as contributing to this iron lack.

Deficiency secondary to poor dietary intake of iron is very rare in adult men or post-menopausal women. Given normal or even reduced iron stores, it is virtually impossible to develop anemia since excretion of iron is 1 mg or less per day. The investigation of an adult case of iron deficiency should never be delayed or abandoned on the excuse that the patient's anemia is due to a poor diet.

Clinical Manifestations

The symptoms of iron deficiency anemias are the same as for any anemia (see p. 22). Often the anemia is accompanied by no or few symptoms. Fatigue, weakness, shortness of breath, and symptoms of heart failure may occur. Some gastrointestinal symptoms may be seen with iron deficiency: glossitis manifested by inflammation and soreness of the tongue; in children, *pica,* or craving and ingestion of strange substances such as dirt or paint (often containing lead); and in adults, desire to eat ice (*pagophagia*) or clays or starches.

The physical findings include those associated with any anemia, e.g., pallor and tachycardia. There may be atrophy of the tongue papillae. Fingernails rarely may assume the shape of the head of a spoon, with central depression and raised borders (*koilonychia*). There may be cracking of the lips, *cheilosis,* and inflammation of the corners of the mouth, *angular stomatitis.* Very rarely patients with iron deficiency anemia manifest the *Plummer-Vinson syndrome,* with a web of mucosa at the junction of the hypopharynx and esophagus. Another rare, unexplained finding in iron deficiency is splenomegaly. Currently, these findings are very uncommon, probably because iron is used so readily to treat various anemias, whether or not they are due to iron lack.

Associations between iron deficiency, atrophic gastritis, and histamine-fast achlorhydria are well known, but the reasons for these associations are not. After stimulation of an iron-deficient patient's stomach parietal cells with intramuscular histamine, little or no hydrochloric acid is detected. Younger patients may have a return of HCl secretion after treatment of their iron deficiency.

The peripheral blood findings are most helpful. The red cell indices reveal a low MCV (55–74 fL) and MCHC (25–30 gm/dL). Red cell morphology is characterized by microcytosis, smaller than normal cells, hypochromia, cells with central pallor, and in some cases, cells with only a rim of hemoglobin near the cell wall (Plate 18.) Target cells (Plate 19), characterized by pink centers and periphery with a clear ring in between, are often found along with elliptical and teardrop-shaped erythrocytes and other abnormal erythroid shapes referred to as *poikilocytes*. Generally, the more severe the anemia, the greater the abnormalities of the shape. Indeed, the red blood cell indices are normal in some patients with iron deficiency anemia, particularly when it is mild. The reticulocyte count is variable, sometimes less than 1 percent, in other cases 2 to 3 percent. The reticulocyte production index is low. Platelets may be normal, decreased, or often increased in number.

The bone marrow examination is helpful in making a diagnosis, since Prussian blue staining of marrow aspirates or clot sections will show an absence or near absence of both normoblast and reticuloendothelial (storage) iron. Fewer than 10 percent of normoblasts will have Prussian blue–staining siderotic granules in their cytoplasm.

With Wright staining poorly hemoglobinized normoblasts with scant cytoplasm are seen in cases of severe iron deficiency; these are sometimes called *tissue paper normoblasts*. Mild erythroid hyperplasia with a decreased myeloid-to-erythroid cell (M : E) ratio is common.

As expected, serum iron levels are low (< 50 μg/dL). These are assayed by a chemical reaction between ferrous iron and a chelating agent that turns pink when complexed with iron. Total iron-binding capacity is usually elevated (> 400 μg/dL), and saturation of this protein is less than 15 percent and in many cases less than 10 percent. Total iron-binding capacity is determined by incubating serum with excess iron, separating unbound iron, and then determining by the previously described chemical method the amount of iron bound to protein.

Serum protoporphyrin levels are high, and serum ferritin levels are low (< 10 μg/L) in iron-deficient patients. When both iron deficiency and inflammation are present, the levels of ferritin may be misleading. If the serum ferritin level is low, iron deficiency is usually present; however, the level of ferritin may be in the normal or slightly elevated range even in the presence of iron deficiency if the patient also has chronic inflammatory, infectious, or neoplastic disease.

One of the best and least expensive tests for iron deficiency is a trial performed with therapeutic amounts of oral iron. In 5 to 10 days after starting therapy, the reticulocyte count rises to 3 to 10 percent, proportional to the severity of the anemia. The hematocrit should rise in 3 weeks and reach normal values in about 2 months.

Sequence of Development of Iron Deficiency Anemia

The first response to negative iron balance is the utilization and diminution of iron stores. Tissue iron stores, including those in the bone marrow, are reduced, and serum ferritin levels fall ($<$ 10 μg/L). With exhaustion of iron stores and reduction of marrow sideroblasts to fewer than 10 percent, serum iron falls, and total iron-binding capacity begins to rise. Initially there is a normochromic, normocytic anemia. With continued reduction in hemoglobin synthesis, hypochromic and microcytic erythrocytes are produced. Finally, the tissue changes seen in iron deficiency anemia may appear in mucus membranes and nail beds.

As an explanation for the microcytic and hypochromic character of this anemia, it has been observed that when the transferrin saturation falls below 15 percent, iron availability for hemoglobin production is critically reduced and poorly hemoglobinized cells result. An extra normoblastic mitotic division is hypothesized to occur in response to the low MCHC, leading to the production of small red cells.

Therapy

Therapy for iron deficiency anemia is almost always the administration of iron salts such as ferrous sulfate. Three hundred milligrams of the hydrated salt of ferrous sulfate contains approximately 60 mg of elemental iron. Because many patients have gastrointestinal intolerance to iron, it is often best to start off with 300 mg of ferrous sulfate per day and slowly increase the dose to the point where the patient is taking one tablet three times per day.

Allowing for the fact that iron absorption will decrease as the iron deficiency anemia is corrected, a minimum of 6 months of therapy is required to correct the anemia and replenish iron stores. Common side effects of iron therapy include heartburn, nausea, abdominal cramps, constipation, and diarrhea. These side effects can be counteracted by decreasing the dose of iron salt, by having the patient ingest the tablets immediately after or with meals, or by switching to a different iron preparation such as ferrous gluconate, ferrous fumarate, or ferrous succinate. Patients should be warned that their stools will turn black while they are taking iron salts. Since iron is severely toxic when ingested in large doses, tablets must be stored in "childproof" bottles out of reach.

Failure to respond to replacement therapy may be due to one of the following:

1. Incorrect diagnosis
2. Continued loss of iron, usually secondary to continuing blood loss
3. Chronic infection or inflammatory conditions suppressing marrow productivity
4. Failure to take iron-containing medication
5. Use of sustained-release preparation that fails to release iron into duodenum
6. Malabsorption of iron (rarely seen)

Parenteral iron therapy with iron-dextran complex (Imferon) and iron sorbitol citrate (Jectofer) should be instituted only for one or more of the following reasons:

1. Inability to tolerate side effects of oral therapy
2. Presence of inflammatory bowel or peptic ulcer disease
3. Failure to take iron tablets
4. Malabsorption of iron
5. Too-rapid loss of iron (e.g., hereditary hemorrhagic telangiectasia) due to bleeding

A formula that allows for both hemoglobin and storage iron replenishment is generally used to calculate the dose of parenteral iron:

$$\text{Iron to be injected (mg)} = (15 - \text{Hgb}) \text{ (gm/dL)} \times \text{body weight (kg)} \times 3$$

The available parenteral preparations contain 50 mg of iron per milliliter. A test dose should be given to test for sensitivity, since anaphylactic, sometimes fatal, reactions can occur. The solution is given by a special injection technique to prevent leakage of fluid from the buttock into the skin, which can leave a permanent stain.

The added cost and risks of parenteral injection make parenteral injection of iron salts a procedure to be avoided if possible. Generally, adequate study of the patient or a change in oral iron salt dose or method of administration will eliminate the need for parenteral therapy. The rapidity of response to therapy is similar with oral and with parenteral treatment.

Intravenous rather than intramuscular iron may sometimes be necessary, for example, when the number of painful intramuscular iron injections would be poorly tolerated. Intravenous iron administration may be preferable in such settings despite concerns regarding the increased risk of anaphylactic and other reactions. It is unclear that such reactions are actually more common with IV than IM iron.

Although single-dose total iron replacement therapy has been safely administered, side effects can be minimized by use of a test dose, limiting each dose to 100 mg per administration, and diluting the iron in 250 to 500 mL fluid.

Porphyrias

Heme Synthesis

The biosynthesis of heme is a complex process. A simplified outline of this process is presented in Figure 3-2 in order to explain the pathophysiology of the porphyrias and other hematologically relevant diseases. Succinyl coenzyme A (CoA) and glycine condense in the presence of pyridoxal phosphate (vitamin B_6) and the inducible, rate-limiting enzyme Δ-aminolevulinic acid (Δ-ALA) synthetase to form Δ-ALA. The activity of Δ-ALA synthetase is controlled in part by its ultimate product, heme. Another enzyme, Δ-ALA dehydrase, helps form porphobilinogen (PBG), a monopyrrole with a heterocyclic structure. Four PGB molecules are assembled into a large ring-shaped molecule, uroporphyrinogen III. Further changes in the side chains of the pyrroles culminate in the formation of protoporphyrin IX, which chelates with iron under the influence of heme synthetase, or ferrochelatase, to form heme. The final and initial steps in heme production occur primarily in the mitochondria of erythroid cells; the intermediate steps take place in the cytoplasm.

Pathophysiology

Although the porphyrias are not associated with hypochromic anemia, their pathophysiology is related to that of the sideroblastic anemias and lead poisoning. Three porphyrias of concern to hematologists are discussed here.

Acute intermittent porphyria (AIP), an inherited, autosomal dominant disease, is characterized by acute attacks of abdominal pain sometimes accompanied by severe neurologic deficits, including motor and respiratory paralysis, or by severe psychiatric disturbances. AIP usually has its onset in early adulthood. It is the only porphyria not typically associated with skin manifestations. Acute attacks may be precipitated by barbiturates, sulfa drugs, ergot, estrogens, griseofulvin, alcohol, and many other drugs. Most drugs that precipitate attacks create an increased demand for hepatic heme by inducing cytochrome P-450. This induces hepatic ALA synthetase. Increased quantities of ALA and PBG are found in the urine. Increased urinary excretion of PBG is revealed by the Watson-Schwartz test. Urine, sodium acetate, and Ehrlich's reagent are mixed, and in the presence of PBG a red compound forms. To confirm its identity as PBG, the reaction mixture should be extracted

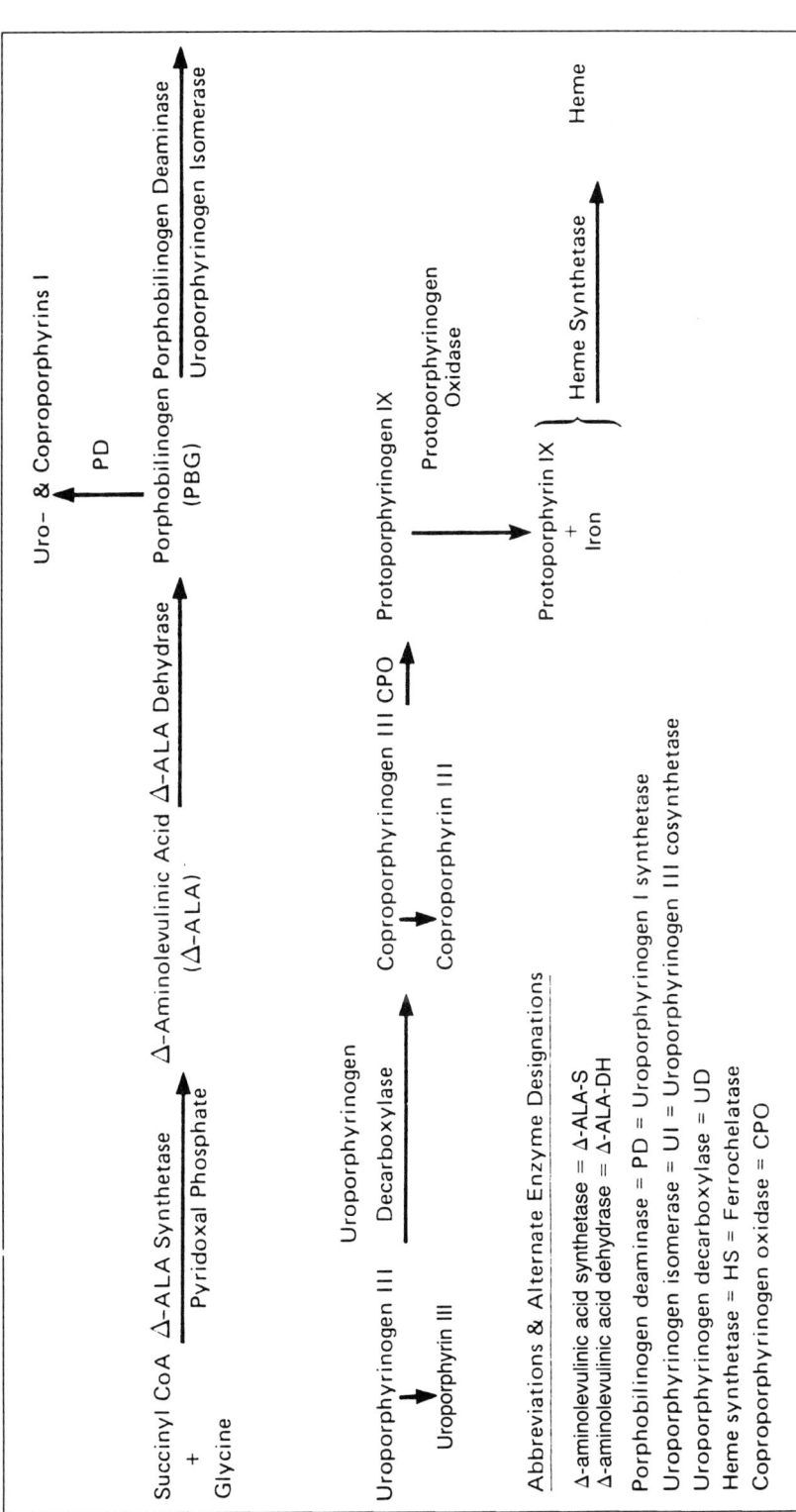

Fig. 3-2 Biosynthesis of heme (simplified).

with chloroform. PBG will remain in the upper aqueous layer, while urobilinogen will be extracted into the lower chloroform layer. A further butanol extraction step will remove other Ehrlich-reacting compounds, leaving only PBG in the aqueous layer. Chromatographic methods for determining PBG levels in urine are available and less subject to false results than the Watson-Schwartz test.

The primary abnormality in AIP is a defect in porphobilinogen deaminase (PD) activity. Presumably this defect would interfere with heme production and lead to a compensatory rise in Δ-ALA synthetase activity. Enough heme would be synthesized to prevent anemia, but Δ-ALA and PBG would be overproduced. There would be no increase in porphyrin excretion, since PD also catalyzes the conversion of PBG to porphyrins. These pathophysiologic mechanisms do not account for the neurologic manifestations of AIP. It is likely that ALA is a neurotoxin, and this, or a critical deficiency of heme in neuronal tissue, is doubtless the cause of symptoms in these patients. Treatment includes avoidance of drugs and carbohydrate deprivation. In some afflicted women, suppression of ovulation has given relief from attacks. Phenothiazines, codeine, and other narcotics can be used to treat symptoms. Hematin (ferric heme) given intravenously is used therapeutically to suppress ALA synthetase, and thereby ALA and PBG formation, in patients with severe attacks.

The second clinically important type of hepatic porphyria is variegate porphyria. The symptoms (abdominal pain and neurologic symptoms, sometimes associated with ingestion of barbiturates) are similar to those in AIP except that these patients usually also have light sensitivity, suggesting that light-sensitizing porphyrins are present in their plasma in addition to non–light-sensitive ALA and PBG. ALA and PBG are elevated in the urine during acute attacks, and increased levels of protoporphyrin and coproporphyrin are continually excreted in the feces. The disease runs in families, is found particularly in South Africa, and is inherited as an autosomal dominant. Decreased activity of protoporphyrinogen oxidase, which catalyzes the oxidation of protoporphyrinogen IX to protoporphyrin IX, is the primary metabolic defect. Treatment is similar to that given for AIP along with protection from sunlight.

Acquired symptomatic porphyria or porphyria cutanea tarda is associated with alcoholic or toxic liver disease and dermal photosensitivity. Increased amounts of porphyrins are excreted in urine and feces, but there is no increased excretion of ALA or PBG. A partial defect in uroporphyrinogen decarboxylase activity is the basis of this disorder. This may be inherited or apparently acquired, although even acquired cases may have a genetic basis. Many patients with the enzyme defect remain asymptomatic throughout life. Expression of the disorder is usually associated with iron build-up in the liver and this iron further inhibits uroporphyrinogen decarboxylase activity. In some patients hepatic accumulation of iron secondary to alcoholism may lead to clinical expression of a borderline congenital enzymatic defect. Abstention from alcohol is therefore advisable, as is avoidance of estrogens, since both of these may precipitate the clinical disorder. Protection from the sun can reduce the skin manifestations. Removal of iron by phlebotomy or iron chelating agents may induce a clinical remission.

A fourth disorder of porphyrin metabolism, protoporphyria, an autosomal dominant disorder, is associated with dermal photosensitivity and occasionally liver disease. Free erythrocyte protoporphyrin (FEP) levels, measured fluorometrically, are elevated. Increased FEP levels are also found in iron deficiency anemia and lead poisoning. Decreased activity of heme synthetase is the primary defect in protoporphyria. Induction of carotenemia reduces photosensitivity, since carotene quenches photo-excited oxygen and scavenges free radicals. Sunscreens and cholestyramine, which binds and therefore enhances the excretion of protoporphyrin, may also be of benefit.

Sideroblastic Anemias

The second major type of hypochromic anemia is associated with tissue iron overload. These anemias (see p. 52) have the following characteristics:

1. Impaired erythropoiesis related to defective heme synthesis and not to iron deficiency
2. Usually increased plasma iron, saturation of transferrin ($>$ 50%), and serum ferritin
3. Presence of ringed sideroblasts (Plate 17) in the marrow, usually associated with increased reticuloendothelial as well as normoblast iron. Defective iron utilization within erythroblasts is often most marked in the latter stages of erythroblast development and results in ineffective erythropoiesis.
4. Often a dimorphic peripheral blood picture with normal-sized or small cells seen along with macrocytes—only some of the cells appear hypochromic

The following classification has been found helpful in differentiating between the various types of sideroblastic anemia.

Hereditary (Sex-linked) Sideroblastic Anemia

Hereditary sideroblastic anemia is usually inherited as an X-linked recessive disease and therefore primarily affects males, although there can be partial expression in females. The diagnosis is usually made in adolescence and is characterized by a mild-to-moderate

---

Classification of sideroblastic anemias

I. Hereditary (X-linked) sideroblastic anemia*
II. Acquired
   A. Primary
     1. Acquired sideroblastic anemia
   B. Secondary
     1. Alcoholism
     2. Chronic disease and infections
     3. Drugs, including isoniazid, cycloserine, chloramphenicol
     4. Hemolytic anemia
     5. Lead poisoning
     6. Leukemia
     7. Megaloblastic anemia
     8. Thalassemia

---

* Some are pyridoxine-responsive.

anemia with all the features of an iron-loading anemia. In some patients partial improvement of the anemia results from treatment with large doses of vitamin B_6, pyridoxine. Liver and spleen enlargement and a clinical picture resembling hemochromatosis have also been described.

The iron-loading seen in these patients has been attributed to two factors: decreased utilization of iron for heme synthesis and increased gastrointestinal absorption of iron. The latter is often seen in disorders associated with ineffective erythropoiesis. If normoblast heme concentration regulates iron absorption, impaired heme production would explain why iron continues to enter the normoblast despite the cellular iron overload. The excess iron is deposited in mitochondria, thereby rendering them relatively immobile and fixing them in the perinuclear position that they assume during mitosis. These normoblasts are called *ringed sideroblasts* (Plate 17) and are the sina qua non for the diagnosis of sideroblastic anemia.

Decreased activity of key enzymes in heme synthesis, most commonly Δ-aminolevulinic acid synthetase (Δ-ALA-S), has been implicated as the primary defect in hereditary sideroblastic anemia. Pyridoxal phosphate, formed from pyridoxine, is the active coenzyme for Δ-ALA-S and stimulates the low Δ-ALA-S activity, measured in vitro, in some patients with hereditary sideroblastic anemia. This observation may explain the occasional responsiveness of this disease to high doses (100 mg three times per day) of pyridoxine. However, true vitamin B_6 deficiency has never been documented in conjunction with this disease.

The variability of response to vitamin B_6 reflects the variability of defects found to affect mitochondrial Δ-ALA-S in sideroblastic anemias. Hereditary X-linked sideroblastic anemias may or may not be pyridoxine-responsive.

Besides treatment with pyridoxine, therapeutic phlebotomies to remove excessive tissue iron stores have been tried as treatment for inherited sideroblastic anemia when the anemia is mild. Rises in red cell mass may follow the removal of 10 gm or more of iron. This observation suggests that relieving mitochondrial iron overload sometimes improves heme synthesis. However, the basic defect in heme synthesis remains despite phlebotomy.

Primary Acquired Sideroblastic Anemia

Primary (or idiopathic) acquired sideroblastic anemia is usually a disease of the elderly. It presents with the usual symptoms of anemia, which may be mild or quite severe. It should be suspected when an elderly patient has a hypochromic anemia but is not iron deficient and does not have evidence of chronic disease. Except for pallor and occasionally splenomegaly the physical findings are unremarkable. This disorder is one of the five entities that comprise the myelodysplastic syndrome.

The laboratory features of this disease lead to its diagnosis. The peripheral blood smear reveals a population of hypochromic cells, many normal or small, and others that are macrocytic. Macrocytic cells usually predominate and lead to the confusing picture of a high MCV and hypochromia. Staining peripheral blood cells for iron may reveal iron-containing inclusions (Plate 20) in mature red cells, which are then called *siderocytes*. These siderocytes can also be seen after Wright staining (Plate 21), when they appear as clusters of small, irregular inclusions called Pappenheimer bodies. Such inclusions are seen in a number of disorders besides iron-loading anemias, including hyposplenism and some hemolytic anemias. Other blood abnormalities in acquired sideroblastic anemia may include neutropenia, immature red and white cells, and mild thrombocytopenia or thrombocytosis.

The pathognomonic finding in the bone marrow is the presence of ringed sideroblasts on iron stain. The rings are due to iron in mitochondria surrounding the nucleus of erythroblasts. Characteristically erythroid hyperplasia is present, often with changes such as those observed in megaloblastic anemia. In certain cases there may be abnormalities in the myeloid series, with a "shift to the left"; in others dysplastic changes may occur. These are abnormalities that may be associated with the various myelodysplastic syndromes, which previously were considered to be parts of the spectrum of the syndrome of "preleukemia."

The saturation of the total iron-binding capacity is usually 50 percent or more and is often 100 percent. Serum ferritin is elevated. Besides the iron-loading anemias discussed in this chapter, severe hemolysis, extensive blood transfusions, hepatic necrosis, recent oral ingestion of iron tablets, and marrow hypoplasia may cause saturation of the total iron-binding capacity with iron.

This anemia is usually resistant to all forms of therapy. In most cases folic acid (1 mg/day) is tried, since in a number of patients the serum folic acid level is low and there may be megaloblastic changes in the bone marrow. Anemia is improved in a few cases, but in most, folic acid has little effect. Patients are treated with blood transfusions as needed, and often live for many years without a significant change in transfusion requirements. Pyridoxine, in a dose of 100 mg three times per day, and an androgen such as oxymethalone (50 to 100 mg/day) are often prescribed but are usually unsuccessful. Treatment with adrenocorticosteroids or splenectomy is not advised. A minority of patients may respond to therapy with erythropoietic. Patients with sideroblastic anemia who are transfusion-dependent have a worse prognosis, and problems related to iron overload from multiple transfusions may develop. A minority of sideroblastic anemias evolve into acute myelocytic leukemia. Unfortunately, these leukemias are usually resistant to therapy and are often rapidly fatal. Chromosomal abnormalities similar to those seen in myelodysplastic diseases have been reported.

Pyridoxine-responsive Sideroblastic Anemia

The clinical findings of pyridoxine-responsive sideroblastic anemia are similar to those of hereditary sideroblastic anemia. Occasionally patients with acquired sideroblastic anemia have some response to pyridoxine. Because of this, the only way to make the diagnosis is to treat all patients suffering from unexplained sideroblastic anemias with large doses of pyridoxine. Those who respond are labeled as having *pyridoxine-responsive sideroblastic anemia.* A rare patient will respond to pyridoxal phosphate, but not pyridoxine, suggesting that a defect in the conversion of pyridoxine to its active coenzyme form, pyridoxal, may be a cause of this anemia.

Secondary Sideroblastic Anemia

The association of ringed sideroblasts with chronic diseases, infections, leukemia, and hemolytic or megaloblastic anemia is unusual and unexplained. In megaloblastic anemia, if the vitamin B_{12} or folic acid deficiency is successfully treated, the sideroblastic changes will disappear. Similarly, the successful treatment of any other primary underlying disease usually results in disappearance of ringed sideroblasts and other evidence of iron overload.

Drugs such as cycloserine or isoniazid have been associated with iron-loading anemia. Isoniazid interferes with pyridoxine metabolism, and this adverse effect can be prevented by simultaneous administration of pyridoxine. Chloramphenicol (an inhibitor of ferrochelatase, or heme synthetase) also may cause sideroblastic anemia.

The anemia associated with the inherited disease thalassemia is primarily due to a defect in globin rather than heme synthesis. Iron-loading is a prominent finding in thalassemics, but ringed sideroblasts are found infrequently. The presence of iron in the bone marrow, family history, and presence of increased quantities of hemoglobins such as A_2 and F distinguish thalassemias from both iron deficiency and sideroblastic anemias.

Lead Poisoning

Anemia secondary to lead intoxication is a form of drug-induced sideroblastic anemia and is characterized by hypochromic red cells, hyperferremia, ringed sideroblasts, ineffective erythropoiesis, and mild hemolysis. The last may be a result of inhibition of membrane cationic pumps. Additionally, in the peripheral blood there is an increased number of coarsely stippled red cells (Plate 22). The stippling is produced by aggregations of altered mitochondria and ribosomes. As a result of the inhibition by lead of sulfhydryl-containing enzymes Δ-ALA DH, coproporphyrinogen oxidase, and heme synthetase in the heme synthetic pathway, there is impaired conversion of Δ-ALA to PBG, coproporphyrinogen to protoporphyrin, and protoporphyrin to heme. As a result, patients with lead intoxication excrete in the urine large amounts of Δ-ALA and coproporphyrin, and free erythrocyte protoporphyrin is increased. In contrast to acute intermittent porphyria, PBG excretion is not increased. Other effects of lead on cellular metabolism include damage to mitochondria and impaired globin synthesis.

Symptoms of lead poisoning include abdominal colic, peripheral neuropathy, and neuropsychiatric disorders, and may resemble those of acute intermittent porphyria in which Δ-ALA levels are also increased. Poisoning is confirmed by lead levels of 70 μg per deciliter or greater in the blood, or greater than 50 μg per day in the urine. Mass screening programs detect either elevations in the red cell protoporphyrin levels or increased serum or urine lead levels. It should be recalled that free red cell protoporphyrin levels will be elevated not only in lead intoxication but also in iron deficiency anemia and the anemia of chronic disease.

Chelating agents, such as dimercaprol (BAL) or sodium ethylene-diamine-tetraacetate (EDTA), and removal of the patient from exposure to lead are the only available treatment. Children in lower socioeconomic classes are particularly affected by this disease, since lead-containing paint chips that they ingest are readily available in their environment. They are especially likely to have an iron-deficient diet and an iron deficiency may develop that is associated with "pica" or ingestion of paint chips.

Alcoholism

Abnormal heme metabolism contributes to the anemia found in alcoholics. Disordered heme synthesis is manifested, particularly after "binge" drinking, by vacuolization of erythroid precursors, ringed sideroblasts, and increased reticuloendothelial iron stores. These disappear after withdrawal of alcohol and within ten days reticulocytosis and a return of hematocrit to normal are seen. The mechanism of the production of ringed sideroblasts is unclear.

Anemia of Chronic Disease

A moderate anemia often accompanies infection, inflammatory disease, cancer, or tissue necrosis. This third major type of hypochromic anemia also interferes with the response of the bone marrow to replacement therapy in the presence of iron, folic acid, or vitamin B_{12} deficiency. The hematocrit usually ranges between 30 and 36, and the anemia is generally normochromic and normocytic. It may occasionally be hypochromic and microcytic, and because it involves disordered iron metabolism, it must be considered in the differential diagnosis of hypochromic anemia. The anemia of chronic disease is characterized by low serum iron, low total iron-binding capacity, normal or low transferrin saturation, and normal or elevated serum ferritin levels. Although the bone marrow is morphologically normal and is filled with storage iron, the red cell production index is either decreased or not increased enough considering the severity of the anemia.

The low serum iron that characterizes the anemia of chronic disease (ACD) results from altered iron metabolism with impaired release of iron from macrophages to transferrin in the serum. The macrophages are filled with Prussian blue–staining iron (hemosiderin) while iron in the normoblast is reduced. Although the exact mechanism of the defective iron metabolism is not known, it appears related to lactoferrin, a protein that, like transferrin, binds iron. Lactoferrin is released into the serum in increased quantities during inflammatory states, and competes with transferrin for iron. Iron just released from macrophages after red cell death preferentially binds to lactoferrin, which diverts it back to macrophages— cells rich in lactoferrin receptors—instead of binding to transferrin, which delivers it to developing red cells. It has been suggested that this pathway has evolved as a host defense mechanism against infection since low plasma iron levels inhibit bacterial growth.

Other factors may contribute to the ACD, including a slightly decreased red cell life span and an inadequate reticulocyte response. The cause of the shortened RBC survival is not known, but may be a consequence of nonspecific stimulation of macrophages and a resultant increase in red cell destruction. The inadequate reticulo-cyte response is mediated in part by the impairment in iron availabil-ity to red cell precursors, and in part by a relative underproduction of erythropoietin in relation to the degree of anemia.

Total iron-binding capacities may be helpful in distinguishing the anemia of chronic disease from iron deficiency anemia. In both cases, serum iron is quite low, even less than 20 µg per deciliter and transferrin saturation may be less than 15 percent. However, the total iron-binding capacity is usually elevated in iron deficiency anemia and decreased in anemia of chronic disease. If there is doubt, bone marrow examination can easily distinguish between the two entities. In iron deficiency, reticuloendothelial iron is absent, and fewer than 10 percent of the normoblasts contain Prussian blue–staining inclusions. In anemia of chronic disease, reticuloendothe-lial iron is plentiful, even though there is a reduction in normoblast iron. Serum ferritin levels assayed by radioimmunoassay are low in iron deficiency but normal or elevated in patients with ACD. In practice there is another way of distinguishing these diseases—by a trial of iron therapy. Patients with the anemia of chronic disease respond little, if at all, to therapeutic amounts of iron. Iron-deficient patients show a rise in peripheral blood reticulocyte count and hematocrit.

Anemia associated with chronic disease rarely demands therapy, since the anemia is usually not severe. Even if therapy is required, there is none available except supportive treatment with trans-fusions. These patients require only red cells, not plasma volume; therefore, packed red cells, and not whole blood, should be used for transfusion therapy. Treatment with iron is obviously not indicated. It has recently been demonstrated that treatment with erythropoi-etin can improve anemia in ACD.

Thalassemias

The normal adult carries three types of hemoglobin, A (96–98%), F (2–3%), and A_2 (2–3%). Two types of hemoglobin F exist, one whose γ-chains have glycine in position 136, the other with alanine in this position. After birth the γ-loci are switched off, and β- and δ-loci are fully activated. The α-chains combine with β- and δ-chains to produce hemoglobin A and A_2, respectively. In the thalassemias genetic defects result in decreased synthesis of α- or β-globin chains.

Normal Human Globin Gene Organization

α-Chain genes are situated on human chromosome number 16, and there are two α-chain genes on each haploid DNA strand, yielding a total of four loci. Human chromosome number 11 carries single $^G\gamma$ (gamma chain for fetal hemoglobin having glycine at amino acid residue 136), $^A\gamma$ (gamma chain for fetal hemoglobin with alanine at residue 136), δ (delta) and β (beta) genes per haploid strand. The loci are arranged in the order listed reading from the 5' to 3' end of the chromosome (Fig. 3-3). Structural similarities exist between these genes and even α-chain genes suggesting that they are descended from a single, primitive heme-containing polypeptide chain. Gene reduplication and segregation to different chromosomes probably account for the present globin gene organization.

In thalassemia, a genetic defect results in decreased synthesis of either α- or β-globin chains. Impaired production of αβ tetramers results in defective cells that often never leave the marrow, resulting in ineffective erythropoiesis. Red cells that do enter the circulation are small and poorly hemoglobinized, and have abnormal shapes and a markedly shortened survival. Excessive unbound globin chains (whether due to decreased α or β production) form aggregates, and these cytoplasmic inclusions damage the red cell, contributing to their destruction both in the marrow and in the circulation. The imbalance of globin chain synthesis and the aggregation of these chains is crucial to the red cell pathophysiology noted in the thalassemias. For instance, in certain forms of the disease γ-chain production partially compensates for decreased β-chain production. In this thalassemia variant, the α- and γ-chains form stable fetal hemoglobin, associated with a more benign clinical course.

α-Chain and β-chain genes, like other genes, contain two segments of DNA: nonprotein encoding regions termed *introns* located between the regions that are transcribed (exons) and code for globin chains (polypeptides). In the nucleus, precursor globin messenger RNA (mRNA) is transcribed from these DNA templates. The intervening introns are spliced from mRNA and the mRNA moves to the cytoplasm for translation into globin chains. As is discussed later, many forms of β-thalassemia are caused by incorrect splicing of the introns from mRNA, resulting in a decreased or absent translation product. Variations in splicing errors, in addition to a variety of mutations in the DNA sequences necessary for efficient transcription, account for the broad diversity of clinical phenotypes in β-thalassemia.

α-Thalassemia most often results from a deletion of all or part of the gene that codes for the α-chain. In contrast to β-thalassemia, its clinical presentation is usually straightforward, reflecting simply the number of α-genes deleted.

The science of molecular biology has added new techniques for the study of thalassemia. These methods, along with new knowledge concerning the synthesis, translocation, and stability of mRNA, now allow us to better understand the nature of the gene defects in the various thalassemia syndromes.

Fig. 3-3. Simplified diagram of non-embryonic human globin genes and their deletions in non–α-thalassemias. In the β-globin gene, introns are represented as dark areas and exons are light. HPFH, hereditary persistence of fetal hemoglobin.

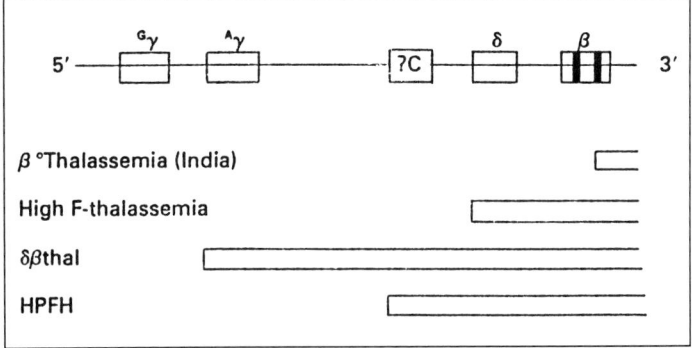

DNA from large segments of the human genome can be digested by restriction enzymes that "recognize" and cleave double-stranded DNA at specific sequences. The resulting DNA fragments can be separated by size in an electrophoretic gradient and transferred to a DNA-binding membrane. Specific sequences of DNA can be identified by binding with complementary DNA of known origin (a "probe"). This technique, known as a Southern hybridization or "Southern blot," has been utilized to identify the loss of genes associated with α-thalassemia.

Fragments or entire genes identified by Southern blots can be inserted into self-replicating vectors (plasmids) that allow DNA fragments to be reproduced or cloned in significant quantity for DNA sequencing. Globin chain DNA fragments from normal and thalassemic individuals have been analyzed by these techniques and have been used to define the molecular basis of both α- and β-thalassemia.

Genetic Defects in Thalassemia

Although gene deletions explain the decreased α-chain synthesis in most α-thalassemia syndromes, nondeletion α-gene defects are also known to cause α-thalassemia syndromes, such as hemoglobin H disease (see pp. 63–64).

Several molecular deficits can lead to β-thalassemia. Most commonly β-thalassemia results from defective removal of introns, producing reduced or absent β-globin chain production. A well-documented abnormality that can cause the defective splicing is a single base pair mutation in one of the introns at the intron-exon junction or splice site in the β-globin gene. The enzyme (s) responsible for removal of the intron cannot recognize the correct break point in the resultant precursor mRNA, and it remains trapped in the nucleus, unable to be translated to globin chains in the cell cytoplasm. A small amount of mRNA may undergo normal splicing, resulting in reduced but not absent β-globin chain production. In general, mutations closer to splice sites have more profound effects in decreasing translation efficiency.

Mutations in the gene at sites other than introns can also result in reduced β-globin chain production. Mutations have been identified in an upstream noncoding region of the chromosome important for globin gene regulation. Mutations in or near this region, called the promoter, generally do not result in severe disease. Efficient translation of mRNA also depends on cleavage of the end of the mRNA followed by attachment of a long string of adenines (polyadenylation). Mutations affecting polyadenylation that reduce β-chain production by as much as 90 percent have been detected in certain β-thalassemia kindreds.

Single base pair mutations within the coding region (exons) of the β-thalassemia gene have a profound effect on globin chain production. In contrast to mutations in regulatory or splice sites, these mutations often lead to premature chain termination and a nonfunctional gene product. Insertions and deletions in coding regions have also been identified as rare causes of β-thalassemia.

Gene deletions are a less common cause of β-thalassemia. However, when deletions occur in the β-gene locus on chromosome 11, all or part of the δ-chain gene on the same locus also may be deleted. This genetic phenotype may cause increased expression of the γ-chain locus and therefore increased production of hemoglobin F, resulting in hereditary persistence of fetal hemoglobin, which has a benign clinical course (see later in text).

β-Thalassemia Syndromes

Three clinical types of β-thalassemia are recognized. These syndromes are clinical descriptions and do not directly relate to specific genetic defects. In general, thalassemia major is the result of mutations associated with severely reduced β-globin expression on both chromosomes (e.g., β^{thal0}, β^{thal0}). These mutations might be chain termination mutations, uncommon gene deletions, or a point mutation in an intron that has profound effect on translation. Intermediate clinical disease usually is also due to homozygous or doubly heterozygous mutations that are associated with moderate reductions in globin chain expression from both chromosomes (e.g., β^{thal+}, β^{thal+}). Thalassemia minor results from a reduction in β-globin synthesis from one chromosome but not the other (e.g., β^{thal0}, normal β). The designation β^{thal0} indicates that the mutation in that globin gene, whatever its nature, completely prevents the formation of β-globin chains; the designation β^{thal+} is used to denote a mutation that reduces but does not fully suppress β-chain production.

THALASSEMIA MAJOR

The most severe type is *β-thalassemia major*. This disease is usually recognized during the first years of life. Small size, poor weight gain, severe anemia (4–6 gm per deciliter), jaundice, chronic leg ulcers, mongoloid facies—flattened nose and wide-apart eyes with bossing of the skull, hypertrophy of the upper maxillae, and prominent malar eminences—characterize affected children. X-rays of the skull show dilatation of the space between the tables of bone with a series of radiating striations, giving a *hair-on-end* appearance. The long bones are thin, and fractures are not uncommon. These patients do not develop normally physically and may not be normal mentally. Sexual development is delayed and may not appear at all. Hepatosplenomegaly, with massive enlargement of the spleen, is common. Infections of the bones, gallbladder (gallstones are common), and sinuses occur less commonly. Examination of the bone marrow shows intense erythroid hyperplasia, and in many patients there are megaloblastic changes because of folate deficiency. Some patients die as a result of infections or iron deposition in tissues, such as the myocardium, leading to organ failure. The iron overload is due to both transfusions and increased iron absorption.

THALASSEMIA INTERMEDIA

The second clinical type is *thalassemia intermedia*. These patients have similar abnormalities to thalassemia major in their hemoglobin patterns but suffer only a moderate degree of anemia and require intermittent or no transfusions. They may live with chronic disease into adult life.

THALASSEMIA MINOR

The third type is *thalassemia minor* or *trait*, in which there is little in the way of symptoms, and the diagnosis is made on the basis of family studies or on examination of the peripheral blood, which shows substantial microcytosis and marked abnormalities in the face of only mild anemia.

Anemia in β-Thalassemia

Anemia in β-thalassemia is a result of (1) decreased synthesis of the β-globin chains of hemoglobin and (2) precipitation and subsequent removal of excess α-globin chains, which in turn lead to ineffective erythropoiesis and hemolysis. Hypochromia, microcytosis, fragmented forms, and basophilic stippling are found in blood from thalassemia patients (see Plates 23 and 24). Many target cells are also common.

The hypochromia is a result of decreased cellular content of hemoglobin, a major defect in thalassemia. The bone marrow is hyperplastic but the reticulocyte count only moderately increased. The production abnormality is due to ineffective erythropoiesis, that is, destruction of immature erythroid cells in the bone marrow. In addition, there is hemolysis of erythrocytes in the peripheral blood. Both this intramedullary and extramedullary destruction of erythroid cells appear to be due largely to the presence of Heinz bodies—in this case, excess α-chains—and to the process by which these excess α-chains are removed from the cells. These Heinz bodies deform the cells and membrane abnormalities occur when the Heinz bodies are "pitted" from the cells by mononuclear phagocytes of the reticuloendothelium. In the bone marrow this leads to ineffective erythropoiesis, in the peripheral blood to hemolysis. Pitting of circulating erythrocytes occurs particularly in the spleen. The splenic reticuloendothelial cells may first deform cells into teardrop shapes while plucking out the inclusions. Further injury leads to decreased plasticity of the red cell membrane and formation of fragmented forms. Triangular forms, target cells, tiny microcytes, teardrop forms, and other shape abnormalities are commonly seen. Basophilic stippling, polychromatophils, and nucleated red cells are also present. Supravital staining or phase microscopy reveals Heinz inclusion bodies and pits or craters in the cell membrane, indicating where Heinz bodies have been removed. The Heinz bodies are most numerous after splenectomy and in patients with severe anemia.

The anemia stimulates the bone marrow to maximum activity, resulting in expansion of the bone marrow cavity and the skeletal abnormalities previously described. Iron is abundant, and small numbers of ringed sideroblasts may be found.

In milder forms of thalassemia, microcytosis, hypochromia, and an abnormal blood smear are present in a patient with minimal or mild anemia.

It is possible for the β^{thal0} or the β^{thal+} gene to interact with a sickle mutation. Patients with $\beta^S\beta^{thal0}$ genes have virtually all sickle hemoglobin and no HbA, whereas patients with $\beta^S\beta^{thal+}$ genes have some HbA present. The patient with $\beta^S\beta^{thal0}$ will usually have less severe disease than a patient with $\beta^S\beta^S$ (homozygous sickle cell disease) because of the decreased cellular hemoglobin content (i.e., hypochromia) in the former disorder.

Hemoglobin Lepore (Hb$_{Lepore}$) Syndromes

As a result of a structural defect in hemoglobin, a thalassemia-like picture can be produced in patients who carry genes for Hb_{Lepore}. This hemoglobin results from an unequal crossover between the closely linked β- and δ-chain gene loci, creating a fusion gene. It has the electrophoretic mobility of hemoglobin S, a δ-chain sequence at one end, and a β-chain sequence at the other. Patients with two Hb$_{Lepore}$ genes synthesize hemoglobin at a reduced rate, presumably because they lack a normal β-chain gene. The clinical findings resemble those of thalassemia major. Patients with a single Hb$_{Lepore}$ gene have the clinical picture of thalassemia minor.

In high F thalassemia or homozygous δβ-thalassemia, patients do not produce hemoglobin A or A_2, but compensate by persistent γ-chain production making fetal hemoglobin. In the usual patient with β-thalassemia, although HbF levels are elevated, HbF is confined to a small population of cells (heterogeneous distribution). The HbF-containing cells survive longer because the γ-chains can bind α-chains and prevent Heinz body formation. Therefore, the clinical severity of the disorder depends on the number of cells producing HbF.

Hereditary Persistence of Fetal Hemoglobin

A variant of this disorder found primarily in the black population is called hereditary persistence of fetal hemoglobin (HPFH). These patients exhibit higher levels of γ-chain synthesis that effectively compensate for reduced β-chain expression. In HPFH, HbF is present in all the red cells (homogeneous distribution). Hemoglobin can be demonstrated using a Kleinhauer-Betke or acid elution stain of a peripheral blood smear after treatment with citrate-phosphate buffer (pH 3.2), which elutes HbA and leaves HbF behind. In HPFH, there is a clear-cut failure to suppress γ-chain synthesis postnatally. Since the deletion of chromosome 11 is more extensive in HPFH than in high F thalassemia, it may be that the deletion affects a region of the chromosome regulating γ-chain synthesis. The location of the genetic "switch" that affects γ-chain synthesis is currently under investigation. This system is of great interest since increasing fetal hemoglobin production can ameliorate the clinical severity not only of β-thalassemia but also of sickle cell disease.

α-Thalassemia

In contrast to the two β-chain loci, four gene loci (two closely linked genes on each chromosome) exist for synthesis of globin α-chains. Mutations may affect one or all four of these gene loci. Different clinical pictures result, depending on the number of gene loci affected (i.e., deleted).

The four main α-thalassemic syndromes in order of increasing severity are the silent carrier trait, α-thal trait, hemoglobin H disease, and hemoglobin$_{Bart's}$ (γ_4) or hydrops fetalis. Patients with the silent carrier trait are clinically normal and have normal hematologic findings. These patients have a deletion of one of the four α-chain loci. α-Thal trait is characterized by two abnormal loci, which may exist on the same chromosome or on both chromosomes. Genetically α-thal trait can result from two defective genes on one chromosome received from one parent or one defective α-chain gene on the chromosome received from each parent. In either case there are mild hematologic abnormalities (mild anemia, low MCV and MCH, and hypochromia) compatible with thalassemia trait. Hemoglobin H disease results from three deleted α-chain loci. It is clinically characterized by the clinical picture of thalassemia intermedia and by variable amounts of hemoglobin H, a β-chain tetramer. The most severe form of α-thalassemia occurs in severely anemic, edematous, stillborn infants whose hemoglobin composition is almost all hemoglobin$_{Bart's}$. These patients have deletion of all four α-chain loci and therefore can produce in the fetal state only γ-chains, which polymerize to form Hb$_{Bart's}$. The amount of Bart's hemoglobin in a fetus or newborn has a direct correlation with the number of thalassemic α-chain loci, so that 1 to 2 percent is found in fetuses with the silent carrier state, 5 to 6 percent in α-thal minor, 25 percent in HbH disease, and greater than 80 percent in hydrops fetalis.

An interesting nondeletion α-chain structural mutant is hemoglobin$_{Constant\ Spring}$ (HbCS). This hemoglobin is characterized by an α-chain elongated at the C-terminal end by 31 amino acid residues. It arises from mutation of the terminating codon of the normal α-gene. This gene is similar to Lepore hemoglobin in that it has a thalassemia-like effect causing reduced synthesis of the α-CS chain. Double heterozygosity for α-thalassemia trait (two affected α-chain loci) and HbCS result in a picture similar to that of hemoglobin H disease but with a small percentage of HbCS also present.

HbH ($β_4$) is electrophoretically fast, unstable, and thermolabile and has an oxygen affinity ten times normal (no heme–heme interaction). Anemia results from Heinz body formation in marrow and peripheral blood erythrocytes. These inclusion bodies can be demonstrated, particularly after splenectomy, by incubation of red cells with brilliant cresyl blue for 20 minutes. This dye oxidizes free thiols in the HbH molecules, thereby causing HbH to precipitate. Presumably, newly produced erythrocytes contain soluble HbH, which precipitates during the cell's life, and the Heinz body formed is pitted from the cell by mononuclear phagocytes in the bone marrow, spleen, and elsewhere in the reticuloendothelial system. The increased oxygen affinity of HbH further complicates the anemia by preventing normal release of oxygen to tissues. Luckily the majority of the hemoglobin present in patients with HbH disease is HbA. Microcytosis, hypochromia, target cells, stippling, and poikilocytes are found on examination of peripheral blood smears.

Treatment of Thalassemia

Transfusion remains the mainstay of treatment for patients with thalassemia major or Cooley's anemia. Patients maintained on a vigorous transfusion regimen from an early age may have more normal growth and development, and less skeletal deformity, heart failure, and hepatosplenomegaly. The higher hematocrit decreases erythropoietin production and thus dampens the severe erythroid hyperplasia of the bone marrow. In some patients splenectomy may be necessary to decrease the transfusion requirement and to reduce the discomfort that results from a large spleen. However, splenectomized thalassemic children appear particularly susceptible to both postsplenectomy sepsis and an increased tendency for iron overload and therefore it is best to avoid splenectomy as long as possible.

Transfusions and ineffective erythropoiesis lead to an increased load of systemic iron. Thus, these patients develop hemochromatosis and may die of the resulting heart or liver disease. Iron chelation therapy administered through continuous infusion of subcutaneous desferrioxamine has been extremely useful in removing large quantities of iron from these patients, particularly those receiving transfusion therapy. It is not yet certain, however, that chelation therapy reduces heart failure from iron overload, the major cause of death in patients with thalassemia.

In addition to chelation therapy, supplementation with folic acid is necessary to support increased erythroid activity of the marrow. Vitamin C therapy may enhance the efficacy of chelation therapy. Oral iron therapy, often mistakenly administered because of a low MCV, should be avoided.

Bone marrow transplantation has been successfully utilized in severely affected thalassemic patients and may be employed with increasing frequency in the future as it becomes a safer procedure.

Newer therapies have been directed toward increasing synthesis of HbF. The chemotherapeutic agent, 5-azacytidine, can increase γ-chain synthesis; initially, it was thought that it did so by altering methylation in the regulatory region of this gene. Use of this agent has proved too toxic in the short term, and there have been additional concerns about its carcinogenic potential in the long term. Cell cycle specific agents such as hydroxyurea along with growth factors such as erythropoietin are being employed to increase HbF production by "stressing" erythropoiesis in the bone marrow, and may prove useful for treatment of thalassemia and sickle cell disease in the future. 5-Azacytidine doubtless works through a similar mechanism.

The genes for α- and β-globin have been cloned and the marrow compartment is accessible for genetic manipulation, making gene replacement therapy theoretically possible. However, major technical problems must be overcome before gene therapy becomes a reality.

Diagnosis of Thalassemia

The diagnosis of thalassemia major is usually made from a family history of thalassemia, skeletal and facial abnormalities at birth, and the presence of a severe microcytic and hypochromic anemia (Plate 24) with evidence of ineffective erythropoiesis. Confirmation comes from measuring hemoglobin A_2 and hemoglobin F levels. Most forms of β-thalassemia are associated with an increase in hemoglobin A_2 levels, sometimes accompanied by an increase in hemoglobin F. In the hemoglobin$_{Lepore}$ and δβ-thalassemia syndromes, hemoglobin A_2 levels are normal or decreased but hemoglobin F levels are elevated. Hemoglobin A_2 and F levels are usually normal in the different forms of α-thalassemia. Hemoglobin A_2 is generally determined by starch block electrophoresis or diethylaminoethylcellulose (DEAE) column chromatography. Hemoglobin F is measured by addition of potassium hydroxide to a hemoglobin solution. In this method denatured HbA is precipitated by ammonium sulfate and removed by filtration. The alkali-resistant HbF remains in the supernatant. The proportion of alkali-resistant hemoglobin F is expressed as a percentage of the total hemoglobin present. Normal hemoglobin A_2 levels are 2 to 3 percent and hemoglobin F levels are 0 to 2 percent.

In some cases family studies will be necessary to determine a thalassemic patient's genotype; rarely, special globin chain separation procedures are required to confirm the diagnosis of thalassemia, as follows: Reticulocytes from a patient are incubated with radiolabeled amino acids, and the newly synthesized hemoglobin purified. After separation of the hemoglobin chains, it is possible to measure, by assaying radioactivity, the amount of nascent α- and β-chains. In β-thalassemic patients the ratio of β-chain production to α-chain production is reduced 50 percent in the heterozygote and considerably more in the homozygote. In α-thalassemics increased β-chain-to-α-chain synthesis ratios are found.

In the adult the diagnosis of thalassemia intermedia or minor is usually suspected in patients of Mediterranean ancestry with microcytic anemia. Examination of their peripheral blood (Plate 23) shows microcytosis, hypochromia, target cells, and poikilocytosis. These patients usually have a normal or near-normal hematocrit in the case of thalassemia minor and are moderately anemic in the case of thalassemic intermedia. The discrepancy between the severe microcytosis, abnormalities of shape, and the mild or moderate anemia should suggest the diagnosis of thalassemia minor.

Some thalassemic patients come to attention because of their extremely low MCV—75 femtoliters or less by the Coulter counter. Iron deficiency may cause MCV values this low, but an MCV of 75 fL or less would then be associated with severe anemia. The following calculation serves as rule of thumb: MCV(fL)/PCV(L/L) × 0.1. A value of less than 13 suggests the diagnosis of thalassemia rather than iron deficiency anemia.

α-Thalassemia heterozygotes are detected by unexplained micro-cytosis in black, Southeast Asian, or Chinese populations. Hemo-globin H disease may be suspected and supravital staining for the characteristic erythrocyte inclusions performed in such patients with moderate degrees of anemia. Hb$_{Bart's}$ disease should be suspected in Asian women with a history of repeated hydropic stillbirths.

Prenatal Diagnosis

Defining the molecular basis of α- and β-thalassemia has been enor-mously useful not only in understanding gene expression but also in providing genetic information useful for the prenatal diagnosis of thalassemia. Chorionic villus sampling allows fetal blood to be ana-lyzed in the first trimester. Genetic detection methods can be utilized in prenatal diagnosis of thalassemia from either this fetal blood or amniocentesis specimens.

Prenatal diagnosis of α-thalassemia is usually straightforward since the cause of this disease is most often gene deletion. Southern blot hybridization studies using α-chain DNA as a probe are usually sufficiently informative. Identification of a fetus at risk for homo-zygous β-thalassemia is more difficult. In some cases family studies can be useful in determining if there is an alteration in the restriction enzyme digestion pattern in the region of the non–α-globin gene cluster. Identification of a particular base pair substitution mutation is possible using a battery of oligonucleotide probes and, if neces-sary, the polymerase chain reaction.

Approach to Patient with Microcytic Anemia

On the basis of the historical and physical findings, serum iron, total iron-binding capacity (TIBC), serum ferritin, and bone marrow examination, it is usually possible to distinguish anemias due to iron lack, sideroblastic anemia, chronic disease, or thalassemia.

The characteristic low serum iron and high TIBC distinguish iron deficiency anemia from sideroblastic anemia and thalassemia, with saturation of iron-binding capacity. Anemia of chronic disease may be confused with iron deficiency, since serum iron levels may be quite low in both. However, in ACD the TIBC is low or normal, with normal or increased marrow iron stores, and there is evidence of a chronic disease such as infection or cancer. Serum ferritin determi-nations usually separate iron deficiency from anemia of chronic disease. Ferritin levels are normal or elevated in the face of chronic disease but low in iron-deficient patients. Ferritin levels are typically elevated in sideroblastic anemia and thalassemia.

Approach to patient with microcytic anemia

I. History
   A. Adults
      1. Menstrual: menorrhagia, metrorrhagia
      2. Pregnancy: deliveries, miscarriages
      3. Blood loss
         a. Gastrointestinal: peptic ulcer symptoms, change in bowel habits, hematemesis, melena, hematochezia
         b. Drug-induced: aspirin, indomethacin (Indocin), phenylbutazone
         c. Urinary: hematuria, hemoglobinuria
         d. Respiratory: hemoptysis
      4. Chronic disease
         a. Infections
         b. Inflammatory diseases
         c. Malignancy
         d. Fever, weight loss
      5. Diet
      6. Family history: thalassemia, hereditary hemorrhagic telangiectasia, sideroblastic anemia
   B. Infants and children
      1. Diet
      2. Perinatal: prematurity, multiple births, maternal iron lack
      3. Blood loss: gastrointestinal
      4. Chronic disease
      5. Family history
II. Physical examination
   A. Mucus membranes: cheilosis, angular stomatitis
   B. Tongue: glossitis, atrophy
   C. Skin: telangiectasia, koilonychia (nails)
   D. Breasts, abdomen, pelvic, rectal, etc.: evidence of infections, inflammatory or malignant disease
   E. Splenomegaly (thalassemia)
III. Laboratory tests
   A. Blood counts and smear (Wright stain)
   B. Reticulocyte count and production index
   C. Stool examination for occult blood
   D. Serum iron and total iron-binding capacity
   E. Bone marrow examination for iron stores
   F. Serum ferritin
   G. Erythrocyte sedimentation rate
IV. Special tests
   A. Gastrointestial x-rays or endoscopies
   B. Stool examination for parasites
   C. Urine or sputum stained for hemosiderin
   D. Tests for malabsorption syndromes
   E. Hemoglobins A_2 and F for β-thalassemia
   F. Therapeutic trial with oral iron supplementation
   G. Therapeutic trial with pyridoxine (sideroblastic anemia)

In some cases bone marrow examination of hemosiderin stores is required for differential diagnosis. Adequate iron stores rule out iron deficiency anemia, and ringed sideroblasts are characteristic of sideroblastic anemias. In ACD iron is seen in macrophages but not in RBC precursors.

Once the diagnosis of iron deficiency anemia is established, the possibility of blood loss, usually from the intestine or uterus, must be investigated. Only after blood loss has been ruled out should such rare causes of iron lack be considered as malabsorption syndrome, hemoglobinuria secondary to intravascular hemolysis, and pulmonary hemosiderosis (a disorder associated with microhemorrhages and hemosiderin-laden macrophages in the lungs).

Sideroblastic anemias are subclassified on the basis of family history, response to pyridoxine, and the presence of primary diseases or drugs known to cause ringed sideroblast formation.

Usually when anemia of chronic disease is suspected, malignant, inflammatory, or infectious diseases are generally apparent. Occasionally none of these can be readily demonstrated, but the *erythrocyte sedimentation rate (ESR)* is often elevated.

Case Development Problem: Microcytic Anemia

A 60-year-old man who underwent removal of the lower half of his stomach for ulcers 10 years ago was seen and treated yesterday at his neighborhood health center for acute kidney infection and has been referred to you for further examination.

His hematocrit was 0.21 (21%); hemoglobin, 5.0 gm/dL; red blood cell count, 3.2×10^{12}/L; and reticulocyte count, 3 percent.

1. Calculate and interpret his red cell indices. What would you find on his peripheral blood smear?

   Mean corpuscular volume: 70 fL
   Mean corpuscular hemoglobin: 16 pg
   Mean corpuscular hemoglobin concentration: 24 gm/dL
   You would expect to find microcytosis, smaller than normal cells, and hypochromic, pale-staining cells whose ring of hemoglobin would extend less than two thirds of the distance between the cell's membrane and center.

2. His peripheral blood smear shows no polychromatophilia. Calculate his reticulocyte production index and interpret the value obtained.

   Reticulocyte production index $= (3 \times 21/45)/1 =$ approximately 1.5

The production index indicates his bone marrow is 1½ times more active than normal. Considering his very low hematocrit, this response is inadequate. What appears to be an elevated reticulocyte count really represents an inadequate response to his anemia.

After an appropriate history and physical examination are obtained, you order determinations of serum iron and total iron-binding capacity and a stool examination. Three different sets of laboratory values are listed below. For each, describe what you would most likely find in the patient's bone marrow.

a. Serum iron: 20μg/dL
Total iron-binding capacity: 450μg/dL
Stool for occult blood: positive
Bone marrow examination would reveal erythroid hyperplasia with many poorly hemoglobinized erythroid precursors. The stain for iron would show no reticuloendothelial (extracellular) iron or normoblast (sideroblast) iron.

b. Serum iron: 190μg/dL
Total iron-binding capacity: 200μg/dL
Stool for occult blood: negative
Serum ferritin: 500 ng/mL
Bone marrow would show erythroid hyperplasia.
Sideroblastic and extracellular iron would both be increased, and there might be ringed sideroblasts. (The patient could have sideroblastic anemia or thalassemia.)

c. Serum iron: 10μg/dL
Total iron-binding capacity: 100μg/dL
Stool for occult blood: negative
Serum ferritin: 300 ng/mL
Bone marrow examination would be unremarkable, except that intracellular normoblastic iron might be low relative to the normal or increased stores of extracellular iron (anemia of chronic disease).

The serum iron and ferritin of the patient referred to you was low, and his total iron-binding capacity very high. His bone marrow revealed mild erythroid hyperplasia and absent stainable iron.

3. What findings are likely on physical examination?

This patient has iron deficiency anemia, so signs of anemia including pallor of skin, nails, and mucus membranes are present. Angular stomatitis, cheilosis, glossitis, tongue atrophy, and koilonychia may be present if the iron deficiency is long-standing. It is also important in such a case to look for a source of blood loss. It is common in this age group for a colonic or stomach neoplasm to present with bleeding and iron deficiency anemia.

Gastrointestinal x-rays done on your patient revealed a recurrent ulcer at the site where his duodenum had been reattached to the remnants of his stomach. It is believed that he has had intermittent bleeding from this site. No neoplasm or other lesion is demonstrated. Ferrous sulfate, 300 mg orally three times per day, is begun.

4. What response would you expect to these therapeutic doses of iron?

In most cases an elevation in the reticulocyte count begins 3 to 5 days after oral iron therapy is started and reaches a peak in 7 to 10 days. The reticulocytosis depends on the severity of the anemia. Severely anemic patients often have reticulocyte counts above 10 percent. Within 2 to 3 weeks his hematocrit should rise.

Your patient has started iron therapy and has an initial reticulocyte response. However, his hematocrit fails to rise.

5. In this patient, what possible explanations exist for failure to respond adequately to therapy?

First, he may not be taking his iron pills. Stools will turn black if adequate amounts of iron have been ingested. Second, he may be bleeding again and therefore losing blood as fast as he is making it. A follow-up examination of his stools, looking for blood, should be done. Third, his urinary tract infection may prevent adequate response of the bone marrow. Fourth, some patients, particularly those who have undergone gastrectomy, inadequately absorb iron. If this is true of this patient, it may be necessary to treat him with intravenous or intramuscular iron. However, postgastrectomy patients usually absorb iron salts well, although they may malabsorb food iron.

Your patient makes a complete recovery from his iron deficiency anemia and his ulcer heals. Ten years later he again presents with a hypochromic anemia, but this time his serum iron is 200μg/dL and his TIBC is 210μg/dL. A bone marrow specimen, after staining with Prussian blue, reveals small blue cytoplasmic inclusions surrounding the nuclei of normoblasts. Serum ferritin is 700 ng per milliliter.

6. What is the most likely diagnosis? How should he be treated?

This patient has developed sideroblastic anemia. A close study of his bone marrow for leukemia is necessary. If a complete workup reveals no etiology, then treatment with pyridoxine should be undertaken. A few patients will respond to this with an elevated hematocrit and reduced blood transfusion requirement, but for the great majority the only treatment is blood transfusion.

Topics for Discussion: Microcytic Anemias

Gastrointestinal absorption of iron

Role of hydrochloric acid, phytates, chelating agents, ascorbic acid, and molybdenum in iron absorption

Red cell inclusions (stippling, Pappenheimer bodies, etc.)

Ferrokinetics

Mechanism of action and use of desferrioxamine

Iron storage compounds, ferritin, and hemosiderin

Heme and hemoglobin synthesis

Tissue changes in iron deficiency anemia

Achlorhydria and atrophic gastritis in iron deficiency anemia

Subtotal gastrectomy and its effects on iron absorption

Pathophysiology of secondary sideroblastic anemias

Anemia of chronic disease

Alcohol and sideroblastic anemia

Porphyrin synthesis

Lead poisoning

Selected Readings

Finch, C. A. Clinical aspects of iron deficiency and excess. *Semin. Hematol.* 19 : 1, 1982.

General Considerations

Jandl, J. H. The Hypochromic Anemias and Other Disorders of Iron Metabolism, Section 6. In J. H. Jandl, *Blood: Textbook of Hematology.* Boston: Little, Brown, 1987. p. 181.

Williams, W. J. (Ed.). Synthesis of Heme (Chap. 32), Iron Deficiency Anemia (Chap. 48), and Anemia of Chronic Disorders (Chap. 51). In *Hematology* (4th ed.) New York: McGraw Hill, 1990.

Iron Metabolism

Finch, C. A., and Huebers, H. A. Iron metabolism. *Clin. Physiol. Biochem.* 4 : 5, 1986.

Woods, S., Demarco, T., and Friedland, M. Iron metabolism. *Am. J. Gastroenterol.* 85 : 1, 1990.

Worwood, M. An overview of iron metabolism at a molecular level. *J. Intern. Med.* 226 : 381, 1989.

Iron Deficiency Anemia

Cartwright, G. E. et al. Association of HLA-linked hemochromatosis with idiopathic refractory sideroblastic anemia. *J. Clin. Invest.* 65 : 989, 1980.

Cook, J. D. Clinical evaluation of iron deficiency. *Semin. Hematol.* 19 : 6, 1982.

Dagg, J. H., and Goldberg, A. Detection and treatment of iron deficiency. *Clin. Haematol* 2 : 365, 1975.

Finch, C. A. Drugs Effective in Iron-Deficiency and Other Hypochromic Anemias. In A. G. Gilman, L. S. Goodman and A. Gilman (eds.), *The Pharmacological Basis of Therapeutics* (6th ed.). New York: Macmillan, 1980.

Irie, S., and Tavassoli, M. Transferrin-mediated cellular iron uptake. *Am. J. Med. Sci.* 293 : 103, 1987.

Jacobs, A., and Worwood, M. Ferritin in serum: Clinical and biochemical implications. *N. Engl. J. Med.* 292 : 951, 1975.

Wheby, M. S. Effect of iron therapy on serum ferritin levels in iron-deficiency anemia. *Blood* 56 : 138, 1980.

Porphyria

Goldberg, A., and Moore, M. R. (eds.). The porphyrias. *Clin. Haematol.* 9 : 227, 1980.

Tschudy, D. P. Acute intermittent porphyria: Clinical and selected research aspects. *Ann. Intern. Med.* 83 : 851, 1975

Sideroblastic Anemia

Beris, P., Graf, B. J., and Miescher, P. A. Primary acquired sideroblastic and primary acquired refractory anemia. *Semin. Hematol.* 20 : 101-113, 1983.

Bottomley, S. S., and Muller-Eberhard, U. Pathophysiology of heme synthesis. *Semin. Hematol.* 25 : 282-302, 1988.

Cartwright, G. E., and Deiss, A. Sideroblasts, siderocytes, and sideroblastic anemia. *N. Engl. J. Med.* 23 : 185-193, 1975.

Kushner, J. et al. Idiopathic refractory sideroblastic anemia: Clinical and laboratory investigation of 17 patients and review of the literature. *Medicine* (Baltimore) 50 : 139, 1971.

May, B. K., Bhasker, C. R., and Cox, T. C. Molecular regulation of 5-aminolevulinate synthase: Diseases related to heme biosynthesis. *Mol. Biol. Med.* 7 : 405-421, 1990.

Nusbaum, N. J. Concise review: Genetic bases for sideroblastic anemia. *Am. J. Hematol.* 37 : 41-44, 1991

Promelli, S. Lead Poisoning. In D. G. Nathan and F. A. Oski (eds.), *Hematology of Infancy and Childhood.* Philadelphia: Saunders, 1981.

Robinson, S., and Glass, J. Disorders of Heme Metabolism: Sideroblastic Anemia and the Porphyrias. In D. G. Nathan and F. A. Oski (eds.), *Hematology of Infancy and Childhood.* Philadelphia: Saunders, 1981.

Weatherall, D. J. et al. Iron loading in thalassemia: Five years with the pump. *N. Eng. J. Med.* 308 : 456, 1983.

Weintraub, L., Conrad, M., and Crosby, W. Iron loading anemia. Treatment with repeated phlebotomies and pyridoxine. *N. Engl. J. Med.* 275 : 169, 1966.

Woods, S., Demarco T. and Friedland M. Iron metabolism. *Am. J. Gastroenterol.* 85 : 1-8, 1990.

White, J. M., and Selhi, H. S. Lead and the red cell. *Br. J. Haematol.* 30 : 133, 1975.

Anemia of Chronic Disease

Barret-Conner, E. Anemia and infection. *Am. J. Med.* 52 : 242, 1972.

Cartwright, G. The anemia of chronic disorders. *Semin. Hematol.* 3 : 351, 1966.

Thalassemia

Bank, A. Globin gene structure in disorders of hemoglobin. *Prog. Hematol.* 12 : 25, 1981.

Bunn, H. F. Evolution of mammalian hemoglobin function. *Blood* 58 : 189, 1981.

Burns, A. L. et al. Isolation and characterization of cloned DNA: The δ and β globin genes in homozygous β^+ thalassemia. *Blood* 57 : 140, 1981.

Cao, A., Carcassi, U., and Rowley, P. T. (eds.). *Thalassemia: Recent Advances in Detection and Treatment*. New York: Alan R. Liss, 1982.

Forget, B. G. Molecular genetics of human hemoglobin synthesis. *Ann. Int. Med.* 91 : 605, 1979.

Hanash, S. M., and Rucknagel, D. L. Clinical implications of recent advances in hemoglobin disorders. *Med. Clin. N. Am.* 64 : 775, 1980.

Kan, Y. W. Prenatal diagnosis of hemoglobin disorders. *Prog. Hematol.* 10 : 91, 1977.

Kronenberg, H. M. Looking at genes. *N. Engl. J. Med.* 307 : 50, 1982.

Leder, P. Mechanisms of gene evolution. *J.A.M.A.* 248 : 1582, 1982.

Ley, T. J. et al. 5-azacytidine selectively increases β-globin synthesis in a patient with β thalassemia. *N. Engl. J. Med.* 307 : 1469, 1982.

Nienhuis, A. W., and Propper, R. D. The Thalassemias: Disorders of Hemoglobin Synthesis. In D. G. Nathan and F. A. Oski (eds.), *Hematology of Infancy and Childhood*. Philadelphia: Saunders, 1981.

Pearson, H. A., and O'Brien, R. T. The management of thalassemia major. *Semin. Hematol.* 12 : 255, 1975.

Pirastu, M. P. et al. Alpha-thalassemia in two Mediterranean populations. *Blood* 60 : 509, 1982.

Pressley, M. B. et al. A new genetic basis for hemoglobin-H disease. *N. Engl. J. Med.* 303 : 1383, 1980.

Stamatoyannopoulos, G., and Nienhuis, A. W. (eds.). *The Organization and Expression of Globin Genes*. New York: Liss, 1981.

Weatherall, D. J., and Clegg, J. B. *The Thalassemia Syndromes* (3rd ed.). St. Louis: Mosby, 1981.

Weatherall, D. J., and Clegg, J. B. Hereditary persistence of fetal haemoglobin. *Br. J. Haematol.* 29 : 191, 1975.

Wintrobe, M. M. et al. The Thalassemias and Related Disorders—Quantitative Disorders of Hemoglobin Synthesis. In M. M. Wintrobe et al. (eds.), *Clinical Hematology* (8th ed.), Philadelphia: Lea & Febiger, 1981.

Wood, W. G., Clegg, J. B., and Weatherall, D. J. Developmental biology of human hemoglobins. *Prog. Hematol.* 10 : 43, 1977.

4 Macrocytic Anemias

Paul R. Reich
Stephen H. Robinson

As shown in Table 4-1, macrocytic anemias are divided into those that are associated with megaloblastic changes in the cells of the marrow and peripheral blood and those that are not. This chapter is devoted primarily to the megaloblastic anemias. However, several forms of macrocytosis are not accompanied by megaloblastic changes and some of these are relatively common.

The anemia of liver disease is usually associated with mild to moderate macrocytosis, with mean cell volumes (MCV) often in the range of 100 to 110. The reason for the macrocytosis of liver disease is unclear. It is to be distinguished from the swelling of the red cell membrane that accounts for target cells in some patients with obstructive jaundice. Some authors believe that it is the result of the reticulocytosis that accompanies the hemolytic component of the anemia associated with liver dysfunction. Similarly, macrocytosis, often in the absence of anemia, is seen in patients who consume large amounts of alcohol, and this is sometimes used as a criterion for the diagnosis of chronic alcoholism.

Anemia associated with hypothyroidism can have various morphologic characteristics, but is sometimes macrocytic in nature, for reasons that are not entirely clear. The postsplenectomy state is often associated with mild macrocytosis, in addition to the formation of some target cells and acanthocytes; these changes are due to the fact that young red cells normally undergo a process of surface remodeling, with loss of some of their redundant red cell membrane, within the spleen, and thus splenectomy may be associated with cells containing excessive plasma membrane material. Erythrocytes during the neonatal period are normally macrocytic and are then replaced by cells of normal size.

The macrocytosis that accompanies "stress" erythropoiesis deserves some attention. In the presence of high serum levels of erythropoietin stimulated by anemia and the attendant hypoxemia, there is early release of immature red blood cells from the bone marrow, that is, a "shift" of immature bone marrow reticulocytes into the peripheral blood. These immature cells are larger than normal and they are also usually polychromatophilic (gray in color)

Table 4-1. Causes of macrocytosis

Nonmegaloblastic
  Liver disease, alcoholism
  Hypothyroidism
  Postsplenectomy
  Neonatal macrocytosis
  "Stress" erythropoiesis (with expanded or compromised erythropoiesis
    in the marrow)

Megaloblastic
  Vitamin B_{12} deficiency (multiple causes)
  Folic acid deficiency (multiple causes)
  Other causes (antineoplastic drugs, metabolic disorders, neoplastic
    erythropoiesis)

(Plate 25) because they still contain relatively large amounts of RNA (which is blue in stained blood films) and have not yet completed the process of hemoglobin synthesis (they are not yet fully "pinked up"). Thus, the MCV is typically moderately elevated with the reticulocytosis and polychromatophilia that accompany the erythroid hyperplasia of the bone marrow in response to hemolysis or bleeding. Macrocytosis of mild degree is often seen as well in conditions in which the anemia is due to a decrease in erythropoietic tissue in the bone marrow, for example, aplastic anemia, pure red cell aplasia, or the bone marrow suppression caused by chemotherapy. In these situations there is also a high titer of erythropoietin in the plasma, and this causes a rapid rate of ingress of young red blood cells into the peripheral blood. However, the total number of such young cells emerging from the bone marrow is limited. The reticulocyte count is usually normal and there is generally no polychromatophilia in the peripheral blood. Thus, it appears that the relatively few cells that emerge early from the bone marrow in these states of marrow compromise lose their RNA (and hence their staining properties as reticulocytes) before they lose their excess surface membrane via splenic remodeling. In contrast, both macrocytosis and an elevation of the number of reticulocytes occur in parallel when there is a marked increase in the number of immature erythrocytes emerging from the bone marrow, as with the response to hemolytic anemia or hemorrhage.

Major causes of macrocytic anemia that are megaloblastic in nature are vitamin B_{12} or folic acid deficiency, both of which have multiple causes, as is described later in this chapter. In addition, there are other relatively uncommon causes of megaloblastic erythropoiesis, including those caused by antineoplastic drugs that directly interfere with DNA synthesis (e.g., 6-mercaptopurine or

Table 4-2. Typical findings in megaloblastic anemia

High-grade macrocytosis (MCV usually > 110 fL)
Oval macrocytes in an otherwise heterogeneous peripheral blood smear
Hypersegmented granulocytes (polys)
Pancytopenia
Marrow cells showing delayed nuclear maturation
Ineffective hematopoiesis: High serum LDH, unconjugated bilirubin reflects
 ineffective erythropoiesis

cytosine arabinoside), drugs that compete with folic acid utilization (e.g., methotrexate), and rare metabolic disorders such as orotic aciduria. Finally, the dyserythropoietic changes that occur in certain neoplastic disorders such as the myelodysplastic syndromes and erythroleukemia have many features in common with megaloblastosis.

Table 4-2 lists several of the laboratory findings that indicate that macrocytosis is megaloblastic in nature. In megaloblastic, as compared with nonmegaloblastic, causes of macrocytosis, the MCV is usually quite high, exceeding 110 femtoliters. However, it should be kept in mind that the MCV in some patients with magaloblastic anemia may not be very high or may even be in the normal range because of the severe degree of red cell fragmentation that occurs with megaloblastic anemia, or in some instances because of coexisting iron deficiency or thalassemia minor. The macrocytes in megaloblastic anemia are typically oval and the peripheral blood smear usually contains a heterogeneous array of red cell shapes and sizes that may initially obscure the oval macrocytes; in nonmegaloblastic macrocytosis the macrocytes are more commonly round and, when the macrocytosis is due to stress erythropoiesis, conspicuous polychromatophilia may be seen on the peripheral blood smear.

Megaloblastic anemia is characteristically associated with hypersegmentation of neutrophils, with many five- and some six-lobed forms. The metabolic defect in megaloblastic anemia typically affects the production of white cells and platelets as well as red cells, so that a depression of all cell counts in the peripheral blood (pancytopenia) is a common finding. Thus, it is sometimes possible to make a diagnosis of megaloblastic anemia by simple inspection of the peripheral blood smear. However, it is usually necessary to examine the bone marrow, which will demonstrate delayed nuclear as compared to cytoplasmic maturation of erythroid cells and giant early white cell forms with abnormal nuclear configurations. Finally, a patient with megaloblastic anemia frequently has a high serum level of lactic dehydrogenase (LDH) and unconjugated bilirubin, the result of the ineffective erythropoiesis that is characteristic of this pathophysiologic condition.

Pathophysiology of Megaloblastic Anemia

The basic underlying defect in megaloblastic anemia is defective DNA synthesis and cell division. This results in ineffective erythropoiesis, that is, death of immature erythroid cells before release from the bone marrow, associated with some early destruction of circulating erythrocytes as well. It is not entirely clear, however, how the deficiency in vitamin B_{12} or folic acid leads to defective DNA synthesis or how defective DNA synthesis results in premature cell death. (The biochemical events that result from vitamin B_{12} and folic acid deficiency are discussed under those headings, pp. 80 and 92.) It is known that a state of unbalanced growth exists in the marrow cells of patients with megaloblastic anemia. The megaloblasts contain a substantially increased amount of RNA and a normal or slightly increased amount of DNA. This imbalance comes about because there is a delay in cell division due to impaired synthesis of one or more deoxyribonucleotides, the precursors of DNA, while RNA production proceeds normally. It is possible that premature cell death results from this unbalanced cell maturation—a concept that, although not yet experimentally confirmed, is helpful in understanding the morphologic and clinical manifestations of megaloblastic anemia. Presumably the degree of impairment of DNA synthesis varies from cell to cell and is more prominent among erythroid cells than among granulocyte and platelet precursors.

Laboratory Findings

As a result of ineffective erythropoiesis, granulopoiesis, and thrombopoiesis, and premature destruction of defective cells in the peripheral blood, it is unusual to find a patient with megaloblastic anemia who does not have depression of all three cell lines in the peripheral blood. Despite this pancytopenia, the bone marrow is hyperplastic—reflecting the fact that ineffective production of blood cells with early death in the marrow is the major pathophysiologic mechanism in megaloblastic anemia.

The megaloblastic bone marrow produces macrocytic, oval red cells. Their MCH and MCV are both increased, and the MCHC is normal. Macroovalocytosis (Plate 26), as seen in the peripheral blood smear, is a hallmark of megaloblastic anemias. The reticulocyte count is usually less than 1 percent. Occasionally it is 2 to 3 percent, but the reticulocyte production index is low, a reflection of a functionally defective marrow.

Marked abnormalities in the shape of red cells also occur in megaloblastic anemias. It has been suggested that these abnormalities result from fragmentation of the abnormal large red cells as they pass through small arterioles. Although this explanation is not accepted by everyone, it is clear that, as the megaloblastic anemia becomes more severe, bizarre shapes such as triangles and helmets increase proportionately. In severe megaloblastic anemia the poikilocytosis approaches that seen in microangiopathic hemolytic anemias due to mechanical fragmentation of erythrocytes.

The megaloblastic process also leads to abnormalities in white cells. Cell size and average number of lobes in the mature granulocyte *(poly)* are increased. Normally no more than 1 percent of polys have six nuclear lobes, but in megaloblastic anemia many have six or more, even ten, lobes (Plate 27). There is disagreement about how lobes should be counted. Most observers insist that there be a definite constriction between separate lobes, with only a thin chromatin strand separating them. The hyperlobulation is presumably due to abnormal nuclear development.

Elevated levels of serum lactic acid dehydrogenase (LDH), bilirubin, and fecal and urinary urobilinogen are due to ineffective erythropoiesis. The LDH isoenzyme that is elevated in patients with megaloblastic anemia is characteristic of bone marrow erythroid precursors. Serum LDH elevation is secondary to premature destruction of red cell precursors within the bone marrow. Similarly, the increase in serum bilirubin is a reflection of an increase in heme degradation due largely to marrow destruction of erythrocyte precursors. Radiolabeled heme is produced in bone marrow cells after injection of radioactive glycine. In patients with megaloblastic anemia, a markedly enlarged "early peak" of radiolabeled bilirubin appears within a few days after the glycine is given, indicating early destruction of hemoglobin-containing erythroid cells. This is a direct manifestation of the process of ineffective erythropoiesis in megaloblastic marrows.

Studies of iron kinetics also indicate ineffective erythropoiesis. Plasma iron turnover and marrow iron uptake are both increased despite decreased incorporation of iron into mature red cells. Elevated plasma iron levels, which transiently fall to low values after successful treatment with vitamin B_{12} or folic acid, are characteristically found in patients with megaloblastic anemia.

Hemolysis, or premature death of mature erythrocytes in the peripheral blood, as measured by radioiron or radiochromium red cell life span assays, also occurs in megaloblastic anemia. Despite hemolysis the reticulocyte production index is reduced because of the ineffective erythropoiesis in the bone marrow.

Megaloblastic anemia is characterized by megaloblastic erythropoiesis and giant myeloid forms in the bone marrow. Morphologically, the megaloblastic erythropoiesis (Plates 28 and 29) is characterized by the presence of large cells, with asynchronism between nuclear and cytoplasmic development. This morphologic appearance—an immature nucleus associated with mature cytoplasm—parallels the biochemical abnormality whereby DNA synthesis and maturation of the cell nucleus are impaired while cytoplasmic RNA and hemoglobin synthesis proceed normally. The nuclear–cytoplasmic dissociation is best recognized in the late, hemoglobinized normoblast, for in the early basophilic normoblast the nucleus is normally immature. Concomitant iron deficiency, resulting in delay of hemoglobinization, may make it difficult to recognize megaloblastic erythropoiesis. Transfusions and inappropriate treatment—for example, the use of folic acid to treat vitamin B_{12} deficiency—may also obscure or normalize the nuclear–cytoplasmic dissociation, thereby making the diagnosis of megaloblastic anemia difficult or impossible.

Giant white cell precursor forms (Plate 30), abnormal megakarocytes, and hypercellularity of all three cell lines are also features of megaloblastic marrows. The increased size of the granulocytes is most noticeable at the metamyelocyte and band stages. These granulocytes also have open chromatin patterns and bizarre lobulations or twists to their nuclei. These cells are precursors of hypersegmented polys. Megakaryocytes may be distinctly abnormal, with many lobes to their nuclei. The platelets produced by these megakaryocytes tend to be large and sometimes functionally abnormal.

Vitamin B_{12} Deficiency

The metabolism of vitamin B_{12} and pathways by which its deficiency may interfere with DNA synthesis are reviewed here. Since vitamin B_{12} is common in human diets, almost all deficiencies of vitamin B_{12} are a result of malabsorption, and for this reason we discuss in some detail the normal absorption of vitamin B_{12}. Clinical features of vitamin B_{12} deficiency, its common causes, and an approach to its diagnosis are also described.

Biochemistry of Vitamin B_{12}

In simplest terms vitamin B_{12} is made up of a porphyrinlike structure attached to a nucleotide. This structure is analogous to the porphyrin structure of heme, with the position of the heme iron being occupied by a cobalt atom. *Cobalamin* refers to a vitamin B_{12} that lacks a ligand covalently bound to the cobalt atom. Cyanide binding yields a compound called *cyanocobalamin,* and if a hydroxyl group is bound to cobalt, it is called *hydroxycobalamin*. Vitamin B_{12} is usually isolated by first stabilizing the molecule with cyanide. Cyano- and hydroxycobalamin are probably inactive and must be converted to active compounds such as 5'-deoxyadenosylcobalamin or methylcobalamin.

Three reactions dependent on vitamin B_{12} may be important to human metabolism. In bacteria and mammalian tissues, deoxyadenosylcobalamin (and methylmalonyl CoA mutase) is required for conversion of methylmalonyl CoA to succinyl CoA. The excretion of methylmalonic acid is increased in vitamin B_{12}–deficient humans. In certain bacteria the reduction of purines and pyrimidines to deoxypurines and deoxypyrimidines requires vitamin B_{12} as well as ribonucleotide reductase. This requirement for vitamin B_{12} for the synthesis of DNA precursors has not been demonstrated in man but has been found in the organisms previously used to assay vitamin B_{12}, namely, *Lactobacillus leichmannii*. Vitamin B_{12}–starved organisms undergo unbalanced growth and acquire forms that are analogous to the megaloblasts of human vitamin B_{12} deficiency. Methylcobalamin is required for the synthesis of methionine in bacteria and probably in man. This synthesis of methionine also leads to the conversion of N^5-methyltetrahydrofolate (N^5-methyl-FH_4) to tetrahydrofolate (FH_4):

$$\text{Homocysteine} + N^5\text{-methyl-}FH_4 \xrightarrow[\text{methylcobalamin}]{\text{methyltransferase}} \text{methionine} + FH_4$$

Unless methylcobalamin is present, N^5-methyltetrahydrofolate will accumulate, leading to a deficiency of tetrahydrofolate, which is required for thymidine synthesis (Fig. 4-1). This would lead to a defect in DNA synthesis. This entrapment of methyltetrahydrofolate in the absence of vitamin B_{12} may account for the defective synthesis of DNA seen in vitamin B_{12} deficiency and for the partial reversal by folic acid of the megaloblastosis associated with vitamin B_{12} deficiency. Again, it should be emphasized that only the methylmalonic CoA-to-succinyl CoA metabolic pathway has been conclusively demonstrated in animal tissues. Thus the role of vitamin B_{12} in the production of megaloblastic erythropoiesis is not yet fully defined. Futhermore, none of these metabolic pathways adequately accounts for the defective myelin synthesis and neurologic symptoms prominent in severe human vitamin B_{12} deficiency.

Vitamin B_{12} Requirements and Stores

The ultimate source of vitamin B_{12} in man is from microbial synthesis. The vitamin B_{12} synthesized by microbes is deposited in animal tissues, such as liver, eggs, and milk, and is therefore plentiful in fish and meat products. The average diet contains 5 to 30 µg of vitamin B_{12} daily, 1 to 2 µg of which usually is absorbed and retained. In the adult a storage pool of 3,000 to 5,000 µg is present, of which 1,000 to 3,000 µg is stored in the liver. There is some disagreement about the human minimum daily requirement for vitamin B_{12}. It once was put at 0.6 to 1.2 µg, but, according to studies of the loss of

Fig. 4-1. Simplified metabolic pathways for dU and THF.

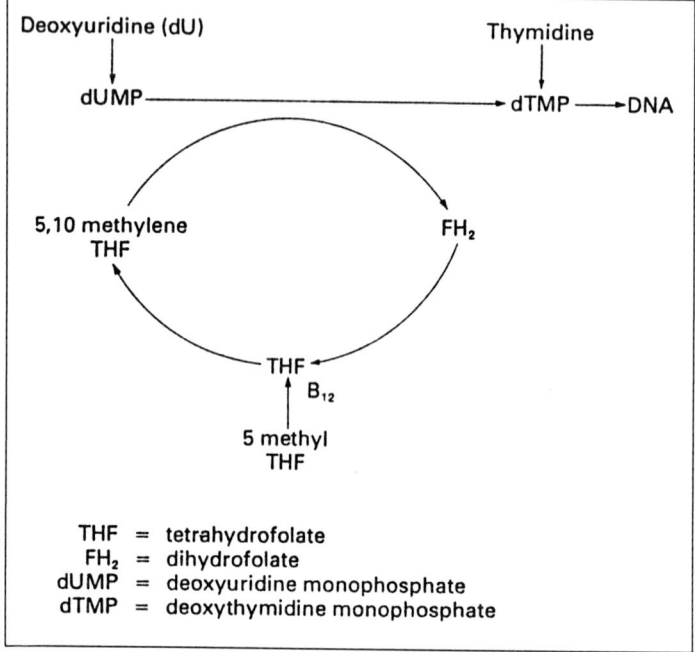

vitamin B_{12} in feces and urine and of the amount of vitamin B_{12} required to completely correct megaloblastic anemia due to vitamin B_{12} deficiency, a higher value of 2 µg or somewhat more may represent the true daily requirement. The amount of vitamin B_{12} lost per day has been reported as 0.1 percent of total body stores. This might account for the variability in the reported amounts of vitamin B_{12} required daily. These numbers are clinically important for two reasons. First, it is clear that the average American diet contains enough vitamin B_{12}, so that deficiency should not result unless there is a defect in absorption of this vitamin. Also, it is clear that should malabsorption of vitamin B_{12} occur, it will take 2 to 5 years before body stores are exhausted and megaloblastic erythropoiesis supervenes.

Vitamin B_{12} Absorption

Since vitamin B_{12} deficiency is almost always due to malabsorption, it is necessary to understand the normal physiologic mechanisms involved in the intestinal absorption of this vitamin. In brief, vitamin B_{12} binds with a glycoprotein called *intrinsic factor* (IF), which is secreted by the parietal cells located in the body of the stomach. The intrinsic factor–B_{12} complex is absorbed in the distal ileum, and the IF removed. Vitamin B_{12} without IF is then transferred to a binding protein in the plasma, which transports the vitamin to the liver, where it is stored. The most common disease associated with vitamin B_{12} malabsorption, *pernicious anemia*, is caused by failure to secrete adequate amounts of IF.

Human gastric IF is secreted by the same cell that produces hydrochloric acid. This parietal cell can be stimulated into producing acid and IF by histamine and the histamine analogue betazole hydrochloride and by insulin and gastrin. Healthy subjects secrete about 900 to 8,300 units (1 unit binds 1 nanogram of vitamin B_{12}) per hour, with a mean of 3,000 units. With a single 0.5-mg dose of histamine given parenterally, the concentration of IF increases from 36 to 44 units per milliliter and approximately 4,500 units is produced per hour. Intrinsic factor reaches a peak in the first 15 minutes following injection of histamine, while acid and pepsin secretion reaches a peak in 30 to 45 minutes after histamine stimulation. In general the output of IF is paralleled by the amount of acid secreted. Approximately 500 to 1,000 units of IF is required for maximal absorption of 1 μg of vitamin B_{12}.

In humans vitamin B_{12} is absorbed only in the lower ileum. Removal of as little as 2 feet of ileum may impair vitamin B_{12} absorption, and when more than 6 feet is removed, absorption is invariably abnormal. The uptake in the ileum is 70 percent of dietary vitamin B_{12} to a limit of 10 μg per day. The vitamin IF–B_{12} complex attaches to the microvilli of the brush border of the cells lining the ileum. Calcium ions and neutral pH must be present, but there appears to be no energy requirement. Transport through the mucosal cell is poorly understood but probably involves an energy-requiring step. Vitamin B_{12} enters the mitochondria of the mucosal cell, remains there for 6 hours, and then appears in the blood unattached to IF.

In the absence of IF there is a second mechanism by which vitamin B_{12} can be absorbed through the ileum. Large oral doses of 1,000 μg per day can reverse the hematologic and neurologic abnormalities found in patients with IF deficiency. The mechanism for this nonphysiologic absorption of large doses of vitamin B_{12} is probably simple diffusion from a high concentration in the intestine into the mucosa. It is probably this mechanism that accounted for responses to oral, high-dose, liver therapy in patients with pernicious anemia who were treated before vitamin B_{12} was available for therapy.

Transport of Vitamin B_{12} in Plasma

Three to four hours after oral ingestion, vitamin B_{12} is detected in the blood. A peak level is obtained in 8 to 10 hours. The vitamin is attached to three protein binders named transcobalamin (TC) I (an α_1-globulin present in granulocytes), TC II (a β-globulin), and TC III. Transcobalamin I has a half-life of 9 to 10 days, as opposed to TC

II, which is cleared rapidly in hours. Studies also suggest that transcobalamin III and transcobalamin I are immunologically related. From studies in man it appears that transcobalamin II is most important physiologically, since infants lacking this protein develop severe megaloblastic anemia. It is probably responsible for all vitamin B_{12} transportation in the body. TC I, to which most vitamin B_{12} is bound, serves a storage rather than a transport function. It has been suggested that at least some of these vitamin B_{12} protein binders are produced in leukocytes, which explains their elevation in myeloproliferative diseases and other diseases associated with leukocytosis.

Schilling Test

One of the most useful means of making the diagnosis of vitamin B_{12} deficiency and determining its etiology is the Schilling test, which measures the absorption of orally administered radiolabeled vitamin B_{12}. The simplest and most commonly employed method is to give the patient a 0.5- or 1-μg dose of radiocobalt-labeled cyanocobalamin and either immediately or 2 hours later to administer a 1-mg dose of nonradioactive cyanocobalamin intramuscularly. This "flushing" dose is used to saturate vitamin B_{12} binding sites in the plasma and liver. A 24-hour collection of urine is begun after the radioactive B_{12} has been ingested. Normal subjects will excrete in their urine 7 percent or more of the radioactivity taken orally, whereas patients with pernicious anemia or other causes of vitamin B_{12} malabsorption will excrete well less than 7 percent. Renal insufficiency or incomplete collection of urine may result in a spuriously low excretion rate.

Certain precautions must be observed. If the patient's renal function is not normal, a 48-hour or 72-hour collection of urine will be required, since the excretion of vitamin B_{12} will be delayed. If the patient uses a bedpan, contamination with fecal material can sometimes give artefactually high recoveries in the urine collection. If, for one reason or another, a urine collection cannot be obtained, then either whole body radioactivity counting is done, or a serum radioactive B_{12} is obtained approximately 8 hours after an oral dose of radiolabeled vitamin. In the latter case the normal values depend upon the dose of vitamin B_{12} given and the time at which blood samples are drawn. These must be standardized, and normal values made available to the clinician. If whole body radioactivity or plasma radioactivity is measured, a flushing dose of vitamin B_{12} is not used. Some patients with vitamin B_{12} deficiency following a partial gastrectomy or vagotomy give normal or near-normal results in the Schilling test. These patients can absorb crystalline B_{12} in the Schilling test but cannot liberate B_{12} adequately from food in their regular diet. It should be remembered that this test can be used to measure abnormal vitamin B_{12} absorption even after the patient has been treated for B_{12} deficiency and has fully recovered. On the other hand the administration of the 1-mg flushing dose will treat the megaloblastic anemia and make the hematologic findings revert rapidly toward normal.

The second part of the Schilling test is performed only if the first part gives abnormal results. In the second part 60 mg of hog IF is given orally along with the radioactive vitamin B_{12}. If there is a defect in the absorption of the vitamin IF-B_{12} complex, then abnormally small amounts of B_{12} will be excreted. However, if the patient's gastric secretions lack IF, the addition of hog IF to the vitamin B_{12} oral dose leads to normal urinary excretion of the vitamin B_{12}. Thus, the part one and part two Schilling tests distinguish IF deficiency from ileal malabsorption of IF-B_{12} complex. A third part of the Schilling test may be performed to determine if the patient suffers from malabsorption of the IF-B_{12} complex secondary to small-intestinal bacterial overgrowth. In part three of the Schilling test a 2-week course of antibiotic therapy with tetracycline, 250 mg four times per day, is prescribed. If bacterial overgrowth was responsible for the abnormal second part of the Schilling test, then tetracycline treatment should normalize vitamin B_{12} absorption. In practice, the third part of the Schilling test is seldom performed.

Clinical Findings in Vitamin B_{12} Deficiency

Anemia secondary to vitamin B_{12} deficiency is associated with low serum vitamin B_{12} levels, abnormal Schilling test results, response of the anemia to physiologic doses of vitamin B_{12} and, sometimes, neurologic defects. *Subacute combined system disease* is due to degeneration of myelin in the dorsal and lateral columns of the spinal cord in association with vitamin B_{12} deficiency. It is characterized by paresthesias or tingling in the extremities and by decreased vibratory and position sense. An abnormal gait and loss of bladder and rectal control are characteristic of the chronic, severe form of this disease. In modern times it is unusual to encounter more than the paresthesias and loss of position and vibratory senses, probably because most patients with pernicious anemia are detected and treated early. Occasional patients may have combined systems disease in the absence of noticeable anemia. Other nervous system abnormalities include changes in the patient's personality, giving rise to *megaloblastic "madness."* The patient may be demented, disoriented, irritable, or depressed, or have memory and intellectual impairment.

The ability to assay the concentration of serum vitamin B_{12} has greatly simplified the diagnostic approach to patients with megaloblastic anemia. The first reliable tests utilized organisms such as *Euglena gracilis* or *Lactobacillus leichmannii,* which require vitamin

B_{12} for growth. Today most vitamin B_{12} assays are done by radio-isotope dilution methods. Aliquots of serum containing vitamin B_{12} binders are incubated with radiolabeled vitamin B_{12} and increasing amounts of unlabeled vitamin B_{12}. The more unlabeled B_{12} present, the more radioactive vitamin B_{12} will be released from the B_{12} binders and then absorbed by charcoal or DEAE-cellulose (diethylaminoethyl cellulose). The amount of radioactivity remaining bound is inversely proportional to the amount of unlabeled vitamin B_{12} present in the serum sample. By plotting known amounts of vitamin B_{12} added against radioactivity remaining after absorption with charcoal or DEAE-cellulose, a curve is obtained from which the amount of vitamin B_{12} in a serum sample can be determined. In normal sera, 200 to 1,000 ng per liter is detected.

Serum methylmalonic acid and total homocysteine levels are useful in cases in which serum vitamin B_{12} assays are equivocal, or increased cobalamin-binding proteins are present, for example, in patients with myeloproliferative disorders. These tests are reliable and specific, and are now generally available for the diagnosis of vitamin B_{12} deficiency.

A therapeutic trial is sometimes undertaken to determine whether patients with megalobastic anemia have vitamin B_{12} or folic acid deficiency. Physiologic amounts—5 μg or less—of vitamin B_{12} are given parenterally each day. If the patient has vitamin B_{12} deficiency, a reticulocytosis is seen in 3 or 4 days and reaches a peak in 5 to 10 days. With a complete response the hematocrit rises to normal, usually within 3 to 4 weeks. The amount of time required to perform this trial inclines clinicians to use, instead, the serum B_{12} assay and Schilling test. It should be emphasized that patients undergoing this therapeutic trial must be on a folic acid–deficient diet. If they were to receive large amounts of folic acid in their diet and were folic acid–deficient rather than vitamin B_{12}–deficient, they would have a reticulocyte response that might be falsely attributed to the parenteral vitamin B_{12}. Large doses of folic acid, 0.4 mg or more, may produce a reticulocyte response in patients with vitamin B_{12} deficiency, but the hematocrit will not return to normal. Moreover, administration of large amounts of folate to patients with pernicious anemia who have neurologic involvement may lead to further neurologic impairment.

Conditions Associated with Vitamin B_{12} Deficiency

The causes of vitamin B_{12} deficiency are listed on page 87.

DIETARY DEFICIENCY

Dietary deficiency of vitamin B_{12} is rare, since foods of animal origin have high concentrations of this vitamin. Strict vegetarians, particu-

Causes of vitamin B_{12} deficiency
Decreased intake
Strict vegetarianism (very rare)
Decreased absorption
Pernicious anemia
Congenital lack of IF production
Gastrectomy
Chronic pancreatitis
Regional ileitis, particularly with ileal resection
Ileal resection
Selective malabsorption of vitamin B_{12}
Sprue
Competition
Fish tapeworm
Blind loop syndromes
Small-intestinal diverticulosis

larly in India, may have a diet so deficient in vitamin B_{12} that megaloblastic anemia develops.

PERNICIOUS ANEMIA

Pernicious anemia is the disease most often associated with vitamin B_{12} deficiency. It is defined as anemia resulting from defective secretion of IF by the gastric mucosal cells associated with chronic atrophic gastritis. Characteristically patients with PA are of Northern European extraction and have fair complexions and blue eyes. Long earlobes, prematurely gray hair, and blood group A are other clinical features that have been associated with PA. The patients are usually elderly, but can be of any age. Not all patients fit this description, and many patients who have these clinical findings do not suffer from PA.

Patients with PA invariably do not secrete hydrochloric acid, even after parenteral stimulation of gastric secretion with histamine or betazole. Their defective IF secretion means that they give abnormal results on part one of the Schilling test and normal results on part two. The correction of the Schilling test by oral IF (in part two of this test) is an important laboratory confirmation of this diagnosis. Two types of antibodies to IF may be detected in the serum or gastric juice of a large percentage of patients. One type of antibody blocks the binding of vitamin B_{12} to IF and is called *blocking antibody*. The second type, *binding antibody*, attaches to and precipitates IF or IF-B_{12} complex, thereby preventing the attachment of the IF-B_{12} complex to the ileal mucosa.

The presence of these antibodies and the ability of corticosteroids to reverse defective parietal cell function early in pernicious anemia (presumably by suppressing antibody production or effect) support the role of an autoimmune process in the etiology of PA. According to this theory, injury to the gastric mucosa leads to production of antibodies directed against the parietal cell or IF. Parietal cell antibodies are relatively common and are found not only in patients with pernicious anemia but also in those with gastritis without PA and in several other diseases. It has been presumed that these parietal cell antibodies are cytotoxic and able to impair parietal cell function. The antibodies to IF are effective in neutralizing IF function, but only when they are present in gastric juice. Seventy-five percent of patients with PA have detectable IF antibodies in the gastric juice, about 50 percent in the serum. This autoimmune theory has not been proved, and autoimmune mechanisms may play only a secondary role in the pathogenesis of PA.

Pathologic examination of the stomach of patients with PA reveals atrophy of the mucosa with some inflammatory cells. Megaloblastic epithelial cells may be present and occasionally are mistaken for neoplasia. For this reason caution should be exercised in examining exfoliated epithelial gastric cells for malignancy before megaloblastic anemia is corrected. There appears to be a small but definite increased incidence of gastric carcinoma in patients with pernicious anemia.

The diagnosis of PA is confirmed by a low serum B_{12} level and typically abnormal results of the Schilling test. A therapeutic trial with minute doses of vitamin B_{12} is useful but often impractical. Assays for antibodies to IF or parietal cells can also be of value. Gastric analysis or the Diagnex Blue test for achlorhydria is readily available, but often unnecessary. Most patients with pernicious anemia are in the elderly age group, and a finding of achlorhydria is not unusual in normal persons who are elderly. If gastric acid is present, however, the diagnosis of pernicious anemia is effectively ruled out. Vitamin B_{12} deficiency can exist in the presence of gastric acidity, but not when PA is the etiology. Gastric hydrochloric acid is measured by determining the pH of gastric juice with a pH meter. Achlorhydria is present if the pH is greater than 3.5 pH units and does not decrease by more than 1 pH unit following maximal stimulation with histamine.

Pernicious anemia has been associated with thyroid disease, particularly Hashimoto's disease, with the presence of thyroid autoantibodies. This association may be part of Schmidt's syndrome, which can include PA, Hashimoto's thyroiditis, vitiligo, diabetes mellitus, and hypoadrenalism, all presumably due to autoimmune assault on different target tissues.

CONGENITAL IF DEFICIENCY

Congenital IF deficiency is a rare disease of children and is characterized by a selective defect in IF secretion. The resultant vitamin B_{12} malabsorption is correctable with oral IF. Gastric mucosa and gastric acidity are both normal. Autoantibodies to IF and parietal cells are not present. Production of a qualitatively abnormal form of intrinsic factor is another very rare congenital cause of B_{12} deficiency.

SELECTIVE VITAMIN B_{12} MALABSORPTION

Selective vitamin B_{12} malabsorption, another rare disorder of children, runs in families and is associated with persistent proteinuria of unknown etiology. IF secretion is normal, and there are no antibodies against IF or against ileal receptors for the IF-B_{12} complex. Recent studies suggest a defect occurring somewhere in the chain of events after IF-B_{12} attaches to the surface of the ileal cell and before the absorbed vitamin binds to transcobalamin II. There is no discernible morphologic lesion, and the absorptive defect does not appear to result from lack of ileal receptors for IF-B_{12} Congenital transcobalamin II deficiency and neonatal vitamin B_{12} deficiency secondary to maternal deficiency, both very rare diseases, can be confused with this disorder.

PARTIAL OR TOTAL GASTRECTOMY

Removal of the stomach in toto eventually results in vitamin B_{12} malabsorption due to lack of IF. Megaloblastic anemia occurs in 3 to 5 years, unless the patient is treated with parenteral vitamin B_{12}. Thus, totally gastrectomized patients should be prophylactically treated with parenteral vitamin B_{12}. Vitamin B_{12} deficiency may also occur in partially gastrectomized patients. Such individuals can develop frank megaloblastic anemia, but in most cases they have only depressed serum B_{12} levels and abnormal results on part one of the Schilling test. Some patients with partial gastrectomies will have difficulty absorbing vitamin B_{12} bound to food but not the purified vitamin. These patients have a normal Schilling test but have depressed serum levels of vitamin B_{12}. The vitamin B_{12} deficiency seen after partial gastrectomy is attributed to surgical loss of IF-producing cells, but another factor may be continued gastritis and loss of parietal cells in the remaining stomach. Although frank megaloblastic anemia develops in only a small percentage of patients with partial gastrectomy, many surgeons administer vitamin B_{12} prophylactically after partial gastrectomy. Iron and folic acid deficiency are both also associated with gastrectomy. (See Interrelationships between iron, folic acid, and vitamin B_{12}, p. 100.)

MALABSORPTION SYNDROMES

Various intestinal defects and diseases can lead to vitamin B_{12} deficiency. These diseases are relatively uncommon compared to pernicious anemia. Nontropical sprue (celiac disease) and tropical sprue are diseases characterized by villous atrophy, which causes malabsorption of various substances, sometimes including vitamin B_{12}. In patients with malabsorption syndromes, both part one and part two of the Schilling test are abnormal.

Chronic pancreatic insufficiency has been associated, in a few patients, with vitamin B_{12} malabsorption. Pancreatic extract reverses this defect, but the precise constituent of the extract that enhances vitamin B_{12} absorption has not been determined.

Vitamin B_{12} malabsorption is sometimes associated with regional ileitis, an inflammatory disease of the ileum of unknown etiology. Most often this occurs after the ileum has been resected as part of the therapy for this disease.

Patients with pernicious anemia often have a somewhat decreased ability to absorb vitamin B_{12}, even in the presence of IF. This ileal defect usually disappears after a few weeks of parenteral therapy with vitamin B_{12}. This malabsorption defect is due to megaloblastosis of the bowel mucosa and may cause a temporary abnormality in part two of the Schilling test. Indeed, for this reason some experts recommend that neither part one nor part two of the Schilling test be performed until any malabsorptive defect has been reversed by at least 2 months of therapy with vitamin B_{12}. Similarly, severe folic acid deficiency can sometimes interfere with vitamin B_{12} absorption by virtue of megaloblastic changes in the intestinal mucosa.

COMPETITION FOR VITAMIN B_{12}

The blind loop syndrome occurs in patients who have a portion of the small intestine surgically isolated from the mainstream of the gut. Isolated duodenal and ileal loops result, respectively, from partial gastrectomies and operative procedures for inflammatory bowel diseases. In these blind loops or in small-intestinal diverticuli (which may occur on a congenital basis), bacterial overgrowth occurs because of stasis of intestinal contents. Although these bacteria do not necessarily require vitamin B_{12} for their growth, binding sites on their cell walls compete with their host's IF for vitamin B_{12}, thereby reducing vitamin B_{12} absorption. The patient's absorption improves after surgical removal of the diverticuli or loop, or after the blind pouch is returned to the main gastrointestinal stream. Antibiotics may also be of value.

A rare but interesting cause of vitamin B_{12} deficiency is fish tapeworm infestation with *Diphyllobothrium latum,* an intestinal parasite present in freshwater fish such as pike. When insufficiently cooked fish is ingested, tapeworms ultimately develop in the intestines. Some Finns and makers of gefilte fish in the United States have a habit of tasting raw fish and thereby become infected by this tapeworm. A newer source is sushi prepared from freshwater fish.

In the intestinal tract the worm competes with the host for vitamin B_{12}. The diagnosis can be suspected on the basis of the patient's history. Confirmation depends on demonstration of tapeworm segments or ova in feces. Once this is demonstrated, appropriate antihelminthic therapy will cure the patient.

Treatment of Vitamin B$_{12}$ Deficiency

Since most vitamin B$_{12}$ deficiency is due to malabsorption of the vitamin, parenteral injection of vitamin B$_{12}$ is required for therapy. For patients who have reversible diseases such as fish tapeworm, sprue, and blind loops, treatment of the primary disease should be undertaken after initial replacement with parenteral vitamin B$_{12}$. If treatment is successful, these patients will not require maintenance therapy. However, the vast majority of patients with vitamin B$_{12}$ deficiency has pernicious anemia or other diseases that cannot be cured by drugs or surgical procedures, and these patients will require lifelong injections of vitamin B$_{12}$.

Initially 100 to 1,000 μg per day of hydroxycobalamin should be injected intramuscularly or subcutaneously for 5 to 7 days. Hydroxycobalamin is preferable to cyanocobalamin, because it binds better to proteins and therefore remains in the body three times longer than cyanocobalamin. Only a small fraction of this material will be retained, but it will begin to replace body stores. Parenteral administration, 100 to 1,000 μg monthly, should then be carried out indefinitely to maintain the hematocrit and vitamin B$_{12}$ level. It is probably easiest to try bimonthly injections. If a patient's hematocrit falls, and the serum B$_{12}$ level is low, then monthly injections should be administered. Pernicious anemia patients will respond to oral treatment with animal IF, but they usually become resistant and ultimately require parenteral vitamin B$_{12}$. A massive dose of 1,000 μg per day of vitamin B$_{12}$ given orally to PA patients who will not accept parenteral therapy gives an adequate hematologic response. However, this treatment cannot be relied upon to maintain normal erythropoiesis, and for this reason it is not recommended.

Transfusion therapy can be dangerous for patients with moderate to severe megaloblastic anemia. These patients often have an increased blood volume and transfusion may cause them to go into severe, irreversible congestive heart failure. Therefore blood should not be given to patients with megaloblastic anemia unless there is evidence of tissue hypoxia manifested by angina or hypoxic symptoms referable to the central nervous system. In most cases it is possible to withhold transfusions and to treat with vitamin B$_{12}$. Patients who need transfusions should be given packed red cells along with a diuretic and their fluid balance should be closely monitored. Alternatively, they can be exchange transfused, removing their low hematocrit blood while transfusing high-hematocrit packed red cells from a normal donor.

Elevated levels of uric acid in serum and urine may occur in response to a physiologic or pharmacologic dose of vitamin B_{12} administered parenterally to deficient patients. In some cases uricosuria is severe enough to precipitate kidney damage. Another very rare complication is sudden death due to potassium levels low enough to precipitate cardiac arrhythmias. It is presumed that the extracellular (serum) potassium level becomes low because of the rapid effective production of new red cells, which requires intracellular potassium. Patients with severe megaloblastic anemia, therefore, require close observation of serum uric acid and potassium levels during therapy.

There is conflicting evidence concerning the association of pernicious anemia with an increased incidence of stomach cancer. There is probably an increased incidence of moderate degree, insufficient to justify regular screening of former PA patients by endoscopy.

Folic Acid Deficiency

Biochemistry of Folic Acid

The terms *folic acid* and *folate* refer to a large group of compounds consisting of three moieties, pteridine, para-aminobenzoic acid, and a variable number of glutamic acid units. The first two moieties in combination are sometimes called *pteroyls*. The number of glutamic acid moieties attached to the pteroyl determines the name of the compound. There are pteroyl monoglutamates, pteroyl triglutamates, and pteroyl polyglutamates. The addition of four hydrogen groups to the pteroyl results in a compound called tetrahydrofolic acid, which participates in many cellular enzymatic reactions. The reduction of folic acid (pteroyl monoglutamate) to dihydrofolic acid and then to tetrahydrofolic acid is catalyzed by an enzyme, dihydrofolate reductase. Compounds structurally resembling folic acid—for example, aminopterin and amethopterin (methotrexate)—may inhibit this enzyme and are called *antifols*.

One-carbon fragments may be bound to various sites on the pteridine moiety of tetrahydrofolic acid. These one-carbon fragments participate in many reactions, particularly those involving the synthesis of purines, pyrimidines, and DNA. Methylation of deoxyuridylate to form thymidylate is effected, in part, by one-carbon transfer from a tetrahydrofolate compound. Limitation of thymidylate synthesis because of impairment of the folate-requiring enzyme, thymidylate synthetase, leads to impairment of DNA synthesis and megaloblastosis (see Figure 4-1).

Folic acid coenzymes are also important in methionine, serine, and histidine metabolism. In regard to the last, an insufficiency in tetrahydrofolic acid leads to the accumulation of formiminoglutamic acid (FIGLU). FIGLU is a product of histidine metabolism and requires tetrahydrofolate for its conversion to glutamic acid. Patients who are folic acid–deficient (and some who are B_{12}-deficient) will excrete elevated amounts of FIGLU, particularly when challenged with large oral doses of histidine. Normal people excrete little or no FIGLU, but no symptoms or abnormalities result from its accumulation in the body. Other enzymatic reactions depend upon folates for their metabolism but are not central to the problem of folic acid deficiency.

Measurement of Folic Acid

Early physiologic and clinical investigations of folic acid metabolism were performed using microbiologic assays with *Lactobacillus casei,* a folic acid–requiring organism. These assays measure all metabolically important folic acid derivatives. Tubes containing culture medium deficient in folic acid are inoculated with *L. casei.* Known amounts of folic acid are added to some of these tubes, and growth, measured by turbidity, is determined after a specified period of time. With these data a standard curve can be drawn that relates concentration of added folic acid to the turbidity or growth of the organisms. This curve can then be used to determine the amount of folate in a serum or tissue sample added to the remaining tubes. In practice serum and red cell folic acid levels are most often determined. For research purposes levels in tissues such as the liver can also be measured. Antibiotics interfere with this microbiologic assay by causing falsely low values.

Recently a folic acid–binding protein (FBP) has been found in condensed milk. Using this folic acid binder and radiolabeled folic acid it is now possible to perform a radioisotope displacement assay similar to that used for vitamin B_{12} measurements. First a standard curve is determined by adding known amounts of unlabeled folic acid to a mixture of binder and radiolabeled folic acid. The amount of radioactivity on the binder is inversely proportional to the amount of unlabeled folic acid added. Serum or tissue homogenates with unknown amounts of folic acid can then be assayed. This method is not affected by antibiotics or other drugs.

Absorption of Folic Acid

Folates are widely distributed in a variety of foods, including green vegetables, liver, kidney, and dairy products. A daily diet contains fifty to several hundred micrograms (normal Western diet, 600–700 μg) of folates. Cooking, particularly boiling, destroys this thermolabile vitamin. Food folate is presented to the intestine largely conjugated to glutamates. The polyglutamates are broken down in the intestinal lumen by *folate conjugases* that convert polyglutamate to monoglutamate. It is not clear whether this cleavage occurs in the brush border of the intestinal cell or within the cell itself. In any case the monoglutamates appear to be absorbed best in the proximal jejunum. Some duodenal, but no ileal or colonic, absorption occurs. Folic acid (monoglutamate) is detected in the serum minutes after an oral dose of unconjugated folic acid, and peak values are obtained in 1 to 2 hours. The peak of activity after an oral dose of conjugated folates (polyglutamate forms) occurs later, at 2 to 3 hours.

The monoglutamate forms of folic acid can be absorbed against a concentration gradient. This suggests the existence of an active transport mechanism. Other data suggest that passive transport occurs as well. There may also be some absorption of folates in the form of diglutamates of triglutamates. During the process of intestinal absorption the folates are converted to 5-methyltetrahydrofolate, which is the main transport and storage form of folate in man.

Folates are excreted by way of the urine and feces and are also destroyed by catabolism, which involves oxidative splitting of the parent molecules into pteridine and para-aminobenzoylglutamic acid. About 50 μg of folic acid is required daily from food to balance these losses. Normally 5 to 20 mg of folic acid is stored in the liver and other tissues. For this reason it takes 3 to 6 months for tissue stores to be completely exhausted in the absence of folate replacement.

Clinical Findings

Experminental folic acid deprivation leads initially to reduced serum folate levels. Hypersegmentation of neutrophils, low red cell folate levels, excretion of FIGLU following histidine administration, macroovalocytosis, megaloblastic bone marrow, and finally anemia develop after $4^{1}/_{2}$ months of deprivation.

Clinically patients with folic acid deficiency present with morphologic features of megaloblastic anemia and low serum and red cell folic acid levels. Often they have diseases associated with folic acid deficiency, such as alcoholism or cirrhosis. Neurologic abnormalities are not caused by folate deficiency but may be present due to alcoholism or liver disease.

The diagnosis is usually confirmed by a finding of low concentrations of serum folate—less than 3 μg per liter (normal, 5–20 μg per liter). The serum levels are a more sensitive test for folate deficiency than red cell levels and fall before the red cell folate levels (normal, 160–640 μg per liter) become depressed. Therefore low serum folate levels indicate folate deficiency, while low red cell folate levels confirm folic acid deficiency as the cause of megaloblastic anemia.

In some diagnostically difficult cases a therapeutic trial with folic acid is performed by first putting the patient on a folic acid–deficient diet, then injecting physiologic doses of folic acid (200 μg/day). A tetrahydrofolic acid compound—folinic acid, or citrovorum factor—is available in a liquid, injectable form that is easily diluted so that 200 μg can be injected each day. In a folic acid–deficient patient the reticulocyte response should occur in 3 to 5 days and reach a peak in 5 to 10 days. A vitamin B_{12}–deficient patient will not respond to this dose of folic acid. Large doses, over 0.4 mg daily, will cause a patient with vitamin B_{12} deficiency to respond with increased reticulocytes, but the anemia will be only partially corrected, if at all. Furthermore it is said that large doses of folic acid administered to patients with pernicious anemia and combined systems disease will lead to neurologic deterioration.

Causes of Folic Acid Deficiency

DIETARY DEFICIENCY

Many individuals have an inadequate dietary intake of folic acid: the elderly person who is unable to obtain proper foods, the chronic alcoholic who rarely eats, the poverty-stricken patient whose diet lacks vegetables, eggs, and meat. Premature infants and children on synthetic diets also have a decreased dietary intake of folic acid. Prolonged cooking of vegetables results in destruction of folic acid compounds, and the person who eats vegetables prepared only in this way may develop dietary deficiency.

ALCOHOLISM AND LIVER CIRRHOSIS

Alcoholics and patients with chronic liver disease suffer from folic acid deficiency, probably because of both poor diet and impaired hepatic storage of folates. Alcohol may cause increased retention of folates in the hepatic cell, thereby preventing normal enterohepatic circulation, and resorption of folate from the intestine. There is some evidence, furthermore, that alcohol and liver disease interfere with absorption and metabolism of folates.

MALABSORPTION SYNDROMES

As in the case of vitamin B_{12} malabsorption, nontropical, gluten-sensitive sprue and tropical sprue may be causes of folate malabsorption and deficiency. Biopsy of the jejunum to look for villous atrophy is indicated if a patient has unexplained folic acid deficiency and symptoms or tests indicative of intestinal malabsorption. The absorption of D-xylose, a nonmetabolizable sugar, by the jejunum has proved to be a valuable screening test for sprue. Fat absorption studies and gastrointestinal x-rays may help to establish the diagnosis. Monoglutamic folic acid, in contrast to food folates, is normally absorbed by patients with malabsorption syndromes. In the case of

Causes of folic acid deficiency
Decreased intake
Poor diet or overcooking of folate-containing foods
Alcoholism (also impairs folate metabolism)
Decreased absorption
Sprue and other malabsorption syndromes
Anticonvulsant and oral contraceptive drugs
Increased requirement
Pregnancy
Erythroid hyperplasia of the marrow (hemolysis, thalassemia)
Leukemias and other neoplastic disorders
Skin diseases such as psoriasis, exfoliative dermatitis
Other causes
Chemotherapy with folic acid antagonists
Renal dialysis
Vitamin C deficiency

tropical sprue, folic acid therapy often improves intestinal symptoms and villous atrophy as well as correcting the folate deficiency.

Folic acid deficiency thought to be secondary to malabsorption has also been found in patients following subtotal gastrectomy, resection of the jejunum, and infiltration of the small intestine by lymphoma, amyloid, or Whipple's disease. It has also been described in association with scleroderma and diabetes mellitus. Treatment of folic acid deficiency due to intestinal malabsorption requires only 1 mg of monoglutamic folic acid orally.

DRUG-INDUCED FOLIC ACID DEFICIENCY

Antifols, inhibitors of dihydrofolate reductase, result in deficiency of active folate compounds, which, if persistent, leads to megaloblastic anemia. The antifols include aminopterin (methotrexate), used in cancer chemotherapy; antimalarial drugs such as pyrimethamine; a diuretic, triamterene; an antiparasite drug, pentamidine; and a drug used for treating urinary tract infections, trimethoprim. Antimetabolites such as hydroxyrurea and cytosine arabinoside, used to treat cancer, cause megaloblastosis by their direct effects on DNA metabolism. These drugs, unlike antifols, do not interfere with folic acid metabolism.

Certain drugs such as the anticonvulsants diphenylhydantoin, phenobarbital, and primidone may also be associated with folic acid deficiency. It is thought that these drugs, along with glutethimide, isoniazid, cycloserine, and oral contraceptives, interfere with folic acid absorption, possibly by inhibiting intestinal folate conjugases.

In the case of anticonvulsant and oral contraceptive users, increased requirements due to catabolic microsomal enzyme induction in the liver, changes in folate-binding protein, and, in the case of oral contraceptives, increased urinary excretion of folic acid have also been proposed as mechanisms of folate deficiency. Folic acid therapy given to patients with anticonvulsant-induced deficiency is said to increase the frequency of seizures, but this phenomenon has not been well confirmed.

FOLIC ACID DEFICIENCY SECONDARY TO INCREASED FOLATE DEMAND

Low folic acid levels are common in pregnancy but are often overlooked because in many nondeficient patients hemoglobin levels may normally fall below 10 gm per deciliter in the third trimester. Lactation, multiple pregnancies, poor diet, and any concurrent conditions that result in abnormal folic acid metabolism further increase the likelihood of folic acid deficiency during pregnancy. Pregnant women should be given 400 µg per day of folic acid, a dose that would not cause a hematologic response if the patient had vitamin B_{12} deficiency. It has been argued that folic acid deficiency leads to maternal complications such as abruptio placentae, spontaneous abortions, and bleeding, but a causal relationship between these complications and folic acid deficiency has not been fully confirmed.

Anemia associated with hyperproliferation of marrow erythroid cells, as seen in sickle cell anemia, congenital spherocytosis, immunohemolytic anemia, and thalassemia may cause folic acid deficiency. This should be suspected when a patient's reticulocyte count has been high but then falls at the same time that the anemia unexpectedly worsens. If folic acid deficiency is the cause, the patient will respond with an outpouring of reticulocytes following folic acid therapy.

Folic acid deficiency may develop in patients with psoriasis and exfoliative dermatitis because of the chronic increase in cell turnover.

Occasionally individuals with neoplastic disease, including carcinoma, leukemia, and lymphoma, will develop reduced levels of serum folate, presumably due to increased demand by tumor tissues and probably also poor diet. In a very few cases, usually when there are other reasons for the development of folic acid deficiency, a frank megaloblastic anemia responsive to folic acid will arise. Similarly, folic acid deficiency may accompany various myeloproliferative diseases, including myelocytic leukemias, but is rarely, if ever, seen in polycythemia vera. Chronic diseases such as rheumatoid arthritis and infections are also associated with folic acid deficiency, which may be due to increased folate requirement as well as poor dietary intake.

Removal of folate from plasma during renal dialysis was a frequent cause of folic acid deficiency until this loss was recognized and routine prophylactic administration of folic acid prescribed.

Therapy of Folic Acid Deficiency

Despite the many causes of folic acid deficiency, 1 mg of oral folic acid per day is sufficient in all cases to restore serum levels and reverse megaloblastic anemia, even in malabsorption syndromes. Parenteral folic acid is seldom used. Folic acid supplementation as prophylaxis against deficiency is indicated for pregnancy, liver disease, hemolytic anemia, thalassemia major, alcoholism, and, if the patient is undergoing dialysis, uremia.

Approach to Patient with Megaloblastic Anemia

In clinical practice megaloblastic anemia is suspected when examination of the peripheral blood smear or Wintrobe indices (MCV > 100 fL), performed as part of an investigation of anemia, suggests that macrocytosis and particularly macroovalocytosis is present. Sometimes a patient comes to the physician because of neurologic signs and symptoms suggestive of vitamin B_{12} deficiency. Historical or physical evidence suggestive of diseases associated with vitamin B_{12} or folic acid deficiency should be obtained. Dietary history, alcohol intake, and history of diarrhea, pregnancy, or drug ingestion are most important. Careful attention must be given to nervous system involvement as manifested by paresthesias, ataxia, difficulty with bladder or bowel, and loss of position or vibratory sense. Peripheral neuropathy with "stocking-glove" sensory loss is not uncommon in association with folic acid deficiency but is due to concurrent alcoholism and nutritional deficiency and not to folate lack.

Careful examination of the peripheral blood usually reveals macroovalocytosis and hypersegmented polys. A bone marrow sample showing megaloblasts and giant myeloid forms may or may not be needed to confirm the diagnosis of megaloblastic anemia. Laboratory studies, such as measurement of serum B_{12} and folate levels and possibly gastric analysis for acid, should be performed to establish etiology. Conditions other than vitamin B_{12} or folate deficiency can also be associated with macrocytosis (see p. 76).

If vitamin B_{12} deficiency is suspected as a cause of megaloblastic anemia, then a Schilling test should be performed, even if the patient has received prior treatment with vitamin B_{12}. The Schilling test should be deferred until the patient has been treated with B_{12} for at least 2 months. Finally, in some cases it may be necessary to follow the reticulocyte and hematocrit responses to small doses of vitamin B_{12} or folic acid. With measurement of serum B_{12} and folic acid levels and Schilling tests readily available, therapeutic trials are now seldom performed.

In a few cases of very severe anemia and tissue hypoxia, particularly if manifested by angina, it may be necessary to treat the patient

---

Approach to patient with megaloblastic anemia

Historical findings
Abdominal operations, particularly if a surgical bypass or blind loop
  was created
Alcohol intake
Ataxia (abnormal gait)
Bladder and bowel dysfunction
Diarrhea or fatty stools
Dietary history
Drug therapy, particularly anticonvulsants, antituberculosis drugs,
  cancer chemotherapy
Glossitis (sore tongue)
Paresthesias
Pregnancy
Physical examination
Evidence of glossitis
Evidence of peripheral neuropathy or combined systems disease
Scleral icterus
Laboratory tests
Tests to establish whether or not anemia is megaloblastic:
  Examination of the peripheral blood
  Bone marrow examination (not always necessary)
  Serum lactic acid dehydrogenase, unconjugated bilirubin levels
Investigations to establish etiology:
  Gastric analysis for acid
  Malabsorption tests, for example, D-xylose absorption
  Serum methylmalonic acid and homocysteine
  Schilling test
  Serum folate
  Serum vitamin B_{12}
Investigations to determine complications:
  Serum potassium
  Serum uric acid

with both folic acid and vitamin B_{12} before the etiology of the deficiency is discovered. By obtaining serum levels and saving extra aliquots in the freezer in case the originals are lost, it is possible to make a definitive diagnosis in retrospect. Even when this fails, a Schilling test can usually be used to separate megaloblastic erythropoiesis due to folate deficiency from that due to vitamin B_{12} deficiency.

Response to Vitamin B_{12} or Folate Replacement Therapy

The changes in symptoms, peripheral blood, bone marrow, and neurologic status associated with treatment of folate or vitamin B_{12} deficiency are as follows:

1. The (elevated) serum iron falls to subnormal levels and then rises to a normal plateau.
2. Serum uric acid level rises and serum potassium falls (48 hours).
3. Bone marrow erythroid morphology reverts to normal (24–48 hours).

4. There are reticulocytosis and increased neutrophil and platelet counts (5–10 days).

5. Macroovalocytes and hypersegmented polys disappear (2–3 weeks or sometimes longer).

6. Evidence of ineffective erythropoiesis, elevated bilirubin, and LDH levels, etc., disappears (a few days).

7. Neurologic improvement occurs (80–90 percent of patients improve in 6 months to 1 year, but some chronic neurologic manifestations of vitamin B_{12} deficiency may be irreversible).

Interrelationships Between Iron, Folic Acid, and Vitamin B_{12}

Chronic iron deficiency is associated with impairment of parietal cell function. Often achlorhydria and occasionally diminished IF secretion are documented in patients with iron deficiency anemia. Patients with iron deficiency may have hypersegmented polys in their blood. These abnormalities are reversed by iron therapy. Occasionally patients develop vitamin B_{12} deficiency in association with iron deficiency.

Vitamin B_{12} deficiency in the gut in some patients leads to difficulty in absorbing the IF-B_{12} complex. This observation explains why some patients with PA have abnormal part two Schilling test results that return to normal after several weeks of parenteral vitamin B_{12} therapy. A few patients with PA have folate malabsorption, which also becomes normal after vitamin B_{12} therapy.

Other Causes of Megaloblastic Anemia

Although most anemias characterized by megaloblastic erythropoiesis are due to either vitamin B_{12} or folic acid deficiency, there are several other causes of megaloblastic hematopoiesis. Some of these diseases are inherited, others are iatrogenic (drug-induced), and some may be neoplastic. All fail to respond to replacement therapy with vitamin B_{12} or folic acid.

Hereditary orotic aciduria is a rare congenital disease secondary to reduced activity of the enzymes required to convert orotic acid to uridylic acid. Because of this defect the synthesis of pyrimidine ribonucleotides, precursors of both RNA and DNA, is impaired. This deficiency is manifested by megaloblastic anemia, growth impairment, and renal excretion of orotic acid in large quantities. Therapy with uridine ameliorates these abnormalities.

Another rare disorder of infancy is due to decreased activity in the liver of formiminotransferase, the enzyme that catalyzes the breakdown of FIGLU. As a result there are excessive urinary excretion of FIGLU, megaloblastic anemia, and extreme elevation of serum folate levels. The very few patients reported appear to respond partially to pyridoxine therapy.

Besides the antifols, a number of antimetabolites used in treating cancer block the synthesis of nucleic acids and lead to morphologic abnormalities indistinguishable from those of megaloblastic anemia. Unlike the antifols, these drugs produce effects that are not reversed by administration of folinic acid. The drugs include the purine analogues, 6-mercaptopurine, thioguanine, and azathioprine, which interfere with the metabolism of nucleic acids by their incorporation into purine nucleotides. This interference leads to the development of megaloblastic changes in the bone marrow that are not reversed by vitamin B_{12} or folic acid therapy but are reversed by discontinuation of the antimetabolite. Cytosine arabinoside and hydroxyurea also cause megaloblastic changes secondary to interference with DNA synthesis.

Megaloblastic "dyserythropoiesis" in the bone marrow may be seen in patients suffering from myelodysplastic disorders, myelocytic leukemias—in particular erythroleukemia—and congenital dyserythropoietic anemias (Plate 31). Dyserythropoiesis is defined by certain morphologic and functional characteristics. A common finding is asynchrony of nuclear–cytoplasmic maturation, along with nuclear lobulation and fragmentation, karyorrhexis, pyknosis, binuclearity, and multinuclearity with budding and internuclear bridging. In some cases there are frank megaloblastic changes. It should be stressed that this megaloblastic dyserythropoietic morphology does not respond to vitamin B_{12} or folic acid administration.

Functionally the dyserythropoietic state is characterized by ineffective erythropoiesis. The marrow appears hypercellular, but the reticulocyte production index is low. Iron kinetic studies reveal rapid plasma clearance of radioiron into the bone marrow but diminished radioiron incorporation into circulating erythrocytes. Increased hemoglobin catabolism is indicated by unconjugated bilirubinemia, increased fecal urobilinogen, and high endogenous carbon monoxide production, which cannot be accounted for by peripheral blood hemolysis. It is therefore assumed that hemolysis is occurring within the bone marrow before release of the mature red cells. In many cases the red cells that are produced are defective and have a shorter than normal survival time in the peripheral blood. In some cases folic acid deficiency may also result because of the hyperactive erythropoiesis.

Recently three types of rare, usually familial, dyserythropoietic anemias have been described. They have in common characteristic morphologic alterations of dyserythropoiesis, ineffective erythropoiesis, increased peripheral erythrocyte turnover, disturbances of iron metabolism usually leading to iron-loading, and nonresponsiveness to the usual hematinics. Although these anemias are often inherited, they may go undetected until adulthood. *Type I* congenital dyserythropoietic anemia (CDA) is characterized by megaloblastoid erythroblasts and erythroblasts with internuclear chromatin bridges—that is, strands of chromatin connecting the nuclei of two adjacent erythroblasts. The anemia is macrocytic in type, chronic, and unresponsive to any known therapy. In some patients it is inherited as an autosomal recessive.

Congenital dyserythropoietic anemia *type II,* sometimes called HEMPAS (*h*ereditary *e*rythroblastic *m*ultinuclearity with a *p*ositive *a*cidified *s*erum test), is characterized by refractory anemia with multinucleated erythroblasts. Anisocytosis and poikilocytosis are found in the peripheral blood, along with inappropriately low reticulocyte counts. In the bone marrow erythropoiesis is essentially normoblastic, but many of the mature normoblasts have two or more nuclei or multilobulated nuclei. There are increased iron stores, but ringed sideroblasts are unusual. In almost all cases the patient's erythrocytes can be hemolyzed by certain sera from normal individuals after acidification of the sera to pH 6.8. This "normal" serum contains a naturally occurring, IgM, complement-binding, cold isoantibody. HEMPAS erythrocytes are strongly agglutinated by antibodies to I and i blood group antigens (reviewed in Chapters 8 and 9), and their cell membranes have an increased sensitivity to complement. Reduced content of sialic acid in their cell membranes has also been described. Large numbers of Gaucher-like (Plate 32) cells are found in the marrow of some HEMPAS patients. This type of CDA is inherited as an autosomal recessive. Although it is the most common type of CDA, it is still extremely rare.

Type III CDA is characterized by erythroblastic multinuclearity and the presence of *gigantoblasts* (Plate 31). These are large, erythroid-appearing cells with multiple or lobulated nuclei and with nuclear–cytoplasmic asynchrony. Neither macrocytosis in the peripheral blood nor internuclear bridging is prominent. There is increased agglutination of the patient's red cells by anti-i and anti-I sera but no lysis by acidified serum. This CDA may be inherited as an autosomal dominant.

Case Development Problem: Megaloblastic Anemia

A 78-year-old man had a subtotal gastrectomy 6 years ago for a benign bleeding gastric ulcer. At that time one half of his stomach was removed and the remaining upper half was joined to the second part of the small intestine, the jejunum. The end of the small intestine that normally connects to the outlet of the stomach was sewn closed. Since then the only medication he has taken is multivitamins containing $1 \mu g$ vitamin B_{12}, 0.1 mg folic acid, and no iron salts. His hematocrit at present is 0.17 (17%); hemoglobin, 4.8 gm per deciliter; mean corpuscular volume, 130 fL; and reticulocyte count, 3 percent.

1. On the basis of the laboratory findings, can you predict the morphologic abnormalities to be found in his peripheral blood smear?

By dividing his mean corpuscular volume into his hematocrit, the red blood cell count is calculated to be 1.3 million per deciliter. Dividing this result into his hemoglobin yields a mean corpuscular hemoglobin of 37 pg. Finally, by dividing his hemoglobin by his hematocrit, a mean corpuscular hemoglobin concentration of 28 gm per deciliter is obtained. Since the MCV is elevated, and the MCHC is low, the peripheral blood smear should reveal macrocytosis and hypochromia.

His peripheral blood smear showed macrocytosis and oval-shaped large erythrocytes. There was hypochromia and variation in the size and shape of his red cells, and an abnormally low number of platelets. A white blood cell count was taken and found low.

2. List the possible causes of his anemia on the basis of the history and laboratory findings and suggest physical findings that would confirm one or more of these diagnoses.

Macroovalocytosis, depression of all three blood counts, and the history of gastrointestinal surgery suggest the diagnosis of megaloblastic anemia. If this is correct, the patient might have lemon yellow skin, which is due to a combination of anemia and hyperbilirubinemia secondary to ineffective erythropoiesis; glossitis; and neurologic disturbances, such as paresthesias, ataxia, and loss of position sense.

The hypochromia seen on the peripheral blood smear and the low MCHC suggest concurrent iron deficiency anemia, which might be manifested by glossitis, cheilosis, angular stomatitis, and spooning of the fingernails.

The high reticulocyte percentage and anemia suggest the diagnosis of hemolytic anemia. Except for hyperbilirubinemia, physical findings do not help confirm this diagnosis. Many cases of hemolytic anemia are associated with an enlarged spleen, and it would be well to look for a mass in the left upper quadrant of the abdomen. However, the reticulocyte count in this patient is actually low in absolute number (reticulocyte % × RBC number), and hemolysis is unlikely.

On physical examination this patient did have lemon yellow skin, atrophy of his tongue papillae, and loss of vibratory sense, but there was no splenomegaly or neurologic findings. There was no exposure to toxins or drugs other than vitamins and no evidence of malignant disease.

Following is a list of tests available at your hospital and the charge for each (billed to the patient).

Bone marrow examination, $125
Serum folate, $15
Serum vitamin B_{12} level, $15
Gastric aspiration for acid, $50
Intrinsic factor assay on gastric contents, $100
Serum antibodies against intrinsic factor and parietal cells, $100
FIGLU test, $30
Schilling test (each part), $30
Hospitalization for therapeutic trials, $850 per day
Serum ferritin, $10
Serum iron and total iron-binding capacity (TIBC), $25

3. Leaving therapeutic considerations aside, what is the most cost-effective approach to diagnosing this patient's anemia?

There is more than one correct answer to this question. One possible approach might be to start with a bone marrow examination, which would make the diagnosis of megaloblastic anemia or iron deficiency anemia, provided the bone marrow was stained for hemosiderin. It would also exclude aplastic anemia and anemia secondary to marrow replacement by fibrosis or tumor. If megaloblastic anemia was found, one would measure the serum vitamin B_{12} level. If this is low, a Schilling test should be performed. The Schilling test would determine whether vitamin B_{12} deficiency was due to lack of IF or ileal malabsorption. Assaying the folic acid level is probably unnecessary, since the patient is taking 100 μg of folic acid per day. In addition a serum iron, and TIBC, or ferritin level might be done to investigate the hypochromia since gastrectomy and duodenal bypass surgery predispose to both vitamin B_{12} and iron deficiency. The total expenditure of funds using this approach would be approximately $210. A therapeutic trial with B_{12}, unless it could be reliably performed at home, would be a very expensive procedure and, unlike the Schilling test, would not determine the mechanisms of any vitamin B_{12} deficiency. Other approaches are certainly possible, and we leave them to the student to consider.

4. This patient's bone marrow revealed changes diagnostic of megaloblastosis. What abnormalities of the red cells, white cells, platelets, and megakaryocytes, other than those previously described, might be found in his bone marrow and peripheral blood?

Often associated with megaloblastosis are pancytopenia and a low reticulocyte production index. The peripheral blood shows hypersegmented polys, and immature red and white cells are sometimes present. Some of the immature red cells are recognizable as megaloblastic. Platelets are decreased and large. Changes in the bone marrow include giant metamyelocytes and myelocytes with characteristic chromatin abnormalities, abnormal megakaryocytes with hyperlobulation of their nuclei, and abnormalities in the normoblasts with an immature chromatin pattern but a relatively well-developed cytoplasm.

This patient had a normal serum folic acid level, a low serum vitamin B_{12} level, abnormal part one Schilling test results, and absent marrow iron stores. Results of the part two Schilling test were entirely normal.

5. What is the most likely diagnosis? Are there any other possibilities? How would you treat the most likely diagnosis?

Almost certainly the patient has acquired absence of IF secretion due to the partial gastrectomy. Loading and then maintenance doses of parenteral vitamin B_{12} will adequately treat the anemia. If angina or other evidence of severe tissue oxygen lack is present, then slow transfusion with packed red cells and concurrent diuretic therapy are indicated. Remember, treatment is actually initiated at the time the Schilling test is done.

Loading doses of vitamin B_{12} were given along with transfusion of two units of packed red cells because the patient developed angina.

6. How would you follow this patient's response to therapy, and what would you consider if he responds only partially?

The reticulocyte count reaches a peak 5 to 10 days following the first injection of vitamin B_{12}. The rise in reticulocyte count might be blunted by the transfusion of 2 units of red cells. Over a period of 3 weeks the hematocrit should rise rapidly toward normal. If the anemia is only partially corrected, then consideration should be given to the following factors: First, there are hypochromia and absent iron stores, so concomitant iron deficiency probably exists. Patients with pernicious anemia often initially have elevated serum iron levels that fall to subnormal levels with treatment but ultimately become normal. In a few cases the serum iron level remains low. Such patients require treatment for iron deficiency. In this patient the concomitant iron deficiency is due to iron malabsorption because of both lack of gastric acid and bypass of the duodenum, the major site of iron absorption from the diet.

Topics for Discussion: Macrocytic Anemia

Biochemistry of vitamin B_{12}
Gastric intrinsic factor
Antibodies to intrinsic factor
Intestinal absorption of vitamin B_{12}
Schilling test and its variants
Vitamin B_{12} binding proteins
Pathogenesis of pernicious anemia
Inherited forms of vitamin B_{12} deficiency
Biochemistry of folic acid
Absorption and malabsorption of folic acid
Drug-induced folic acid deficiency
Neurologic disease and vitamin B_{12}
Malabsorption, gastrectomy, and megaloblastic anemia
Intestinal bacterial flora and megaloblastic anemia
Pregnancy and megaloblastic anemia
Megaloblastic anemia associated with drugs such as anti-
convulsants, birth control pills, and anticancer agents
Dyserythropoietic anemias
Interrelationships between B_{12}, folate, and iron
Hypersegmented poly and its significance
Macrocytosis and its significance
Serum and red cell enzyme changes in megaloblastic anemia
Ineffective erythropoiesis and decreased red cell life span in mega-
loblastic anemia

Selected Readings

General Considerations

Chanarin, I. *The Megaloblastic Anaemias.* Philadelphia: Davis, 1969.
Chanarin, I. et al. Cobalamin-folate interrelations: A critical review. *Blood* 66 : 479, 1985.
Jandl, J. H. Megaloblastic Anemias. In J. H. Jandl, *Blood: Textbook of Hematology.* Boston: Little, Brown, 1987.
Wintrobe, M. M. et al. Megaloblastic and Nonmegaloblastic Macrocytic Anemias. In M. M. Wintrobe et al. (eds.). *Clinical Hematology* (8th ed.) Philadelphia: Lea & Febiger, 1981.

Vitamin B_{12}

Allen, R. H. Human vitamin B_{12} transport proteins. *Prog. Hematol.* 9 : 57, 1975.
Allen, R. H. The plasma transport of vitamin B_{12}. *Br. J. Haematol.* 33 : 161, 1976.
Carmel, R. Macrocytosis, mild anemia, and delay in the diagnosis of pernicious anemia. *Arch. Intern. Med.* 139 : 47, 1979.

Carmel, R., and Johnson, C. S. Racial patterns in pernicious anemia: Early age at onset and increased frequency of intrinsic-factor antibody in black women. *N. Engl. J. Med.* 298 : 647, 1978.

Chanarin, I. New light on pernicious anemia. *Lancet* 2 : 538, 1973.

Cohen, K. L., and Donaldson, R. M. Unreliability of radiodilution assays as a screen for cobalamin (vitamin B_{12}) deficiency. *J.A.M.A.* 244 : 1942, 1980.

Green, R. et al. Masking of macrocytosis by α-thalassemia in blacks with pernicious anemia. *N. Engl. J. Med.* 307 : 1322, 1982.

Hall, C. A. The transport of vitamin B_{12} from food to use within the cells. *J. Lab. Clin. Med.* 94 : 811, 1979.

Lindenbaum, J. et al. Neuropsychiatric disorders caused by cobalamin deficiency in the absence of anemia of macrocytosis. *N. Engl. J. Med.* 318 : 1720, 1988.

Matchar, D. B. et al. Isotope-dilution assay for urinary methylmalonic acid in the diagnosis of vitamin B_{12} deficiency. *Ann. Intern. Med.* 106 : 707, 1987.

Nath, B. J., and Lindenbaum, J. Persistence of neutrophil hypersegmentation during recovery from megaloblastic granulopoiesis. *Ann. Intern. Med.* 90 : 757, 1979.

Norman, E. J., Martelo, O. J., and Denton, M. D. Cobalamin (vitamin B_{12}) deficiency detection by urinary methylmalonic acid quantitation. *Blood* 59 : 1128, 1982.

Sleisinger, M. H. Illuminating the antrum. *N. Engl. J. Med.* 300 : 1436, 1979.

Sullivan, L. W. Vitamin B_{12} metabolism and megaloblastic anemia. *Semin. Hematol.* 7 : 6, 1970.

Tavassoli, M., and Takahashi, K. The tentacles of the cell. *J.A.M.A.* 247 : 1324, 1982.

Thompson, G. T. Evaluation of current criteria used to measure vitamin B_{12} levels. *Am. J. Med.* 82 : 291, 1987.

Folic Acid

Colman, N., and Herbert, V. Total folate binding capacity of normal human plasma and variations in uremia, cirrhosis and pregnancy. *Blood* 48 : 911, 1976.

Herbert, V. Folate forms, functions, and fate. *N. Engl. J. Med.* 286 : 214, 1972.

Hoffbrand, A. V. Synthesis and breakdown of natural folates (folate polyglutamates). *Prog. Hematol.* 9 : 85, 1975.

Rose, M., and Johnson. I. Reinterpretation of the haematological effects of anticonvulsant treatment. *Lancet* 1 : 1349, 1978.

Streiff, R. R. Folic acid deficiency anemia. *Semin. Hematol.* 7 : 23, 1970.

Waxman, S. Folate binding proteins. *Br. J. Haematol.* 29 : 23, 1975.

Wu, A. et al. Folate deficiency in the alcoholic—its relationship to clinical and haematological abnormalities, liver disease and folate stores. *Br. J. Haematol.* 29 : 469, 1975.

5 Normocytic Anemias
Lawrence N. Shulman

Aplastic Anemia

Aplastic anemia is a disease characterized by a decrease in the production not only of red blood cells, but of all nonlymphoid bone marrow elements, red cells, white cells, and platelets. A selective decrease in red cell production is referred to as pure red cell aplasia and is discussed later. Patients with aplastic anemia generally have symptoms characteristic of a particular cellular deficiency. Those with anemia may be fatigued or short of breath, those with neutropenia may manifest serious infection, and those with thrombocytopenia may demonstrate petechiae or bleeding. The diagnosis is suggested by the presence of pancytopenia. A low reticulocyte count suggests underproduction rather than increased loss or destruction of red cells. The diagnosis is confirmed with a bone marrow biopsy that shows a substantial decrease in the number of red cell, white cell, and platelet precursors, and replacement of the usually cellular bone marrow with fat. Aplastic anemia can be mild or severe, and the management of the patient depends on the severity of the illness.

Etiology

Failure of the pluripotential stem cells of the bone marrow to maintain bone marrow cellularity and the production of normal numbers of mature red cells, neutrophils, and platelets characterizes aplastic anemia. See Chapter 1 for a full discussion of stem cell physiology. Failure of the pluripotential stem cell can be caused by many different factors (Table 5-1). In most cases of aplastic anemia, the cause is not known. Even if a careful history is taken, no potentially offending agent can be indentified. These cases are referred to as idiopathic.

Several different toxic agents have been implicated as causes of bone marrow aplasia. One of the best studied in the laboratory and in clinical medicine is radiation. Between 500 and 1,500 R whole body radiation will reproducibly cause total bone marrow aplasia. If left untreated the patient will die of infection and bleeding. Many

Table 5-1. Etiologies of aplastic anemia

I. Idiopathic
II. Radiation
III. Drugs*
    A. Antimicrobials—chloramphenicol
    B. Antiepileptics—carbamazepine, diphenylhydantoin
    C. Anti-inflammatory—phenylbutazone
    D. Antithyroid—methimazole (Tapazole)
    E. Gold compounds
    F. Organic arsenicals
    G. Chemotherapeutic agents—alkylating agents
IV. Toxins*
    A. Solvents—benzene
    B. Insecticides—DDT
V. Viral agents*
    A. Hepatitis B virus
    B. Non-A, non-B hepatitis virus
    C. Epstein-Barr virus

---

*Selected examples of drugs, toxins, and viral agents are shown for the sake of simplicity.

people died in this manner after the atomic bomb explosions in Japan and the nuclear accident at Chernobyl.

Numerous toxic chemicals and drugs are known to cause aplastic anemia. Organic solvents such as benzene reproducibly cause bone marrow damage.

Many agents that cause aplastic anemia, such as benzene and radiation, can on occasion precipitate malignant transformation of the damaged bone marrow stem cells, resulting in the development of acute leukemia. These leukemias are often associated with gross chromosomal abnormalities in the leukemic clones and respond poorly to conventional antileukemic therapy.

The antibiotic chloramphenicol is one of the most widely appreciated etiologic agents in bone marrow injury. All patients, if given high enough doses of this drug, will develop dose-dependent bone marrow suppression and pancytopenia. Fortunately, this almost always disappears entirely when the drug is stopped. Rarely, permanent bone marrow damage and aplastic anemia develop. This is an idiosyncratic reaction. There is no dose dependence and no way to predict in whom this manifestation will develop.

In some patients aplastic anemia appears to develop after viral infections. Many viruses are known to cause transient suppression of the bone marrow. A well-understood example is that of parvovirus, which can cause a transient, severe selective suppression of red cell production. In rare instances viruses can cause severe and permanent bone marrow damage and true aplastic anemia. Hepatitis B virus; hepatitis C virus, the virus that causes most cases of non-A, non-B hepatitis; and Epstein-Barr virus are three that have been associated with the subsequent development of aplastic anemia.

Some cases of aplastic anemia are believed to be caused by immunologic mechanisms. The patient's own T lymphocytes may become cytotoxic to bone marrow stem cells and suppress their normal growth. Evidence for this includes laboratory experiments showing that T lymphocytes from such patients can cause suppression of growth of normal bone marrow in in-vitro culture systems. In other experiments, removal of the patient's T cells allows the bone marrow cells to grow normally in vitro, whereas readdition of the T cells renders growth subnormal once again. Additional evidence comes from the fact that some patients with aplastic anemia treated with immunoglobulin directed against T cells (antithymocyte globulin, or ATG) or other "immunosuppressive" drugs will have an improvement in their blood counts. This is discussed further in the section on treatment.

Diagnosis

The patient generally presents with fatigue, due to a low hematocrit, infection associated with a low white count, and/or bleeding associated with thrombocytopenia. The diagnosis is suspected when all three cell lines are suppressed and pancytopenia is present. The reticulocyte count is low. Generally, no adenopathy or splenomegaly is present. Serum iron, vitamin B_{12}, and folic acid levels are normal or, in the case of iron, often high because of underutilization.

The bone marrow aspirate and especially the biopsy are the keys to the diagnosis. In severe cases very few cells are present in the bone marrow and most of these are lymphocytes and plasma cells. In milder cases red cell, white cell, and platelet precursors are present but in reduced amounts. The marrow is made up primarily of fat. Normally, 50 percent of the bone marrow is fat on histologic examination of the bone marrow biopsy, but in aplastic anemia often 80 to 95 percent is fat.

Prognosis

The prognosis of aplastic anemia is dependent on the severity of the disorder at the time of diagnosis. Patients with mild aplastic anemia may do well for long periods without the need for blood product support and without an increased risk of infection. Patients with severe aplastic anemia have a very poor prognosis without definitive treatment (bone marrow transplantation or ATG). In this group 50 percent of patients will be dead within 6 months of diagnosis and fewer than 30 percent will be alive 5 years after diagnosis. Severe aplastic anemia can be defined in patients with:

I. No significant improvement in blood counts during 3 weeks of observation

II. Two of the following:
  A. Platelet count of fewer than 20,000/cu mm
  B. Neutrophil count of fewer than 500/cu mm
  C. Reticulocyte count (corrected) of less than 1 percent
III. Markedly hypocellular bone marrow

Treatment

ANTIBIOTICS

Patients with neutrophil counts of fewer than 500/cu mm are at high risk for serious infection. Infections that would ordinarily be well contained in a person with a normal neutrophil count can lead to the rapid development of overwhelming sepsis in the neutropenic patient. Infections often arise in the gastrointestinal tract from normal endogenous organisms, but can be caused by essentially any bacteria and affect any organ. Prompt institution of intravenous antibiotics is essential in the management of serious infection in these patients. Often a semisynthetic penicillin such as mezlocillin is used in conjunction with an aminoglycoside such as gentamicin until a specific microorganism has been isolated. In spite of prompt treatment with antibiotics, patients with very low neutrophil counts still have considerable difficulty controlling serious bacterial infections, and these remain the leading cause of death in patients with aplastic anemia.

TRANSFUSION SUPPORT

Patients should only be transfused when absolutely necessary for two reasons. First, many patients with aplastic anemia will be treated with allogeneic bone marrow transplantation, as discussed later, and the likelihood of success of this treatment is reduced by prior exposure to foreign blood antigens through transfusions. In particular, transfusions from family members should be avoided since these may increase the chance of graft rejection after a bone marrow transplant from a histocompatible donor, usually a sibling. Secondly, many patients with aplastic anemia cannot be treated by bone marrow transplantation and will often require blood product support over a long period of time. With increasing numbers of transfusions, the risk of alloimmunization increases. Alloimmunization is the development of antibodies to antigens on blood cells of other people. This is particularly a problem with platelets, for which we are often unable to test for the pertinent antigens. With time patients often become so severely alloimmunized to platelet antigens that platelet transfusions become ineffective. The patient may then have lethal bleeding in spite of repeated platelet transfusions.

Platelet transfusions should not be used until the platelet count is below 20,000/cu mm or even 10,000/cu mm unless significant clinical bleeding is present. When platelet transfusions are necessary, single-donor platelets obtained by plateletpheresis should be used since this type of transfusion will expose the patient to only one set of foreign antigens and transfusion with pooled platelets from random donors will expose the patient to multiple sets of foreign platelet antigens.

Likewise, red cell transfusions should only be used when necessary. One should not attempt to return the hematocrit to normal, but only to maintain it at the lowest level tolerable by the patient.

White blood cell transfusions have been tried in cases of severe neutropenia and infection. They have been of questionable efficacy, are difficult to obtain, and have potentially serious complications. Thus, they are not in common use.

BONE MARROW TRANSPLANTATION

The patient with severe aplastic anemia, as defined previously, has a very poor prognosis and is best treated with allogeneic bone marrow transplantation. As seen in Figure 5-1, the long-term survival of patients with severe aplastic anemia is greatly improved by bone marrow transplantation. Unfortunately, not all patients are acceptable candidates. Patients should be considered for bone marrow transplantation if they meet the following criteria: (1) They must have a confirmed diagnosis of *severe* aplastic anemia as described previously; (2) they must be of an acceptable age—less than 50 or 55 year old—and in good general medical condition; and (3) they must have an acceptable donor—usually a sibling who is human leukocyte antigen (HLA) histocompatible (as described in the following section) and medically able to be a bone marrow donor.

Human Leukocyte Antigen (HLA) System

The HLA system is located in the major histocompatibility complex (MHC) on the short arm of chromosome 6. A patient inherits one chromosome 6 from each parent. Since each parent has two number 6 chromosomes, there are four possible combinations of HLA types from any two parents (Fig. 5-2). Thus, the likelihood of any given sibling being HLA identical to the patient is about 25 percent. Obviously, the more siblings a patient has, the more likely that the patient will have an HLA-identical sibling. During ovum and sperm production, chromosome crossovers can occur that will sometimes cause more complicated genetic schemes. The closer to a "perfect" match of the HLA antigens between donors and recipient, the more likely that the transplant will be successful.

The HLA antigens are only the "major" histocompatibility antigens in humans. We have no way to test for minor histocompatibility antigens except to perform mixed lymphocyte cultures. These tests show reactivity between donor and recipient cells as expressed

Fig. 5-1. Kaplan–Meier estimates of survival according to treatment in the International Aplastic Anemia Study. (From B. M. Camitta, R. Storb, and E. D. Thomas, Aplastic anemia: Pathogenesis, diagnosis, treatment, and prognosis. Reprinted with permission from *The N. Engl. J. Med.* 306 : 714, 1982.)

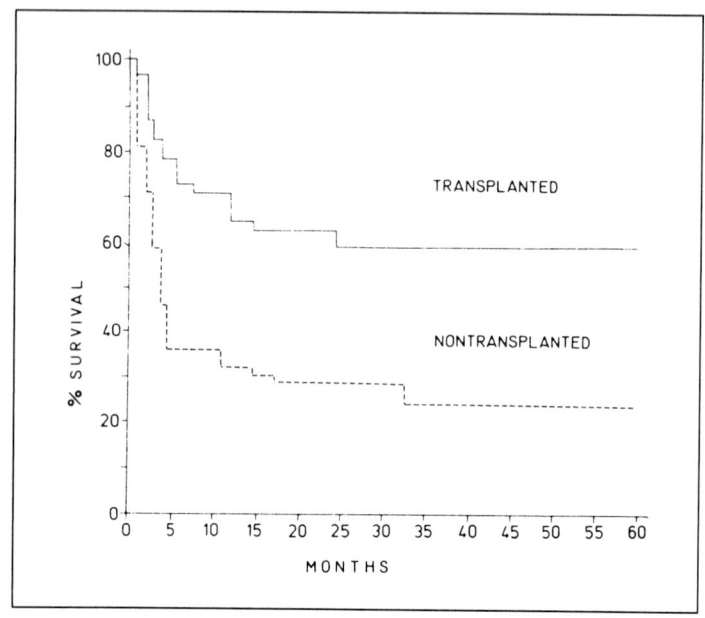

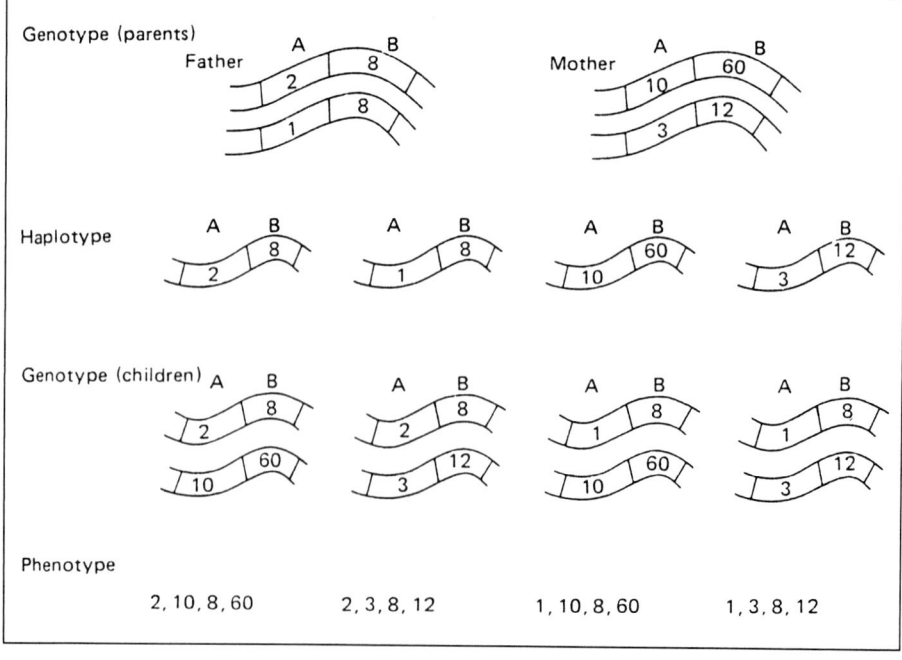

Fig. 5-2. Inheritance of HLA genotypes.

by a lymphocyte cytotoxicity assay and in a general way add to our ability to detect "compatibility" of a donor marrow and a recipient host. It is clear, particularly from the occurrence of graft-versus-host disease, as described in the following section, that minor antigens often cause significant incompatibility.

In patients who do not have an HLA-identical sibling, a few medical centers are performing bone marrow transplants using non-related donors who are HLA identical. The likelihood of finding a donor is small, between 1 in 10,000 to 1 in 50,000, depending on the HLA type of the patient. In addition, the incidence of graft rejection and graft-versus-host disease is much higher with persons who are not related even if they are HLA identical.

Complications of Bone Marrow Transplantation

1. Graft rejection—failure of the donor bone marrow to grow in the recipient. The patient receives the sibling bone marrow cells intravenously as he or she would a transfusion. The donor stem cells find their way to the bone marrow, where they lodge and eventually begin to grow. In general 3 to 6 weeks is required for a transplanted bone marrow to begin to produce mature circulating blood cells. Graft failure can occur because the donor bone marrow is rejected by the patient's immune system, because there are insufficient numbers of stem cells in the donor bone marrow, or because the bone marrow is damaged in the transplantation procedure.

2. Graft-versus-host disease (GVHD). The donor bone marrow lymphocytes recognize the patient's cells as "foreign tissue" and attack them, leading to skin rashes, hepatitis, and gastrointestinal toxicity. This can occur in an acute or chronic form. GVHD can be serious and lead to death. It is more likely to occur and more apt to be severe in the older patient and the patient whose donor is an imperfect HLA match. Except for bone marrow transfusion between identical twins, marrow recipients are routinely treated with immunosuppressive drugs such as methotrexate and cyclosporine in order to suppress GVHD. In patients at high risk for GVHD, the risk can be lowered further by depleting the donor bone marrow of T cells.

3. Infection. The transplanted bone marrow will take 3 to 6 weeks to "take" and produce adequate granulocytes. During this period the patient has no granulocytes and is at risk of serious and potentially fatal infection. Even after recovery of the granulocytes, the patient's lymphocytic system is severely compromised, and he or she is at risk for disseminated infections with cytomegalovirus (CMV), other viruses, and fungi. Infection is a major cause of death in patients treated with bone marrow transplantation.

4. Hemorrhage. While waiting for the donor bone marrow to "take," the patient is very thrombocytopenic. Generally, he or she can be supported with platelet transfusions, but on occasion the patient becomes alloimmunized to transfused platelets, destroying them so rapidly that they cannot protect against bleeding. In these circumstances patients can bleed to death.

5. Venoocclusive disease of the liver. This is an uncommon but potentially life-threatening complication that often causes rapid and severe hepatic failure. The etiology is not clear, but vascular damage due to chemotherapeutic drugs and immunosuppressive agents may be responsible.

Prognosis of Patients Treated with Bone Marrow Transplantation

The overall survival for patients with severe aplastic anemia treated with bone marrow transplantation from an HLA-identical sibling is approximately 75 percent. The major determinant of prognosis is GVHD. In those patients with mild GVHD, the survival is in excess of 90 percent. In patients with moderate to severe GVHD, the survival is less than 50 percent. In particular, younger patients have less GVHD and better survival. Transfusions administered before bone marrow transplantation adversely affect survival and should be kept to a minimum.

TREATMENT WITH ANTITHYMOCYTE GLOBULIN

If a patient is unable to undergo bone marrow transplantation because of age, comorbid disease, or the lack of an acceptable donor, an alternative treatment is ATG. In one of the original bone marrow transplantation patients, ATG was used to suppress the patient's immune system and decrease the chance of rejection of the donor bone marrow. The donor bone marrow did not engraft, but the patient's own bone marrow recovered, probably because of the ATG, which suppressed the aspect of his immune system that was suppressing growth of his own bone marrow cells. Since then ATG has been used in large numbers of patients with aplastic anemia with varied success. Apparently, only a subset of patients have an immunologic cause of their aplastic anemia (as described earlier) and it is difficult to identify these patients. ATG would not be expected to help a patient whose bone marrow has been injured by an exogenous toxic agent such as radiation. Therefore, only a portion of patients with aplastic anemia will respond to treatment with ATG. In addition the responses are often incomplete and temporary. Nonetheless, many patients can have a significant improvement in their blood counts for a significant period in response to ATG.

Antithymocyte globulin is prepared in a variety of ways. Most often human lymphocytes or, specifically, T lymphocytes are repeatedly injected into a horse, causing the horse to produce antithymo-cyte immunoglobulin. The horse's serum is harvested and the immunoglobulin separated. Preparations of ATG vary significantly in their make-up and effectiveness.

OTHER FORMS OF TREATMENT

Many other approaches to the treatment of aplastic anemia have been tried, with marginal or no success. These include high doses of corticosteroids, androgens, or lithium. Though an occasional patient probably has a response to these agents, this is rare and these treatments are generally considered ineffective. There are recent reports of successful treatment of aplastic anemia with cyclosporine, a potent immunosuppressive agent, often used in combination with ATG.

Case Development Problem: Aplastic Anemia

A 48-year-old woman with a history of chronic urinary tract infec-tions presents with acute pyelonephritis (kidney infection) due to an organism that is sensitive only to chloramphenicol. She is treated with this drug in moderately high dosage. At the end of the second week of treatment, her hematocrit has fallen from its previous nor-mal value to 25 percent and her white blood count is 2,800/cu mm with 30% neutrophils. Her platelet count is also reduced at 20,000/cu mm. She has taken no other drugs and has not been exposed to x-irradiation. Her physical examination is entirely normal. Periph-eral blood smear shows reduced platelets and granulocytes but no immature white cells. Red blood cell morphology is normal.

1. What is the likely diagnosis? What laboratory tests would you order and what would the results likely be?

   The most likely cause of her pancytopenia is dose-related, reversible bone marrow suppression caused by chloramphenicol. The reticulocyte count would be low. Serum iron levels would be high, nearly saturating the total iron-binding capacity (TIBC) of the serum. A bone marrow biopsy would reveal normal or reduced cellularity. Erythroid precursors would be vacuolated.

With cessation of antibiotic therapy, her blood counts return to normal. Three months later, however, because of symptoms of an upper respiratory tract infection she medicates herself with leftover chloramphenicol tablets for one week. Six months later she is again found to be pancytopenic. Her hematocrit is 20 percent, the white cell count is 1,000/cu mm with less than 10% neutrophils, and the platelet count is 20,000/cu mm. A bone marrow biopsy shows extreme hypocellularity. The bone marrow is largely replaced with fat, with a few mature lymphocytes and plasma cells seen. There are only rare recognizable red cell, white cell, and platelet precursors.

2. What is the most likely diagnosis? What would you expect to find on the physical examination and laboratory evaluation?

Since considerable time has passed since she has taken the drug the patient most likely has irreversible, idiosyncratic aplastic anemia secondary to chlorampenicol. On physical examination there would be no adenopathy or hepatosplenomegaly. Petechiae would be present, predominantly on the lower extremities. The reticulocyte count would be low. Iron levels would be high, nearly saturating the total iron-binding capacity because of underutilization of iron. If you were to inject radioactive iron intravenously, you would find that there was slow clearance of the iron from the serum, and only small amounts would subsequently appear in peripheral red blood cells. This would indicate an extremely low level of iron utilization and red cell production.

Because of petechiae on the skin and mucus membranes, and because the platelet count is very low, platelets for transfusion are requested.

3. Should platelets be given to the patient, and if so, what guidelines should be followed?

Though there is evidence of minor cutaneous and mucus membrane bleeding, there is no serious clinical bleeding, and a platelet count of 20,000 or more is unlikely to lead to severe bleeding. Since bone marrow transplantation is a potential treatment and exposure to blood antigens through transfusion decreases the likelihood of success with transplantation, transfusions should be avoided unless absolutely necessary. Even if transplantation is not a consideration (because of age or lack of an appropriate donor), transfusions should be minimized because of the risk of progressive alloimmunization (sensitization to foreign blood antigens) and eventual difficulty with accepting future transfusions. If platelet transfusions are necessary, they should be obtained as "single-donor platelets" rather than "pooled random-donor platelets" in order to decrease the number of foreign platelet antigens to which the patient is exposed.

If the patient requires long-term transfusion support, multiple antibodies will probably be formed. If alloimmunization becomes severe, transfused platelets will be destroyed immediately after transfusion and thus have no beneficial effect, leaving the patient in danger of serious or fatal hemorrhage.

The patient is not given platelet transfusions. The platelet count remains at 20,000/cu mm and no serious bleeding occurs. Red cell transfusions are given until the hematocrit is 25 percent. At this level the patient appears comfortable.

4. What should be your next course of action?

You should perform HLA typing on the patient and any siblings who are available as potential donors for bone marrow transplantation. This should be done early in the course of the patient's disease, so that you know what options are available. If the aplastic anemia remains severe for more than 3 weeks, marrow transplantation should be considered for the immediate future.

While the HLA typing is taking place, the patient arrives at the emergency room with a temperature of 105°F. She is having rigors and gives a history of 1 day of urinary frequency and dysuria.

5. What is your suspected diagnosis and treatment?

By history the patient has probably developed a urinary tract infection. Under normal circumstances this is usually a mild illness easily managed with oral antibiotics. In this case the patient's neutrophil count is only 100/cu mm. A normal count is usually greater than 3,000/cu mm and a count below 500/cu mm is extremely dangerous because of the risk of rapid, overwhelming infection. Because of this consideration the patient is immediately admitted to the hospital. Cultures of urine and blood are performed, as well as a chest x-ray. Before any results have returned, the patient is placed on high doses of broad spectrum intravenous antibiotics. Two days later the cultures return, showing *Escherichia coli* in the urine and blood cultures. Antibiotics appropriate for this organism are selected and are continued for 2 weeks.

Family HLA typing reveals that a 42-year-old brother and the patient have identical HLA antigens. Two younger sisters share only half the HLA antigens of the patient (haplotype matches). The brother is healthy and agrees to be a donor. Five weeks after diagnosis the aplastic anemia is still severe. The patient is requiring red cell transfusions once a week. The white count and platelet count remain low. The patient is admitted to the hospital and bone marrow transplantation is performed.

6. What potential problems are most likely in this circumstance? How might you minimize them?

The patient is 48 years old, comparatively old for a patient undergoing bone marrow transplantation. Though her brother is a "perfect match" for the HLA antigens we can test for, he almost certainly differs from the patient in minor antigens, and in addition is of the opposite sex. The age of the patient and the sex mismatch make GVHD a likely possibility. The risk of GVHD can be reduced by depleting the donor marrow of T cells. This increases the risk of graft failure slightly, but is probably advisable in this circumstance.

The patient will have a 3- to 5-week period when her white blood and platelet counts remain very low. During this time she will be at risk for severe infection, and if fever occurs, broad spectrum antibiotics will be administered promptly. Despite this some patients will die of infection during the early transplant period when they are waiting for the donor bone marrow to produce mature peripheral white blood cells. Hemorrhage is another danger, but can usually be prevented by periodic platelet transfusions.

Pure Red Cell Aplasia

Acquired pure red cell aplasia is a rare disorder, usually immuno-logically mediated, in which there is a specific failure of production of red cells. The patient has a normal white blood cell count and normal platelet count. There is severe anemia and a low reticulocyte count. The bone marrow biopsy shows a selective absence of red blood cell precursors, whereas white cell and platelet precursors are present in normal numbers. This disease is sometimes associated with the presence of a thymoma. Antibodies to erythroid precursor cells in the bone marrow are often demonstrable. Treatment is often, though not always, successful with corticosteroids or cyclophos-phamide.

There is also a congenital form of pure red cell aplasia, the Blackfan-Diamond syndrome. These patients often respond to treat-ment with corticosteroids. Recently, stem cell factor (kit-ligand) has been shown to increase red blood cell production in vitro in some patients with this disease. The etiology of this disorder is not clear.

Anemia of Alcoholism and Liver Disease

Anemia of alcoholism and liver disease is common and often complex (Table 5-2). Multiple etiologies can be present and it is important to identify each one, in order to provide appropriate therapy.

Hemodilution

Patients with liver disease often have an expanded plasma volume, leading to lower hematocrit and hemoglobin values than would be commensurate with the actual degree of anemia.

Table 5-2. Etiologies of anemia of alcoholism and liver disease

I. Hemodilution
II. Macrocytic anemia of liver disease, alcoholism
III. Blood loss
   A. Acute or chronic, due to gastritis, ulcer, or esophageal varices
IV. Iron deficiency
   A. Secondary to chronic blood loss and poor diet
V. Folic acid deficiency
   A. Secondary to poor diet
   B. Secondary to decreased absorption
   C. Secondary to hepatic sequestration of body folic acid stores
IV. Direct bone marrow suppression by alcohol
VII. Decreased red cell life span
   A. Secondary to red cell membrane changes with increased membrane cholesterol
   B. Hypersplenism (which helps to account for the macrocytic anemia of liver disease)

Anemia of Liver Disease

Many patients with liver disease have a mild to moderate anemia with mild macrocytosis; the cause of the latter remains unclear and most of these patients do not have the megaloblastic anemia of folic acid deficiency to which patients with liver disease and alcoholism are also prone (see below). The reticulocyte count is usually moderately elevated and studies with chromium 51 have demonstrated shortening of red cell survival and increased red cell destruction in the spleen. There is also a relative decrease in the erythropoietic response of the bone marrow; otherwise the hemolysis would be better compensated. Mild macrocytosis not associated with megaloblastic changes may also be seen in alcoholics without evidence of liver disease. Sometimes the macrocytosis occurs in the absence of anemia.

Blood Loss and Iron Deficiency

Alcoholics commonly suffer from gastritis, which may lead to chronic slow blood loss. Continued blood loss may result in iron deficiency, a problem that may be exacerbated by the fact that an alcoholic's diet may be poor and lack adequate iron. Severe gastritis, gastric ulceration, or, in the case of cirrhosis and portal hypertension, esophageal varices can also cause brisk hemorrhage with often severe anemia and symptoms of hypovolemia, requiring transfusion therapy.

Folic Acid Deficiency

Alcoholics become folic acid deficient for several reasons. Firstly, they often have poor diets, deficient in green leafy vegetables that are rich in folic acid. In addition the effect of alcohol on the intestinal mucosa probably inhibits absorption of what dietary folic acid they do consume. Equally important is the fact that alcohol inhibits the normal hepatic handling of stored folic acid, making it inaccessible to the bone marrow and other organs. The result is that a patient who is drinking actively will rapidly become folic acid deficient on a diet low in folic acid.

Bone Marrow Suppression by Alcohol

Alcohol is a direct suppressant of bone marrow growth, potentially affecting all cell lines. Thus, purely on the basis of heavy alcohol intake, a patient may become anemic with a low reticulocyte count. The bone marrow may show vacuolated early erythroid precursor and there may be ringed sideroblasts, changes that disappear within a few days after alcohol is discontinued. Young healthy volunteers given large amounts of alcohol and plateletpheresed to reduce their platelet counts are unable to increase their platelet counts because of the suppressive effects of alcohol on platelet production. When the alcohol is stopped, their platelet counts return to normal within a few days. Not surprisingly, therefore, mild thrombocytopenia is common among heavy drinkers.

Liver Disease and Hypersplenism

Patients in whom severe liver disease develops, particularly those with cirrhosis, are subject to two problems that shorten red cell life span. Especially with liver disease with a component of biliary obstruction, there is excess unconjugated cholesterol in the plasma, and the cholesterol-phospholipid balance in the red cell membrane is upset, with increased amounts of membrane cholesterol. This leads to excess plasma membrane, with the development of target cells or spur cells. Spur cells are fragile, abnormally shaped cells that are preferentially destroyed in the spleen.

Another problem in liver disease may be portal hypertension, leading to "hypersplenism," that is, an increase in the number of cells sequestered or destroyed, or both, in the enlarged spleen. Hypersplenism may thus lead to a shortening of the red cell half-life and to a decrease in the platelet and neutrophil counts as well. The patient may remain in a compensated hemolytic state, with an elevated reticulocyte count, but when there is concurrent blood loss, iron deficiency, or folic acid deficiency, the shortened red cell survival may become critical. The patient can no longer compensate and progressive anemia ensues. An element of hypersplenism accounts for the shortened red cell survival that contributes to the macrocytic anemia seen commonly in patients with liver disease.

Anemia of Renal Failure

Patients with significant renal disease almost always have anemia. There is only a rough correlation between the degree of renal failure and the degree of anemia. Patients with relatively mild renal failure (serum creatinine = 3–4 mg%) may have severe anemia, and some patients with more substantial renal failure may be only mildly anemic. Patients who require dialysis are almost always severely anemic and need repeated transfusions.

The primary cause of the anemia is a lack of erythropoietin, a hormone necessary for red cell growth and development in the bone marrow. Erythropoietin is made in the kidney. Recently erythropoietin has been cloned by genetic engineering techniques. Dialysis patients given recombinant erythropoietin have a significant improvement in their hematocrits, proving that erythropoietin lack is the primary cause of the anemia of renal failure.

Patients with renal failure also have inhibitors of erythropoietin in their plasma. These inhibitors are dialyzable, explaining why many patients undergoing chronic dialysis experience some improvement in the degree of their anemia.

In addition, there is a shortening of the red cell life span. This probably results from as yet unspecified "toxins" altering the red cell membrane and making red cells more likely to be destroyed by the reticuloendothelial system. Rare patients with anemia have an overt hemolytic disorder of the oxidant type, although they are not deficient in glucose-6-phosphate dehydrogenase (G-6-PD) or other related enzymes.

Patients with anuric renal failure will often become fluid overloaded between dialyses. This intravascular volume expansion can cause hemodilution and thus an element of "relative anemia."

Anemia of Chronic Disease

In cases of chronic systemic inflammation, infection, or malignancy, the anemia of chronic disease (ACD) will often occur. This is frequently a mild to moderate anemia with hematocrits between 29 and 35%. The anemia is usually normocytic and normochromic with a normal reticulocyte percentage. About 40 percent of the time, the anemia is microcytic and hypochromic, usually only mildly so, but occasionally sufficient to cause confusion with iron deficiency anemia. In ACD the serum iron level is low, but so is the TIBC, in contrast to iron deficiency, in which the serum iron is low but the TIBC is usually elevated. The serum ferritin is normal or often elevated in ACD because it is an acute-phase reactant; it is characteristically low in iron deficiency.

Inspection of the bone marrow usually shows abundant iron in reticuloendothelial cells (mononuclear phagocyte system), but little or no iron in red cell precursors. Thus, the patient has adequate iron stores, but is unable to transfer iron from the reticuloendothelial system (RES) storage cells to the red cell precursors that need it to form hemoglobin. The cause of this block in iron reutilization is uncertain (see Chap. 3), and there is no effective treatment other than to correct the underlying chronic disease. In addition to the block in iron reutilization, the pathophysiology of ACD includes mild shortening of the red cell life span and a relative decrease in erythropoiesis in the bone marrow, the latter due to inappropriately low levels of erythropoietin. Indeed, erythropoietin administration may improve the anemia in patients with ACD.

Myelophthisic Anemias

Neoplasms, granulomatous infections, or a fibrotic process can directly replace the bone marrow. This may lead to a "myelophthisic" blood picture (Plates 58 and 59) in which early white cell precursors as well as nucleated red cells are found in the peripheral blood, as are giant platelet forms or megakaryocyte fragments. Mature red cells often display a teardrop appearance. These findings are not always present, but when they are they should immediately alert the physician to the possibility that a malignant, fibrotic, or granulomatous process is present in the bone marrow. A bone marrow biopsy will be diagnostic (Plates 55–57 and 60).

Infectious diseases that may invade the bone marrow include tuberculosis and other mycobacterial infections (including atypical mycobacterial infections in patients with AIDS). All malignancies can involve the bone marrow. Those that commonly cause a myelophthisic blood picture include breast cancer, prostate cancer, and lung cancer.

Anemias Associated with Endocrine Abnormalities

Hypothyroidism

A mild anemia is commonly associated with hypothyroidism. This is usually normochromic and normocytic but may be macrocytic. The reticulocyte count is low, demonstrating that this is a hypoproliferative anemia, though the actual mechanism is not known. Exogenous thyroid replacement will correct the anemia. In addition there is a strong association between Hashimoto's thyroiditis (which often terminates in hypothyroidism) and pernicious anemia.

Hypopituitarism

A mild normochromic, normocytic anemia is associated with hypopituitarism. The mechanism is unclear. The anemia will respond to replacement of thyroid hormone, corticosteroids, and, in men, androgens. Patients with Addison's disease also have a mild normochromic, normocytic anemia that responds to therapy with corticosteroids.

Selected Readings

Aplastic Anemia

Abdou, N. I., et al. Heterogeneity of pathogenetic mechanisms in aplastic anemia: Efficacy of therapy based on in-vitro results. *Ann. Intern. Med.* 95 : 43, 1981.

Champlin, R., Ho, W., and Gale, R. P. Antithymocyte globulin treatment in patients with aplastic anemia: A prospective randomized trial. *N. Engl. J. Med.* 308 : 113, 1983.

Foon, K. A. et al. Immunologic defects in young male patients with hepatitis-associated aplastic anemia. *Ann. Intern. Med.* 100 : 657, 1984.

Gale, R. P. et al. Aplastic anemia: Biology and treatment. *Ann. Intern. Med.* 95 : 477, 1981.

Kagan, W. A. et al. Studies on the pathogenesis of aplastic anemia. *Am. J. Med.* 66 : 444, 1979.

Lynch, R. E. et al. The prognosis of aplastic anemia. *Blood* 45 : 517, 1975.

Marsh, J. C. W. et al. Survival after antithymocyte globulin therapy for aplastic anemia depends on disease severity. *Blood* 70 : 1046, 1987.

Shadduck, R. K. et al. Aplastic anemia following infectious mononucleosis: Possible immune etiology. *Exp. Hematol.* 7 : 264, 1979.

Storb, R. et al. Marrow transplantation in thirty "untransfused" patients with severe aplastic anemia. *Ann. Intern. Med.* 92 : 30, 1980.

Storb, R. et al. Marrow transplantation with or without donor buffy coat cells for 65 transfused aplastic anemia patients. *Blood* 59 : 236, 1982.

Storb, R. et al. Predictive factors in chronic graft-vs-host disease in patients with aplastic anemia treated by marrow transplantation from HLA-identical siblings. *Ann. Intern. Med.* 98 : 461, 1983.

Thomas, E. D., and Storb, R. Acquired severe aplastic anemia: Progress and perplexity. *Blood* 64 : 325, 1984.

Young, N., and Mortimer, P. Viruses and bone marrow failure. *Blood* 63 : 729, 1984.

Zoumbos, N. C. et al. Circulating activated suppressor T lymphocytes in aplastic anemia. *N. Engl. J. Med.* 312 : 257, 1985.

Pure Red Cell Aplasia

Clark, D. A., Dessypris, E. N., and Krantz, S. B. Studies on pure red cell aplasia. XI. Results of immunosuppressive treatment of 37 patients. *Blood* 63 : 277, 1984.

Krantz, S. B. Pure red-cell aplasia. *N. Engl. J. Med.* 291 : 345, 1974.

Secondary Anemias

Budman, D. R., and Steinberg, A. D. Hematologic aspects of systemic lupus erythematosus: Current concepts. *Ann. Intern. Med.* 86 : 220, 1977.

Cowan, D. H., and Hines, J. D. Thrombocytopenia of severe alcoholism. *Ann. Intern. Med.* 74 : 37, 1971.

Eichner, E. R. The hematologic disorders of alcoholism. *Am. J. Med.* 54 : 621, 1973.

Mowat, A. G. Hematologic abnormalities in rheumatoid arthritis. *Semin. Arthritis Rheum.* 1 : 195, 1971.

Straus, D. J. Hematologic aspects of alcoholism. *Semin. Hematol.* 10 : 183, 1973.

Sullivan, L. W., Adams, W. H., and Liu, Y. K. Induction of thrombocytopenia by thrombopheresis in man: Patterns of recovery in normal subjects during ethanol ingestion and abstinence. *Blood* 49 : 197, 1977.

6 Introduction to the Hemolytic Anemias: Heme Catabolism

Stephen H. Robinson

Hemolytic anemia results from an increased rate of destruction of circulating red blood cells. Normally, red cells have an average life span of 120 days and then undergo rapid clearance from the bloodstream and destruction by cells of the mononuclear-phagocyte system. In hemolytic disorders, red cells are destroyed prematurely, usually in a random fashion. If the red blood cell life span is only moderately shortened, the patient will usually have little, if any, anemia because the bone marrow is capable of increasing the rate of new red blood cell production by a factor of 4 to 8. This is known as compensated hemolysis. Since there is little, if any, anemia, it is not clear whether the compensatory erythroid hyperplasia of the bone marrow in these cases is due to increased levels of erythropoietin, which is stimulated by tissue hypoxia; it is possible that, instead, products of increased red cell destruction such as erythrocyte stroma or heme directly account for the augmentation of erythropoiesis. If, in contrast, the red blood cell life span is markedly shortened, the patient will have significant anemia.

In order to understand the clinical and laboratory manifestations of hemolysis, a review of the catabolism of hemoglobin and heme is in order.

Hemoglobin Catabolism

The reasons that red blood cells normally die at about 120 days of age are not well understood. As red cells age their content of glycolytic enzymes, adenosine triphosphate (ATP), and membrane lipids and proteins diminishes, but it is not clear that these changes are critical in limiting the red cell life span. There is evidence that red cell senescence is mediated by naturally occurring autoantibodies to antigenic determinants that develop in the plasma membranes of aging erythrocytes. Decreasing cellular deformability related to changes in membrane and cytoplasmic viscosity apparently also plays a role.

When effete red cells are taken up by cells of the mononuclear-phagocyte system (Fig. 6-1), the globin moiety of hemoglobin is

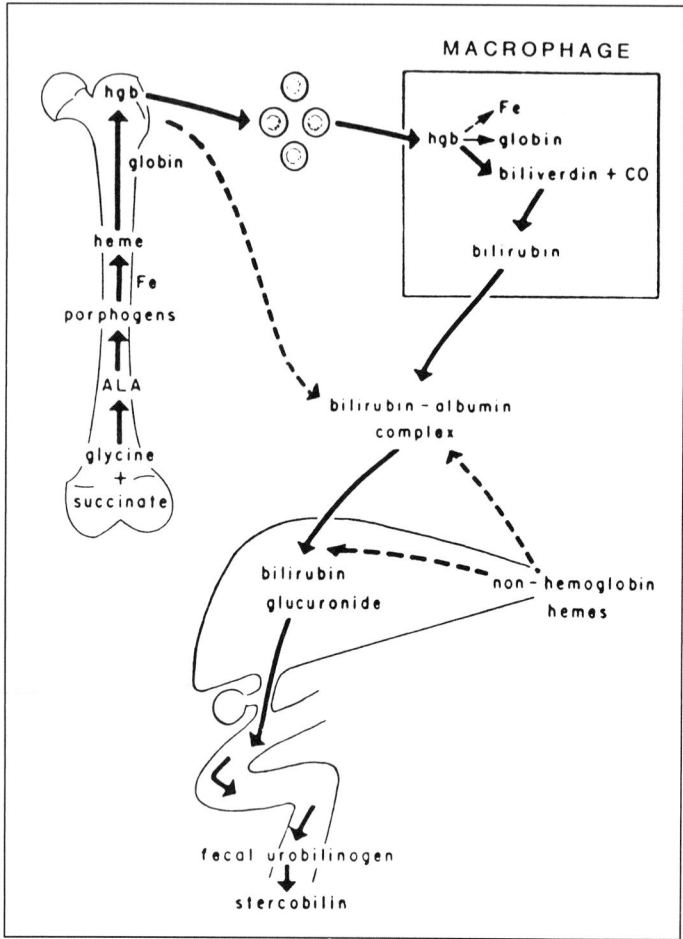

Fig. 6-1. Schematic summary of heme degradation and bilirubin metabolism. The solid arrows show the major metabolic pathway. The dashed arrows indicate the two minor pathways of bilirubin production related to erythropoiesis and turnover of nonhemoglobin hemes. Bilirubin derived from nonhemoglobin sources in the liver may be excreted directly into the bile or may first enter the plasma. ALA, δ-aminolevulinic acid; porphogens, porphobilinogen and the porphyrinogens. (Adapted from S. H. Robinson, Heme Metabolism and the Porphyrias. In W. S. Beck (ed.), *Hematology* (4th ed.), Harvard Pathophysiology Series. Cambridge, MA: MIT Press, 1985. pp. 125–134.)

hydrolyzed to its constituent amino acids, which mix with the general amino acid pool. The iron liberated from heme is efficiently reutilized for new hemoglobin synthesis; iron is taken up from the phagocytic cell by transferrin and transported to developing erythroid cells in the bone marrow, where new heme synthesis is taking place. Some iron remains in the phagocytic cell in a storage form. The heme moiety of hemoglobin is degraded to the bile pigment biliverdin and carbon monoxide, and the biliverdin is then rapidly reduced to bilirubin, which is excreted by the liver into the bile. There are two additional sources of bilirubin and carbon monoxide production. One is related to red cell development in the bone marrow and is markedly increased in disorders associated with ineffective erythropoiesis, that is, the destruction of immature red cell precursors in the bone marrow. The other is related to the turnover of nonhemoglobin hemes, primarily in hepatic cells.

Increased rates of hemoglobin degradation take place with hemolytic anemia, ineffective erythropoiesis, and the resorption of large hematomas. An increase in the production of unconjugated bilirubin may be found under all of these conditions. In addition, as evidenced by depletion of plasma haptoglobin, in all of these situations there is some apparent leakage of hemoglobin into the plasma, a phenomenon that is exaggerated in so-called intravascular hemolysis, when red blood cells are destroyed in the free circulation. Indeed, it has been estimated that 10 to 20 percent of normal red cell senescence involves the release of hemoglobin into the plasma. Thus, when evaluating either normal or accelerated red blood cell destruction, one must understand the metabolic disposition of plasma hemoglobin as well as the production and excretion of bilirubin.

Metabolism of Hemoglobin and Heme in the Plasma (Fig. 6-2)

Hemoglobin in the plasma is bound to the plasma protein haptoglobin. The haptoglobin–hemoglobin complex is carried to the liver, where hepatic cells convert the heme of hemoglobin to bilirubin. If the rate of hemoglobin entry into the plasma is significant, haptoglobin is depleted, and serum haptoglobin levels are typically low in hemolytic anemia because the liver fails to compensate with an increase in haptoglobin synthesis. It should be kept in mind, however, that haptoglobin is also an acute-phase reactant, levels of which rise in various conditions. Thus, the serum haptoglobin concentration may be normal or even increased in patients who have both hemolytic anemia and a coexisting inflammatory, infectious, or neoplastic illness.

The concentration of haptoglobin in plasma is often determined in terms of its hemoglobin-binding capacity, although it may also be measured immunologically. The normal range is 50 to 200 mg/dL. Haptoglobin is composed of both α and β polypeptide chains. Genetic variations in the α-chain account for polymorphisms. Some individuals have haptoglobin isotypes that have a low binding affinity for hemoglobin. Determination of the plasma haptoglobin concentration based on its hemoglobin-binding capacity will give rise to falsely low values in such patients. Moreover, some patients,

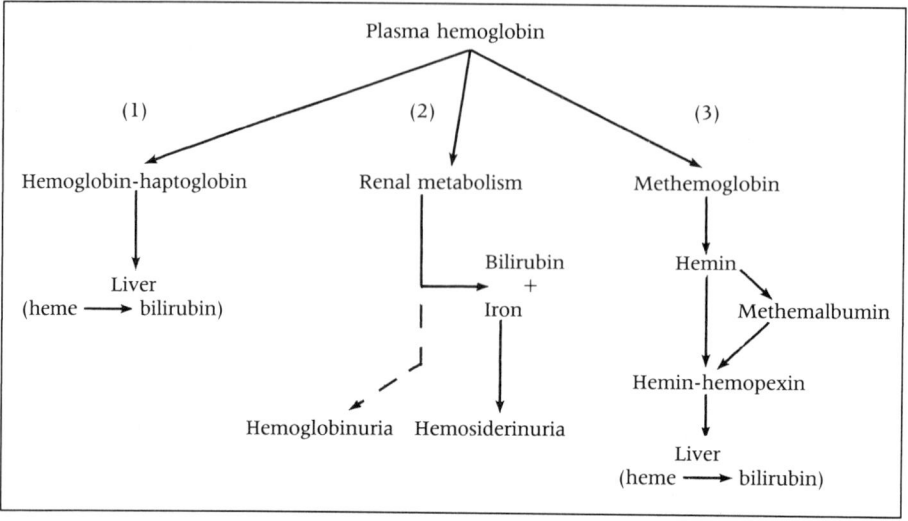

Fig. 6-2. Metabolic disposition of hemoglobin in the plasma. Pathway (1) shows hemoglobin clearance by the liver in the presence of haptoglobin. Pathways (2) and (3) show the fate of plasma hemoglobin after haptoglobin has been depleted. Hemoglobinuria occurs only if the T_{max} for tubular resorption of hemoglobin is exceeded. Hemosiderinuria occurs even in the absence of hemoglobinuria since it is due to heme degradation in renal tubule cells.

particularly blacks, have congenital absence of haptoglobin. These facts should be kept in mind when one interprets laboratory results that indicate a low level of this protein in the plasma. Patients with liver disease may also have low haptoglobin levels, and it is arguable whether this is due to decreased synthesis of this protein by the diseased liver or the hemolysis that is commonly associated with liver disease.

The large size of the haptoglobin–hemoglobin complex prevents its filtration across the glomerulus. When plasma haptoglobin is depleted, unbound hemoglobin readily passes into the glomerular filtrate in the form of $\alpha\beta$-globin chain dimers. These are reabsorbed by proximal tubule cells, but when a T_{max} of about 1.4 mg per minute is reached, hemoglobin is excreted into the urine. Whether or not there is hemoglobinuria, the presence of hemoglobin in the plasma and thus in the glomerular filtrate is manifested by the presence of hemosiderin in the urine. Hemoglobin that has been reabsorbed by renal tubule cells is degraded to bilirubin, with the liberation of iron, some of which enters the plasma but much of which remains in these cells in storage proteins such as ferritin and hemosiderin. When the tubule cells are eventually sloughed into the urine, the presence of hemosiderin can be detected by staining the urine sediment with Prussian blue. This is an easy and inexpensive means of detecting recent intravascular hemolysis.

With depletion of haptoglobin, not only is free hemoglobin in the plasma excreted by the kidney, but some is oxidized to methemoglobin. The oxidized heme moiety (hemin) in methemoglobin is readily dissociated from globin and is bound to hemopexin, another plasma protein synthesized in the liver, the function of which is to bind hemin and convey it to the liver for conversion to bilirubin. Hemopexin is a glycoprotein of the β-globulin class, which binds hemin but not hemoglobin in a 1 : 1 molar ratio. As with haptoglobin, hemopexin is usually depleted in patients with hemolysis. When hemopexin is depleted, free hemin is associated with albumin, also in a 1 : 1 molar ratio, to form methemalbumin. The presence of methemalbumin and hemopexin-hemin imparts a brownish color to the plasma. Clearance of methemalbumin from plasma is slow and appears to involve the transfer of hemin from albumin to newly synthesized hemopexin, by which the hemin is transported to the liver for conversion to bilirubin.

Conversion of Heme to Bilirubin (Figs. 6-1 through 6-3)

The enzymes necessary for converting heme to bilirubin are present in cells of the mononuclear-phagocytic system in the spleen, marrow, and liver, and in parenchymal cells in the liver and kidney. An enzyme system in the microsomal fraction of these cells, known as heme oxygenase, mediates cleavage of the heme ring, with the liberation of biliverdin and carbon monoxide. The biliverdin is rapidly converted to bilirubin by a second enzyme, biliverdin reductase, that is present in the soluble fraction of these same cells. The nature of this enzyme reaction is such that only bilirubin but no biliverdin is detectable in the plasma, even when there is a marked increase in the rate of red blood cell destruction. Cleavage of the heme ring with oxidation of its α-carbon bridge also gives rise to carbon monoxide and represents the only metabolic source of carbon monoxide production in mammals. Carbon monoxide is carried in the blood as carboxyhemoglobin and is then excreted by the lungs.

The major source of bilirubin (and carbon monoxide) formation is destruction of circulating red blood cells at the end of their life span. However, at least two minor sources of bilirubin production have been discerned by studies of radioactive bilirubin or carbon monoxide production. Thus, after administration of glycine-^{14}C or -^{15}N, which is incorporated into the heme molecule at the time of its synthesis, the bulk of radioactive bilirubin is formed between 90 and 150 days later, the time of maximal destruction of senescent red blood cells bearing the radioactively labeled heme molecule (Figs. 6-4 and 6-5). In addition, there is an early-labeled peak of bilirubin formation that is observed within a few hours after labeled glycine administration and lasts for a few days. This early-labeled peak has been demonstrated to originate from two general sources:

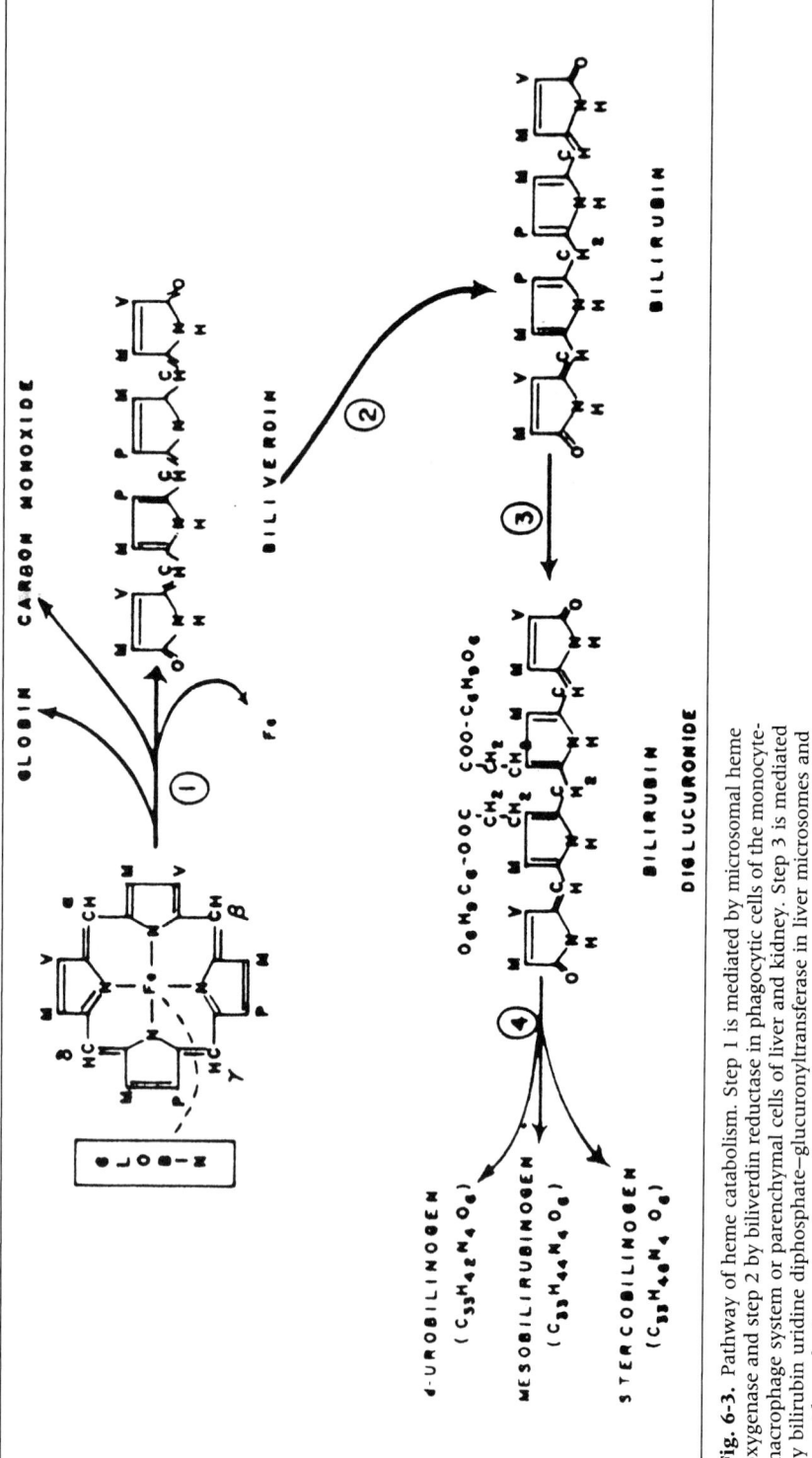

Fig. 6-3. Pathway of heme catabolism. Step 1 is mediated by microsomal heme oxygenase and step 2 by biliverdin reductase in phagocytic cells of the monocyte-macrophage system or parenchymal cells of liver and kidney. Step 3 is mediated by bilirubin uridine diphosphate–glucuronyltransferase in liver microsomes and step 4 by reducing enzymes in intestinal bacteria, leading to the formation of these three major types of "urobilinogen." Side chains on the pyrrole rings are M, methyl; P, propionyl; and V, vinyl. (From S. H. Robinson, Degradation of hemoglobin. In W. J. Williams et al. (eds.), *Hematology* (4th ed.). New York: McGraw-Hill, 1990. pp. 407–414. Reproduced with permission of McGraw-Hill.)

Fig. 6-4. Labeling of blood hemoglobin heme and fecal bile pigment (stercobilin) in a human subject given glycine-^{15}N. (From I. M. London et al., On the origin of bile pigment in normal man. *J. Biol. Chem.* 184 : 351, 1950. Reproduced with permission.)

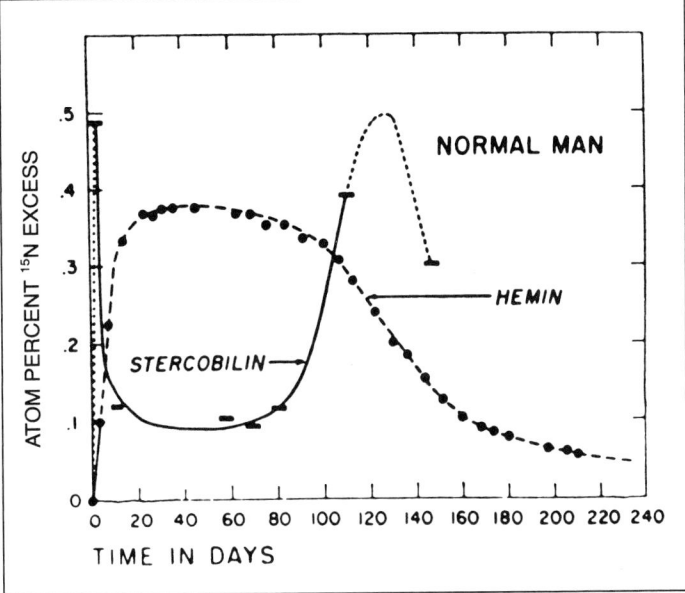

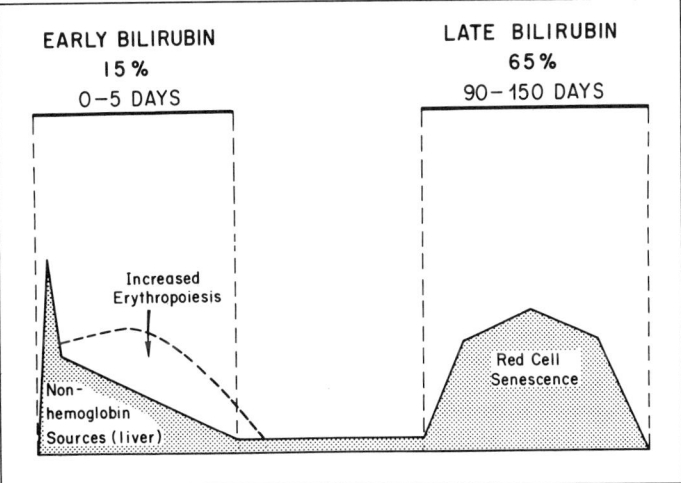

Fig. 6-5. Sources of bilirubin production in humans based on studies with glycine-2-^{14}C. Measurements of bilirubin in plasma and bile have made it possible to measure the kinetics of labeled bilirubin formation more precisely than with studies of bile pigment in the feces. Note that there is some continuing bilirubin production from unknown sources between the early and late peaks. (Adapted from S. H. Robinson et al., Ineffective Erythropoiesis and the Erythropoietic Component of Early-Labeled Bilirubin. In F. Stolhman, Jr. (ed.), *Hemopoietic Cellular Proliferation.* New York: Grune & Stratton, 1970. pp. 180–188.)

the turnover of nonhemoglobin hemes, primarily in the liver, and processes related to the production of red blood cells in the bone marrow. The latter component, which has been referred to as the erythropoietic fraction of bilirubin formation, is probably of diverse origin. It may include a contribution from some hemoglobin that accompanies the nucleus of the immature red blood cell when it is extruded from the cell and probably an element of ineffective erythropoiesis that occurs under normal conditions. This erythropoietic component becomes markedly enlarged and may account for the major fraction of total bilirubin production in patients with hematologic disorders associated with marked ineffective erythropoiesis, such as megaloblastic anemia or thalassemia.

Bilirubin in the plasma is bound to albumin. This pigment is excreted by the liver, a process that is conventionally considered as occurring in three phases: hepatic uptake, conjugation, and secretion. Bilirubin uptake by the liver represents a carrier-mediated transport process involving specific receptors on the liver cell membrane. A significant fraction of the unconjugated bilirubin taken up by the liver cell refluxes back into the plasma, and it is probably this bidirectional flux that accounts for the elevated plasma concentration of unconjugated bilirubin found in hemolytic disorders. Otherwise, the large excretory capacity of the liver would absorb virtually any increment in bilirubin production. A protein known as ligandin, which is identical to the enzyme glutathione S transferase, binds and stores unconjugated bilirubin in the cytosol of the liver cell. Ligandin appears to retard bilirubin efflux back into the plasma, thus helping to regulate the net hepatic uptake of this pigment.

In the second step of hepatic bilirubin excretion, each unconjugated bilirubin molecule is conjugated with either one or two glucuronic acid moieties by an enzyme, bilirubin uridine diphosphate (UDP)-glucuronyltransferase, which is located in the endoplasmic reticulum of the liver cell. The propionic acid side chains of bilirubin are esterified with glucuronic acid, and the nonpolar bilirubin molecule is converted to a polar, hydrophilic molecule, which can be excreted into the bile and then retained within the mucosal barrier of the biliary and intestinal excretory pathways. In the third phase of hepatic bilirubin excretion, conjugated bilirubin is secreted across the canalicular membrane into the bile. This is an energy-dependent process by which large concentration gradients are maintained across the liver cell membrane.

After being excreted into the bile, conjugated bilirubin passes through the intestinal tract and, in the large intestine, is converted to a family of compounds, which collectively are called urobilinogen (see Figs. 6-1 and 6-3). The urobilinogen molecules are derived from bilirubin by a series of reductive steps mediated by the bacteria of the large intestine. These substances are largely excreted in the feces, where they undergo oxidative reactions, leading to the formation of a family of corresponding colored compounds known as urobilin or stercobilin. However, a small fraction of the total urobilinogen in the colon is reabsorbed. It enters the portal circulation, is carried to the liver, and, under normal conditions, is efficiently extracted by the liver and excreted into the bile, thus completing an enterohepatic circulation. A small amount of urobilinogen escapes excretion by the liver, passes into the systemic circulation, and is eliminated in the urine. Measurements of fecal or urinary urobilinogen are sometimes used to estimate the total amount of bile pigment production and, hence, the rate of heme catabolism in states of presumed hemolysis or ineffective erythropoiesis. However, these measurements are cumbersome, unpleasant, and subject to numerous inaccuracies, and thus are currently rarely used.

An increase in the serum level of unconjugated bilirubin may be the result of increased bilirubin production from any of the three major sources described above (see Fig. 6-5), that is, an increased rate of destruction of mature erythrocytes; an increased rate of turnover of tissue hemes, notably in the liver (this is not well established as a cause of clinical jaundice); or an increase in erythropoietic bilirubin production as the result of ineffective erythropoiesis. Bilirubin overproduction may sometimes be associated with resorption of large hematomas. In addition, unconjugated hyperbilirubinemia may result from a defect in the uptake or conjugation mechanisms in the liver. Disorders such as Gilbert's syndrome and the two forms of the Crigler-Najjar syndrome are examples of congenital problems in bilirubin uptake or conjugation, or both. Impairment of secretion of conjugated bilirubin into the bile canaliculi or obstruction of the biliary tree leads to "regurgitation" of conjugated bilirubin into the plasma. In contrast to unconjugated bilirubin, a fraction of conjugated bilirubin is only loosely bound to albumin and this fraction gains entry to the urine. Thus, bilirubin in the urine is a reflection of an increase of the conjugated fraction of this pigment in the plasma and signifies an excretory defect in the liver or in the biliary tract. Bilirubin does not appear in the urine with an increase in the plasma level of unconjugated bilirubin, as observed with bilirubin overproduction or congenital defects in the hepatic uptake or conjugation of bilirubin.

Hemolytic Anemias

Extravascular Versus Intravascular Hemolysis

There are two general sites in which hemolysis may take place (Table 6-1). In intravascular hemolysis, which is uncommon, red blood cells are destroyed directly within the circulatory system,

Table 6-1. Hemolytic anemia

Site of hemolysis		
Extravascular	vs.	Intravascular
Mechanism of hemolysis		
Extracorpuscular	vs.	Intracorpuscular
Extrinsic to RBC		Intrinsic to RBC
Usually acquired		Usually inherited
Morphologic stigmata may or may not be present on blood smear		Morphologic stigmata usually present on smear

Source: Tables 6-1 through 6-4 adapted from S. H. Robinson, Anemia. In E. Braunwald and C. Fanta (eds.), *Intensive Review of Internal Medicine* (3rd ed.). Boston: Brigham and Women's and Beth Israel Hospitals and Nimrod Press, 1988. pp. 46–57.

usually as the result of one of two mechanisms: the lytic action of complement on the red cell membrane or the fragmentation of erythrocytes on abnormal vascular surfaces. Either of these mechanisms leads to rupture of the red cell during its sojourn in the free circulation, with release of hemoglobin into the blood (see Fig. 6-2) and hence into the glomerular filtrate. This may or may not lead to hemoglobinuria, depending on the amount of hemoglobin entering the tubular urine, but it almost invariably leads to hemosiderinuria as the result of the resorption of hemoglobin by proximal tubule cells, which are later sloughed from the kidney. Methemalbuminemia may occur, as well as the usual increase in the plasma level of unconjugated bilirubin.

Extravascular hemolysis is more common than intravascular hemolysis and involves the destruction of red blood cells within mononuclear-phagocytic cells, often in the spleen. Because these cells contain the enzymes, heme oxygenase and biliverdin reductase, that efficiently convert heme to bilirubin, the primary biochemical indicator of hemolysis here is an increase in the serum level of unconjugated bilirubin. However, there must be some leakage of hemoglobin out of the mononuclear-phagocytic cells since haptoglobin is usually depleted in extravascular as well as intravascular hemolysis. Moreover, when the hemolytic rate is very high in extravascular hemolysis, there may be overt hemoglobinemia, hemoglobinuria, and hemosiderinuria, as observed in cases of intravascular hemolysis.

Intracorpuscular Versus Extracorpuscular Defects

In addition to providing a framework for understanding the nature of different forms of hemolysis, the distinction between intracorpuscular and extracorpuscular defects is often used for classifying the many causes of hemolytic anemia (Tables 6-1 through 6-3). Intracorpuscular defects are intrinsic to the red blood cell. They are

Table 6-2. Intracorpuscular hemolytic anemias

Membrane defects
Congenital spherocytosis
Congenital elliptocytosis
Paroxysmal nocturnal hemoglobinuria[a,b]
Metabolic defects
Pentose shunt defects (G-6-PD, GSH, GSH reductase, GSH peroxidase
    deficiency)
Embden-Meyerhof pathway defects (pyruvate kinase, triose phosphate
    isomerase, hexokinase deficiency, etc.)
Hemoglobin defects
Hemoglobinopathies (S, C, unstable hemoglobins, etc.)

---

[a]Acquired defect.
[b]Typically intravascular hemolysis.
G-6-PD = glucose-6-phosphate dehydrogenase; GSH = glutathione.

Table 6-3. Extracorpuscular hemolytic anemias

Immune disorders
ABO incompatibility (transfusion reactions)*
Rh incompatibility (erythroblastosis fetalis)
Autoimmune or immunohemolytic anemias
    Warm   vs.   cold   antibodies
    IgG   vs.   complement Coombs' test
    Paroxysmal cold hemoglobinuria* (Donath-Landsteiner antibody)
Physical damage
Micro- or macroangiopathic hemolytic anemias* (prosthetic valves, DIC, TTP,
    march hemoglobinuria, carcinomatosis, malignant hypertension, etc.)
Burns*
Chemicals, toxins, drugs
H_2O,* *Clostridium welchii* toxin,* spur cell anemia (altered membrane lipids),
    oxidant drugs* (with or without G-6-PD deficiency), drugs causing
    immunohemolytic anemia
Increased activity of reticuloendothelial system
Hypersplenism
Infections (effect usually indirect)
Malaria (hypersplenism, direct lysis*)
Infectious mononucleosis (hypersplenism, autoimmune—often cold type)
Mycoplasma pneumonia (cold hemolytic anemia)
Cl. welchii (hemolytic toxin*)

---

*Typically intravascular hemolysis.
DIC = disseminated intravascular coagulation; TTP = thrombotic thrombocytopenic
purpura; G-6-PD = glucose-6-phosphate dehydrogenase.

usually inherited, and generally (but not always) the abnormality is
observable in the peripheral blood smear, for example, in the form
of spherocytes, elliptocytes, or sickle cells. Intracorpuscular defects
may reside in the red blood cell membrane, its metabolic pathways,
or the nature of the hemoglobin molecule (see Table 6-2). The
exception in this table is paroxysmal nocturnal hemoglobinuria
(PNH), in which the intracorpuscular membrane defect is acquired
rather than inherited. In addition, PNH is usually associated with
intravascular hemolysis because of completion of the complement

sequence on the membrane of the red blood cell, whereas most other intracorpuscular defects are associated with extravascular hemolysis.

Extracorpuscular defects refer to problems in the environment of the red blood cell, not in the red blood cell itself. Examples are autoantibodies to the red blood cell or abnormally functioning prosthetic heart valves leading to fragmentation hemolysis. Extracorpuscular hemolysis is usually acquired and is often but not always discernible in the form of morphologic abnormalities in the peripheral blood smear. As demonstrated in Table 6-3, the extracorpuscular defects are typically classified as due to: (1) immunologic mechanisms; (2) physical damage, with fragmentation of red blood cells; (3) chemicals, toxins, or drugs, a category in which the mechanism is often somewhat indirect [e.g., certain drugs may precipitate hemolysis in patients with glucose-6-phosphate dehydrogenase (G-6-PD) deficiency and other drugs may produce different forms of immunohemolytic anemia]; (4) increased activity of the reticuloendothelial mononuclear-phagocyte system, especially hypersplenism; or (5) hemolysis related to infections, once again often in an indirect manner (see Table 6-3).

These different types of hemolysis are described in greater detail in the following chapters on inherited and acquired forms of hemolytic anemia.

Laboratory Diagnosis of Hemolytic Anemia

The major criteria for the laboratory diagnosis of hemolytic anemia are reticulocytosis and an increase in the serum level of unconjugated bilirubin (Table 6-4). In addition, the serum level of lactic dehydrogenase (LDH) is typically elevated and the serum haptoglobin level decreased. The peripheral blood smear often but not

Table 6-4. Diagnosis of hemolytic anemia

↑ Heme pigments (see below)*
↑ LDH
↓ Haptoglobin
↑ Reticulocytes
↓ Red cell survival by isotopic measurement
Specific morphologic changes of RBCs on smear (not invariable)
Tests for specific types of hemolytic anemia (G-6-PD assay, Coombs' test, etc.)

*Extravascular	*Intravascular or severe extravascular
↑ Unconjugated bilirubin	↑ Unconjugated bilirubin
	Hemoglobinemia
	Hemoglobinuria
	Hemosiderinuria
	Methemalbuminemia

invariably shows morphologic changes in the red blood cells compatible with hemolysis. Moreover, the morphologic abnormality may implicate a specific type of hemolysis. For example, fragmented red cells suggest fragmentation hemolysis, many spherocytes suggest hereditary spherocytosis or immunohemolytic anemia, and sickle cells suggest one of the sickle cell syndromes. The specific type of hemolysis is determined from the patient's history; the nature of the morphologic red cell abnormalities, if any; whether there is evidence of intravascular hemolysis; and, finally, tests for the specific types of hemolysis that are under suspicion, for example, a Coombs' test, G-6-PD assay, osmotic fragility determination, or sucrose hemolysis test.

Many of these laboratory indications of hemolysis may be absent or equivocal. Thus, a patient with hemolytic anemia who also has erythroid suppression of the bone marrow, for example, because of an intercurrent viral illness, may not have reticulocytosis. The serum level of unconjugated bilirubin may not be significantly elevated if the hemolysis is of mild to moderate degree, in view of the large excretory capacity of the liver for bilirubin. The serum haptoglobin level may not be depressed if the hemolysis occurs in the context of an infectious, inflammatory, or neoplastic illness. The serum LDH is a sensitive but not a very specific finding in patients with hemolytic anemia. Finally, red cell morphology may be normal or only minimally abnormal in some forms of hemolysis, for example, PNH and many cases of G-6-PD deficiency.

With intravascular hemolysis, as outlined previously, there are additional findings: hemoglobin in the plasma, imparting a pink color to the plasma; methemoglobinemia, imparting a brownish color to the plasma; hemoglobin in the urine if the T_{max} is exceeded; and hemosiderinuria.

It may be necessary to ascertain whether red urine is due to hemoglobinuria or myoglobinuria, the former a manifestation of intravascular hemolysis and the latter of rhabdomyolysis. Myoglobin is a smaller hemoprotein than hemoglobin and is not bound to haptoglobin in the plasma. Thus, it is readily excreted in the urine. A patient with red urine due to myoglobinuria will have plasma devoid of this red pigment and the serum level of haptoglobin will be normal. In contrast, a patient with hemoglobinuria will have hemoglobin in the plasma and depletion of serum haptoglobin. In addition, if necessary, hemoglobin can be differentiated from myoglobin in the urine by electrophoretic analysis.

Rarely, if it remains difficult to ascertain that a patient's anemia is hemolytic in nature, one can directly measure the rate of red cell destruction using radioactive markers. Most commonly, this is done with chromium 51 (Fig. 6-6). The patient's red cells are incubated with ^{51}Cr, the excess radioisotope washed away, and the labeled

Fig. 6-6. Red blood cell life span determined with ^{51}Cr. The half-time (T$^{1}/_{2}$) of disappearance of ^{51}Cr-labeled red cells from the bloodstream in normal subjects is 25 to 32 days. In contrast, the T$^{1}/_{2}$ shown for a patient with hemolytic anemia is 8 days.

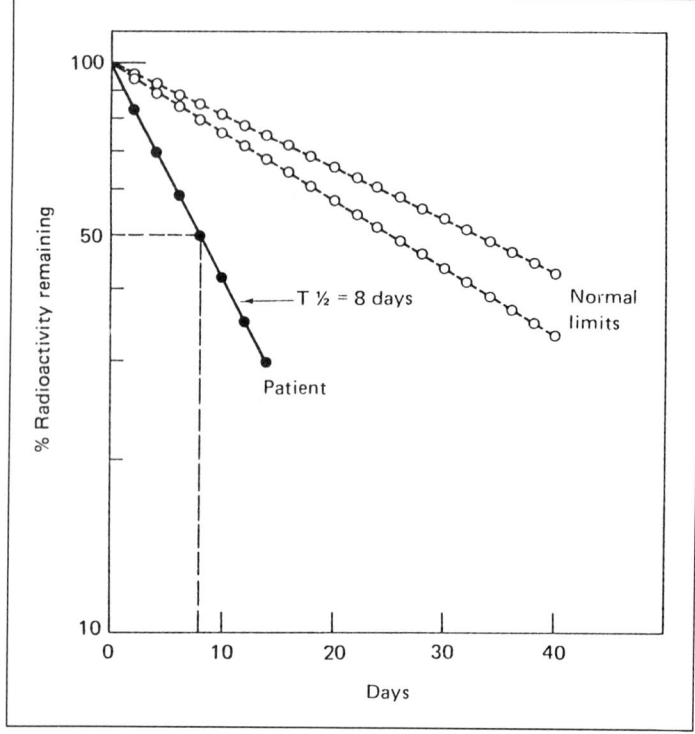

cells injected into the patient. The ^{51}Cr is attached to the β-chain of globin. Serial measurements are made of the ^{51}Cr labeling of the red blood cells. The decrease in labeling with time is due to two phenomena: the rate of red cell destruction and the progressive elution of ^{51}Cr from the remaining red blood cells in the circulation. In patients with normal red blood cell survival, the time for disappearance of half of the original radioactivity from the circulation is 25 to 32 days, and a half-life shorter than this implicates hemolysis. One has to ensure that the patient remains in a steady state during the entire ^{51}Cr red cell survival study since a decrease in the rate of red blood cell production or an increase in the rate of red cell destruction makes analysis difficult. It is sometimes useful to monitor the accumulation of radioactivity over the liver and spleen during a ^{51}Cr red blood cell survival study. Although such analysis is imperfect, a marked increase in splenic as compared to hepatic uptake of ^{51}Cr in a patient with hemolysis can be used as evidence favoring splenectomy as a form of therapy for the hemolytic anemia.

Other radioactive labels can be used in the measurement of red blood cell survival, including ^{59}Fe or glycine-^{14}C or -^{15}N. Unlike ^{51}Cr, which randomly labels red blood cells of all ages, both ^{59}Fe and labeled glycine are so-called cohort labels. They are incorporated into newly synthesized hemoglobin in developing erythroid cells, which then emerge from the bone marrow as reticulocytes and survive as a cohort until the time of red cell senescence (see the hemin curve in Fig. 6-4). Monitoring uptake of radioactivity over the liver, spleen, and bone marrow immediately after administration of ^{59}Fe can also provide information regarding whether extramedullary erythropoiesis is present, whereas monitoring over these organs several days later can provide information about the sites of destruction of mature erythrocytes.

Skeletal Changes

Patients with severe congenital hemolytic anemia or thalassemia often demonstrate changes in bone x-rays because of expansion of the marrow cavity as a result of severe erythroid hyperplasia. This expansion takes place when the patient is very young and the bones are soft and subject to remodeling. In the skull the space between the bony tables is broadened, the intramedullary cavity appears less dense, and the tables may be thinned. Bony trabeculae may develop at right angles to the tables, giving rise to a so-called hair-on-end appearance. The long bones, ribs, vertebrae, and bones of the fingers may also demonstrate widening of the medullary cavity and thinning of the bony cortex. Bone sclerosis as a result of bone infarction may be found in patients with sickle cell anemia. In some children with severe congenital hemolytic anemia or thalassemia, some of these skeletal changes may be demonstrable on physical as well as radiologic examination. These patients may have "chipmunk facies" due to marrow hyperplasia of the facial bones, and elongation of the skull, giving rise to a so-called tower skull.

Approach to the Patient with Hemolytic Anemia

The patient's past history and family history are important in order to determine whether the anemia is inherited or acquired. It is worth asking whether the patient or his or her family members have a history of anemia, jaundice, early development of gallstones, or splenomegaly. A drug history is always of importance in view of the fact that many drugs can incite different forms of hemolysis, for example, in provoking oxidant hemolysis in the presence (or sometimes in the absence) of G-6-PD deficiency and in producing a variety of forms of immunohemolytic anemia. On physical examination the physician should give particular attention to evidence of jaundice and splenomegaly, although neither of these findings is highly specific for hemolytic anemia. The laboratory approach to documenting the presence of hemolytic anemia and then ascertaining the nature of the hemolysis has already been outlined. On the basis of the patient's history, laboratory manifestations, morphologic abnormalities in the peripheral blood smear, presence or absence of intravascular as compared to the more common extravascular form of hemolysis, and tests for specific types of hemolysis, it should be possible to arrive at a precise diagnosis in most patients. The classification of hemolytic anemia provided in Tables 6-2 and 6-3 should serve as a guide in this evaluation. These different forms of hemolysis are discussed more fully in the subsequent chapters on this subject.

Case Development Problems

1. An anemic patient has the following laboratory findings: hematocrit, 21 percent; reticulocyte count, 0.8 percent; serum bilirubin, 2.5 mg/dL (elevated), mostly unconjugated; serum LDH, 400 IU (normal, up to 200); and serum haptoglobin, 40 mg/dL (depressed). Provide two possible explanations for these findings.

The elevated serum levels of unconjugated bilirubin and LDH and the decrease in haptoglobin implicate an increased rate of destruction of hemoglobin-bearing cells, that is, erythroid cells. This could be the result of hemolytic anemia or ineffective erythropoiesis (the premature destruction of erythroid precursor cells in the bone marrow or soon after release into the circulation as reticulocytes). The low reticulocyte count suggests ineffective erythropoiesis. On the other hand, it is possible that the patient has a hemolytic anemia but the erythroid response of his or her bone marrow is temporarily suppressed, perhaps by a viral illness. An alternative explanation is that the patient has sustained an internal hemorrhage that is producing the anemia, and that the findings compatible with an increased rate of heme degradation are related to the resorption of a large hematoma. However, this should have produced a reticulocytosis. How would one distinguish among these possibilities?

Clearly, a large hematoma should be implicated on the basis of the patient's history and physical examination; one might have expected that the patient would have a history of physical trauma or might be anticoagulated in order to sustain a hematoma of sufficient size to cause these chemical abnormalities. The distinction between hemolytic anemia with erythroid suppression of the marrow and ineffective erythropoiesis could be made by marrow examination. In effective erythropoiesis one would find erythroid hyperplasia in the bone marrow, but at least relative reticulocytopenia in the peripheral blood. If the marrow were turned off by viral infection, drug effect, or other cause, the marrow should show a decrease in erythroid activity, although this might be only transient. In addition, the peripheral blood smear might demonstrate morphologic changes, such as spherocytes, sickle cells, or the like, that would implicate a preexisting hemolytic anemia.

2. A patient is sent to see you because of anemia, with hematocrit 25 percent, and is found to have a reticulocyte count of 9 percent. The chemistry laboratory has lost the other tubes of blood so that other laboratory values are unavailable. The physical examination is relatively unremarkable and the patient's stools are negative for occult blood. He returns the following week for a repeat appointment and his hematocrit and reticulocyte count are found to be roughly the same. What is the likely cause of the patient's anemia?

A persistent reticulocytosis without a rise in the hematocrit represents the response to increased red cell loss on a chronic, ongoing basis. The loss might be due to either hemorrhage or hemolysis. In the absence of evidence of gastrointestinal blood loss, the patient in all likelihood has a hemolytic anemia. If the reticulocytosis were due to response of the anemia to specific therapy, for example, folic acid or iron, or to the withdrawal of a marrow-suppressive agent (e.g., alcohol), the hematocrit should have increased from the time of the first to that of the second visit. In essence, the persistent elevation of the reticulocyte count in the presence of persistent anemia signifies a steady state of increased red cell turnover; an increase in the production rate without an increase in the hematocrit must be the result of an equivalent chronic increased loss of red blood cells from the circulation.

Topics for Discussion

Genetics and biochemistry of haptoglobin

Sources of bilirubin production, including the erythropoietic component of the early-labeled fraction

Causes of unconjugated hyperbilirubinemia

The mechanism of the erythroid hyperplasia that accompanies compensated hemolysis, that is, in the absence of anemia and apparent tissue hypoxia

Renal handling of hemoglobin

Selected Readings

Arias, I. M. et al. Chronic nonhemolytic unconjugated hyperbilirubinemia with glucuronyl transferase deficiency. *Am. J. Med.* 47 : 395, 1969.

Bunn, H. F., Esham, W. T., and Bull, R. W. The renal handling of hemoglobin. *J. Exp. Med.* 129 : 909, 1969.

Foulk, W. T. et al. Constitutional hepatic dysfunction (Gilbert's disease): Its natural history and related syndromes. *Medicine (Baltimore)* 38 : 25, 1959.

Giblett, E. R. Haptoglobin. *Semin. Haematol.* 1 : 3, 1968.

Hershko, C. The fate of circulating hemoglobins. *Br. J. Haematol.* 29 : 199, 1975.

Lessin, L. S., and Rosse, W. (eds.). Diagnosis, mechanisms and treatment of hemolytic anemias. *Mod. Treat.* 8 : 321, 1971.

London, I. M. et al. On the origin of bile pigment in normal man. *J. Biol. Chem.* 184 : 351, 1950.

Marchesi, V. T. The red cell membrane skeleton: Recent progress. *Blood* 61 : 1, 1983.

Muller-Eberhard, U. Hemopexin. *N. Engl. J. Med.* 283 : 1090, 1970.

Prankerd, T. A. J., and Bellingham, A. J. (eds.). Haemolytic anaemias. *Clin. Haematol.* 4 : 1, 1975.

Robinson, S. H. Formation of bilirubin from erythroid and non-erythroid sources. *Semin. Hematol.* 9 : 43, 1972.

Robinson, S. H. Heme Metabolism and the Porphyrias. In W. S. Beck (eds.), *Hematology* (4th ed.), Harvard Pathophysiology Series. Cambridge, MA: MIT Press, 1985. pp. 125–1344.

Robinson, S. H. Anemia. In E. Braunwald and C. Funta (eds.), *Intensive Review of Internal Medicine* (3rd ed.). Boston: Brigham and Women's and Beth Israel Hospitals and Nimrod Press, 1988. pp. 46–57.

Robinson, S. H. Degradation of Hemoglobin. In W. J. Williams et al. (eds.), *Hematology* (4th ed.). New York: McGraw-Hill, 1990. pp. 407–414.

Robinson, S. H. et al. Jaundice in thalassemia minor: A consequence of "ineffective erythropoiesis." *N. Engl. J. Med.* 267 : 523, 1962.

Robinson, S. H. et al. Ineffective Erythropoiesis and the Erythropoietic Component of Early-Labeled Bilirubin. In F. Stolhman, Jr. (ed.), *Hemopoietic Cellular Proliferation.* New York: Grune & Stratton, 1970. pp. 180–188.

Sears, D. A. et al. Urinary iron excretion and renal metabolism of hemoglobin in hemolytic diseases. *Blood* 28 : 708, 1966.

Sjostrand, T. Endogenous formation of carbon monoxide in man under normal and pathological conditions. *Scand. J. Clin. Lab. Invest.* 1L201, 1949.

Tenhunen, R. The enzymatic degradation of heme. *Semin. Hematol.* 9 : 19, 1972.

7 Inherited Hemolytic Anemias

Justine Meehan Carr

Premature destruction of erythrocytes occurs in a variety of conditions as outlined in Chapter 6. In this chapter we focus on congenital hemolytic anemias, some of which present at birth, and others later in life, while still others may remain silent unless a physiologic stress is superimposed. Congenital defects resulting in hemolytic anemia may involve abnormalities in the red cell membrane, red cell enzymes, or hemoglobin.

Membrane Disorders

Hereditary Spherocytosis

CLINICAL FINDINGS

Hereditary spherocytosis (HS) is an autosomal dominant disorder that may become symptomatic shortly after birth, or may not be detected until later life. Most patients with HS have spherocytes, splenomegaly, and jaundice. Family members usually have similar histories and findings.

Occasionally HS is diagnosed at birth. In these cases the diagnosis is usually suspected because of extreme jaundice resulting from increased bilirubin formation from hemolysis superimposed on the physiologic impairment of hepatic glucuronidation by the neonatal liver. The jaundice usually abates with hepatic maturation, despite continued hemolysis. About 20 percent of patients with HS have mild disease, often detected for the first time late in life as a result of routine laboratory evaluation. These patients may compensate sufficiently for hemolysis so that little or no anemia is present. A peripheral smear showing significant spherocytosis combined with mild anemia, splenomegaly, and reticulocytosis may suggest the diagnosis. About 70 percent of HS patients have moderately severe disease presenting in childhood with hemolysis and splenomegaly, with eventual development of bilirubin gallstones. The remaining 10 percent have debilitating, severe disease. Such patients develop gallstones in childhood and have significant anemia rendering them transfusion-dependent. These patients have the skeletal abnormalities seen

---

The major inherited hemolytic anemias*

Membrane disorders
  Hereditary spherocytosis
  Hereditary elliptocytosis
Red cell enzyme deficiencies
  Glucose-6-phosphate dehydrogenase deficiency
  Pyruvate kinase deficiency
Abnormal hemoglobin
  Qualitative β-globin chain disorders (e.g., HbS, HbC)
  Unstable hemoglobins
  Hemoglobins with altered oxygen affinity

---

*Similar to Table 6-2, Intracorpuscular hemolytic anemias, most of which are due to inherited abnormalities.

in all severe congenital hemolytic anemias, including expansion of the medullary cavity of the skull, with frontal bossing and characteristic facies.

All patients with HS are subject to aplastic crises. These episodes of marrow failure may result from either intercurrent infection, often viral, with marrow suppression or from depletion of folate stores due to overutilization, particularly in the setting of the increased folate demands of growth or pregnancy. The aplasia of a viral syndrome generally resolves after 7 or 10 days and is usually due to infection by parvovirus. Occasionally, children may develop hemolytic crises in which there is acceleration of hemolysis.

LABORATORY FINDINGS

Patients with HS have laboratory evidence of hemolysis, including anemia, reticulocytosis, increased serum lactic dehydrogenase (LDH) level, decreased or absent haptoglobin, and often mild hyperbilirubinemia. Except during hemolytic crises they do not have hemoglobinemia or hemoglobinuria. Examination of the peripheral blood smear shows large numbers of spherocytes (Plate 33), often accompanied by polychromatophils (Plate 25). These cells have a small diameter and are hyperchromic or darker staining than normal. The normal erythrocyte's pale center is absent. Because of their spheroidal shape, which is due in part to loss of membrane area, they are more susceptible to osmotic stress as measured by the *osmotic fragility test* (Fig. 7-1). To perform this test, red cells are suspended in saline solutions of various tonicities. At lower tonicities water enters and swells the red cells, ultimately causing them to lyse. This normally occurs at a sodium chloride concentration of 0.55 percent. In patients with HS and in patients with other diseases in which large numbers of spherocytes are produced, lysis may begin at 0.70% sodium chloride concentration or even higher. This increased susceptibility to osmotic lysis is accentuated by prior incuba-

Fig. 7-1. Osmotic fragility curves, preincubation and postincubation, normal and abnormal.

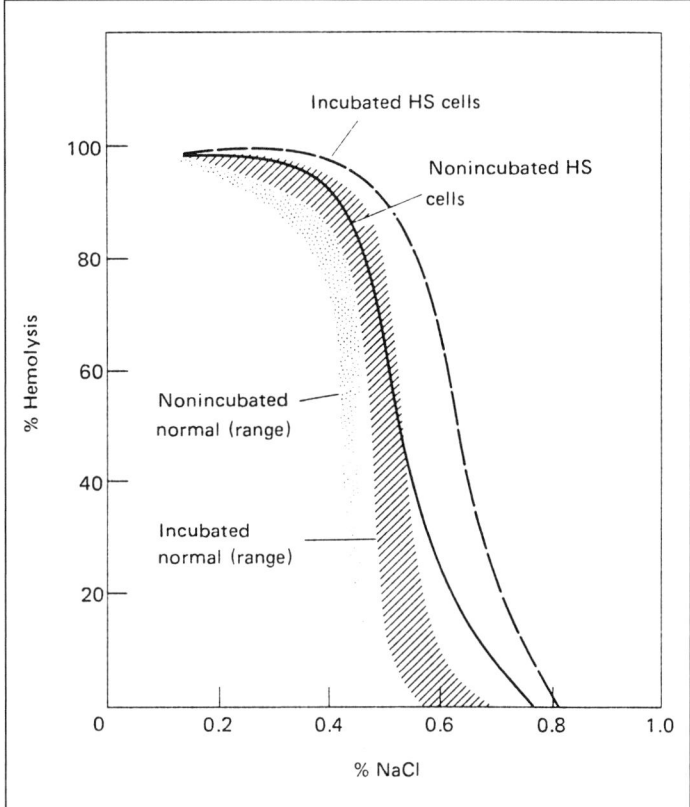

tion of the red cells for 24 hours at 37°C. Both normal subjects and HS patients will have increased osmotic fragility after incubation, but the effect is more marked for the patients with hereditary spherocytosis, whose cells may begin to lyse in 0.80% sodium chloride solution.

The *autohemolysis test,* during which red cells are incubated at 37°C for 48 hours in isotonic sodium chloride, is another stress test of the spherocyte. Because of their metabolic derangement, spherocytes from HS patients will lyse readily. Ten to fifty percent of HS erythrocytes lyse, compared to fewer than 4 percent of normal cells. The addition of glucose or adenosine triphosphate (ATP) will decrease the extent of autohemolysis seen with red cells from HS patients.

Wintrobe indices may be abnormal in patients with HS. The mean corpuscular volume (MCV) may be low normal or, with reticulocytosis, moderately elevated. The mean corpuscular hemoglobin concentration (MCHC) is characteristically high; HS is one of the few causes of an elevated MCHC.

PATHOGENESIS OF THE ANEMIA
IN HEREDITARY SPHEROCYTOSIS

The primary defect in the HS cell is becoming better understood. An intrinsic cellular abnormality by itself is not enough to cause the hemolytic anemia. There must be interaction of the HS cell with the mononuclear phagocytic system of the spleen. Several observations regarding the HS red cell are pertinent:

1. There is a reduction of total membrane lipid content, which returns toward normal after splenectomy.
2. Most patients with HS have a mild decrease in the membrane skeletal protein spectrin. This may be secondary to abnormalities in the other skeletal proteins, such as ankyrin or protein 4.1, and these abnormalities in membrane proteins predispose the cells to lose membrane lipid.
3. There is leakiness of the HS red cells for Na^+. The magnitude of Na^+ flux does not, however, correlate with the rate of hemolysis.

The role of the spleen in causing hemolysis is defined by the following observations: First, HS cells have a decreased life span when transfused into normal subjects whose spleens are intact. After splenectomy, red cell survival in HS patients is almost normal. Further, HS cell survival is also normal when these abnormal cells are transfused into normal subjects who have been splenectomized. Secondly, normal red cells survive normally when they are transfused into nonsplenectomized patients with HS.

In summary, there is an intrinsic defect in the red cell, but its expression depends on the presence of a functioning spleen. The spheroidal, relatively nondeformable shape of the HS cell inhibits its ability to traverse the splenic sinusoids. As a result, the erythrocyte is trapped in a glucose- and oxygen-poor environment, where it becomes metabolically deprived and more spherical, and ultimately lyses after one or more passages through the spleen.

THERAPY

Patients with HS should take daily folate supplementation if splenectomy has not been performed. HS can be cured by splenectomy, with resolution of anemia and prevention of subsequent bilirubin gallstone formation. Failure of resolution of anemia after splenectomy suggests that either the wrong diagnosis was made or that an accessory spleen is present. The decision to perform a splenectomy must be a risk-benefit decision. Patients with very mild HS may be more jeopardized by the small risk of fulminant sepsis after splenectomy than by the risks of mild chronic HS. After splenectomy the appearance of the RBCs is altered somewhat. Spherocytes persist, but microspherocytes, that is, spherocytes conditioned by repeated passages through the spleen, are no longer present. In addition, the usual blood picture of splenectomized patients is evident (see Chap. 8).

Hereditary Elliptocytosis

Hereditary elliptocytosis (HE) is an autosomal dominant disorder characterized by excessive numbers of elliptical cells. HE cells (Plate 34) are biconcave dumbbells with an axial ratio of less than 0.8. In the majority of cases hematocrit levels are normal or near normal with minimal hemolysis; greater than 25 percent (often 75%) of red cells are elliptocytes. In 10 to 15 percent of patients with HE, erythrocyte destruction is substantially increased, leading to all the signs and symptoms of a true hemolytic anemia. The degree of hemolysis does not correlate with the percentage of elliptocytes. Patients with HE who do not have hemolysis usually have normal osmotic fragility and normal autohemolysis tests. These tests may be abnormal, however, in HE patients with overt hemolysis. It should be noted that some elliptical cells also occur in thalassemia, iron deficiency, myelophthisic anemias, sickle cell disease, and megaloblastic anemia. These disorders, however, are accompanied by other characteristic morphologic changes as well. Hereditary elliptocytosis is usually diagnosed in patients with mild or no hemolysis who have large numbers of elliptocytes in their peripheral blood for no apparent reason. Rarely is extensive diagnostic testing or therapy indicated. While most patients require no treatment, patients with severe hemolysis can be effectively treated with splenectomy, as in HS.

PATHOGENESIS

Several defects have been identified in the membrane skeleton of HE cells. The most common defect (20–40% of cases) is the impaired association of spectrin dimers to form tetramers and higher oligomers. Deficiency of protein 4.1 has been identified as the defect in another group of patients with HE. Less common variants of HE have been attributed to other defects, including faulty linkage of spectrin to ankyrin, anomalous protein 4.1, and absent glycophorin C and protein 4.1

Hereditary pyropoikilocytosis (HPP) is a rare congenital hemolytic anemia often included in the discussion of HE. HPP is characterized by severe hemolysis, with virtually all red cells misshapen, including fragments, spheres, and elliptocytes. The MCV is low (55–74 femtoliters) because of the microspherocytes and fragments. Osmotic fragility is increased and autohemolysis is markedly abnormal with or without glucose. HPP cells are extremely unstable when incubated at 45°C. The pathogenesis of this disorder is an instability of spectrin. Symptomatic cases can be treated with splenectomy.

Erythrocyte Enzyme Deficiencies (Congenital Nonspherocytic Hemolytic Anemia)

Hereditary hemolytic anemia has been associated with at least ten red cell enzyme deficiencies. Of these, only three are of clinical significance. The rest occur very rarely and are not described here.

Glucose-6-Phosphate Dehydrogenase Deficiency

Deficiency of the enzyme glucose-6-phosphate dehydrogenase (G-6-PD) is by far the most common inherited erythrocyte enzyme deficiency, affecting more than 100 million people. The gene for G-6-PD is sex-linked. According to the Lyon hypothesis, X-inactivation in cells of female embryos is a random process, indiscriminately inactivating one X chromosome of either maternal or paternal origin. As a result, female heterozygotes with one normal and one abnormal gene will have varying G-6-PD levels. Because of the X-linkage, male patients are more severely affected than female patients.

Also of significance is the fact that over 100 structural variants of this enzyme exist. The two most important have normal enzyme activity (+ sign indicates normal activity, − sign indicates deficient activity). Type B+ is the most common and is found in all populations. Type A+ in addition to B+ is prevalent among blacks. The enzymatic activity of both is normal, but there are differences in their electrophoretic mobility. With the exception of G-6-PD B+, G-6-PD A+, and G-6-PD A−, variants are identified by geographic names.

Glucose-6-phosphate dehydrogenase variants have been subdivided into five classes. Class 1 variants are rare, but have severely deficient enzyme activity and affected individuals have a lifelong hemolytic anemia (congenital nonspherocytic hemolytic anemia). Hemolysis is worsened by febrile illnesses or oxidant drugs. Splenomegaly is common, but splenectomy does not ameliorate the anemia. Heinz body formation is not seen in these patients.

Class 2 and 3 variants are the most common, representing 90 percent of G-6-PD−deficient states. Class 2 and 3 variants of G-6-PD do not manifest hemolysis unless stressed by an oxidant drug, infection, or acidosis. In the Mediterranean variant (class 2), G-6-PD is both unstable and undersynthesized. This variant is seen among Greeks, Sardinians, and Sephardic Jews. The A− variant (class 3) affects more than 12 percent of American black males. Class 4 and 5 variants have no clinical consequences.

PATHOGENESIS OF HEMOLYSIS SECONDARY TO G-6-PD DEFICIENCY

Glucose-6-phosphate dehydrogenase is a key enzyme in the hexose monophosphate pathway (HMP). The HMP is responsible for net production of the reduced form of nicotinamide adenine dinucleotide phosphate (NADPH) from NADP. This cofactor, NADPH, is necessary to maintain glutathione in its reduced state (GSH). GSH helps prevent hemoglobin oxidation and denaturation, maintains reduced sulfhydryl groups in the red cell cytoplasm and membrane, and prevents splitting of essential membrane disulfide bonds.

Drugs that induce hemolysis in G-6-PD–deficient individuals generate forms of activated oxygen, such as superoxide, hydroxyl radicals, and peroxide, which oxidize GSH. GSH in association with glutathione peroxidase is required to detoxify these oxidant species. If the HMP is unable to generate GSH normally because of G-6-PD deficiency, exposure to increased amounts of activated forms of oxygen may result in damage to the red cell membrane and denaturation of hemoglobin. Heinz bodies are intracellular, often membrane-associated, precipitates of denatured hemoglobin. These Heinz bodies cause membrane rigidity and decrease red cell survival. Moreover, these inclusions can then be "pitted" from erythrocytes by macrophages, and the resulting membrane defects further impair red cell deformity and survival. Erythrocytes that have had Heinz bodies pitted out appear as "bite cells" in the peripheral blood (Plate 35).

Drugs and other toxic agents vary in their ability to induce hemolysis, and the severity of enzyme deficiency varies greatly among G-6-PD variants. These two factors account for the different clinical manifestations of G-6-PD deficiency. Glucose-6-phosphate dehydrogenase variants with decreased enzyme activity are due to either acceleration of the enzyme's normal breakdown as the cell ages or reduced activity and abnormal kinetics of the enzyme itself, for example, a low affinity for NADP. At present there are no examples of G-6-PD deficiency due to abnormal regulatory genes that reduce G-6-PD synthesis. Patients with G-6-PD variants who have low intrinsic enzyme activity and unfavorable kinetics are particularly sensitive to oxidant stress and may hemolyze spontaneously.

CLINICAL FEATURES OF G-6-PD DEFICIENCY IN CLASS 2 AND CLASS 3 VARIANTS

Unless specific enzyme or metabolic tests are undertaken, the red cells of affected individuals appear normal. No morphologic abnormality or evidence of hemolysis is seen. However, when stressed by infections, drugs (see p. 153), or acidosis, G-6-PD–deficient individuals may suddenly develop acute hemolytic anemia. Generally, enzyme activity is one fourth of normal before a cell is hemolyzed. Reticulocytosis, manifested by macrocytosis and polychromasia in the Wright-stained peripheral blood, is prominent 1 to 3 days after the metabolic insult. Heinz bodies are found in peripheral blood erythrocytes. Heinz bodies are not visible in Wright-stained blood, but can be seen with special stains such as crystal violet. Alternatively, Heinz bodies may be detected in unstained erythrocytes in saline suspension by phase microscopy; here, they are identified as 1- to 2-μm refractile inclusions. After Heinz bodies are pitted from red cells, telltale bite cells may remain in the circulation for days or weeks (Plate 35).

A screening test for G-6-PD deficiency can be performed using a commercially available kit that is based on the reduction of an oxidized blue dye, changing the dye from blue to red. A red cell hemolysate of patient blood is added to the substrate in a reaction in which the amount of available G-6-PD is the rate-limiting step. As the reaction occurs a by-product is generated that turns the dye from blue to red. When G-6-PD is deficient, the by-product is generated to a lesser extent so that the color change takes longer, or does not occur at all. A caveat to the interpretation of this test is the reticulocyte count. Since reticulocytes are richer in G-6-PD than are older red cells, patients who are G-6-PD deficient may appear normal if they have a reticulocytosis, since the reticulocytes contribute extra G-6-PD to the hemolysate. Patients with reticulocytosis who have apparently normal G-6-PD levels can be further evaluated with the ascorbate-cyanide test.

The ascorbate-cyanide test is used to detect deficiencies in the hexose monophosphate shunt. A defect in any of the limiting enzymes of the hexose monophosphate shunt, including G-6-PD, glutathione peroxidase, and glutathione reductase, or in glutathione synthesis, such as pyruvate kinase, should render a positive test. The test is based on the failure of the patient's cells to detoxify hydrogen peroxide. Hydrogen peroxide is generated by the interaction of ascorbate with oxyhemoglobin, and catalase, which could eliminate the peroxide, is inhibited by cyanide. In the absence of G-6-PD, peroxide attacks hemoglobin, forming brown methemoglobin, whereas normal cells detoxify hydrogen peroxide through the glutathione peroxidase system. Since the test utilizes individual intact cells, it can be used for the detection of the heterozygous state (e.g., in black females) and G-6-PD–deficient cells in the presence of reticulocytosis. Erythrocytes with deficient G-6-PD turn brown, while normal cells remain pink.

Several clinical syndromes are associated with hemolytic anemia due to G-6-PD deficiency. Black male patients with low G-6-PD levels who are given antimalarials prophylactically manifest moderate, self-limited hemolysis that leads to anemia and jaundice. The self-limited nature of this syndrome is due to the fact that young red

Compounds associated with hemolysis in individuals with G-6-PD deficiency*

I. Analgesics and Antipyretics
   A. Acetanilid
   B. Aminopyrine
   C. Antipyrine
   D. Aspirin
   E. Phenacetin
II. Antimalarials
   A. Pamaquine
   B. Primaquine
   C. Quinacrine (Atabrine)
   D. Quinine
III. Nitrofurans
   A. Furadantin
   B. Furadin
IV. Sulfa Drugs
   A. Azulfidine
   B. Gantrisin
   C. Kynex
V. Sulfones
   A. Dapsone
   B. DDS
VI. Miscellaneous
   A. Chloramphenicol
   B. Dimercaprol (BAL)
   C. Fava beans
   D. Isoniazid
   E. Methylene blue
   F. Naphthalene (moth balls)
   G. Phenylhydrazine
   H. Probenecid (Benemid)
   I. Quinidine
   J. Vitamin K analogues

* Hemolysis has been observed in G-6-PD–deficient patients in association with viral or bacterial infections, diabetic ketoacidosis, acute or chronic hepatitis, and nephritis. This list may be reproduced for use by G-6-PD–deficient patients to help them avoid drugs to which they may be sensitive.
Adapted from M. M. Wintrobe et al. *Clinical Hematology* (8th ed.). Philadelphia: Lea & Febiger, 1981. p. 792.

cells have nearly normal G-6-PD levels and are therefore resistant to hemolysis. Even with continued drug therapy, therefore, the hemolytic anemia becomes compensated and the hemoglobin level becomes normal. On the other hand, white patients with severely deficient red cells of all ages (G-6-PD Mediterranean type deficiency) often have severe hemolysis.

Patients with infectious hepatitis and G-6-PD deficiency may undergo a severe, acute hemolytic episode that results in extremely high bilirubin levels. In certain G-6-PD–deficient patients with Mediterranean (not A−) phenotype, life-threatening acute hemolytic anemia develops on ingestion of fava beans. Another factor besides G-6-PD deficiency is involved, since not all patients with similar enzyme deficiencies hemolyze after eating fava beans.

There is no specific therapy for G-6-PD deficiency other than blood transfusion. Splenectomy is of no use. G-6-PD–deficient patients should be given a list of drugs that are likely to cause acute hemolysis (see p. 153). Severe hemolysis with hemoglobinemia and hemoglobinuria can result in shock and renal failure with risk of death. This is particularly true of fava bean–sensitive patients.

Pyruvate Kinase Deficiency

Pyruvate kinase (PK) deficiency is much less common than G-6-PD deficiency. However, it is the second most common erythrocyte enzyme deficiency, with over 300 cases reported. The deficiency is not limited to any particular racial or geographically defined population. Rather than producing acute hemolysis in association with drug ingestion, it causes a chronic congenital nonspherocytic hemolytic anemia.

CLINICAL FEATURES

Manifestations of PK deficiency vary from mild compensated hemolysis to severe hemolysis with onset in the neonatal period. The latter patients often require transfusion support and splenectomy. Cases presenting in older children or adults are generally mild. Natural history and complications in this disorder are comparable to those in other chronic hemolytic anemias. Affected patients have jaundice and splenomegaly, and often develop bilirubin gallstones. Skeletal deformities due to marrow expansion are seen in severely affected patients. Aplastic crises occur with infections, particularly parvovirus infections.

The peripheral blood shows evidence of reticulocytosis with polychromatophilic macrocytes. Irregularly contracted, spiny red cells may be prominent. The unincubated osmotic fragility is normal. The autohemolysis test gives abnormal results, which are poorly corrected by glucose (type II autohemolysis test). The ascorbate-cyanide test is positive. A simple fluorescence test is used to screen for PK deficiency, but the diagnosis rests on determining decreased PK enzymatic activity in the patient's red cells.

Patients with PK deficiency require folate supplementation. Transfusion support is necessary for severe anemia. Splenectomy is beneficial in severely anemic patients. Paradoxically, after splenectomy, reticulocytes may rise from baseline levels of 15 to 20 percent to markedly elevated levels up to 70 percent.

PATHOGENESIS OF ERYTHROCYTE PK DEFICIENCY— ASSOCIATED HEMOLYTIC ANEMIA

The hemolytic anemia of PK deficiency is a result of the mature red cell's inability to produce its energy requirements, most of which depend on anaerobic glycolysis. A deficiency of PK will limit the cell's ability to metabolize glucose and produce energy in the form of ATP by the following reaction:

$$\text{Phosphoenolpyruvate} + \text{ADP} \xrightarrow{\text{PK}} \text{pyruvate} + \text{ATP}$$

Large numbers of mutant PK enzymes are now recognized. They may be abnormal in their catalytic activity, enzyme kinetics, isoelectric points and pH optima, electrophoretic mobility, stability, behavior toward nucleotide cofactors and allosteric modifiers, etc.

Reticulocytes are prominent in the peripheral blood, probably because they have an intact citric acid (Krebs) cycle, which is an efficient energy source. Thus, in severely affected individuals, only the reticulocyte has the necessary metabolic machinery to maintain a viable red cell.

This enzyme deficiency as well as most others, except G-6-PD deficiency, is inherited as an autosomal recessive trait. Homozygotes have hemolytic anemia and splenomegaly, while heterozygotes are hematologically normal. The latter's red cells often have half the normal PK activity.

Pyrimidine-5'-Nucleotidase Deficiency

A chronic hemolytic anemia inherited as an autosomal recessive and characterized by large numbers of erythrocytes with basophilic stippling is due to deficiency in an enzyme, pyrimidine-5'-nucleotidase, which dephosphorylates the ribonucleotides of cytidine and uridine. Since this conversion of ribonucleotides to ribonucleosides is required before these pyrimidines can diffuse from the red cells as waste products, the rate of ribosomal degradation is retarded, causing the observed stippling. Hemolysis may be related to competition between excess pyrimidine nucleotides and the adenine nucleotides, adenosine diphosphate (ADP) and ATP, in metabolically crucial reactions, such as those catalyzed by hexokinase, phosphoglycerate kinase, and pyruvate kinase. Acquired basophilic stippling in lead poisoning may be related in part to red cell pyrimidine-5'-nucleotidase inhibition by lead.

Hemolytic Anemia Due to Other Erythrocyte Enzyme Deficiencies

There are other, rarely encountered, red cell enzyme deficiencies associated with hemolytic anemia as well as some not associated with hemolysis. These rare disorders will not be discussed (see Selected Readings for relevant reviews), but should be suspected in patients who have a clinical picture similar to that of G-6-PD, PK, or pyrimidine-5'-nucleotidase deficiency, but have normal assays for these enzymes. The laboratory diagnosis of the rare erythrocyte enzyme disorders can only be made by specific assays.

Hemoglobinopathies

Mutations in the DNA sequences controlling the synthesis of globin chains in hemoglobin result in either structurally abnormal hemoglobins or reduced globin chain synthesis or, sometimes, both. Generally the term *hemoglobinopathy* is used to signify a structurally abnormal hemoglobin with at least one amino acid substitution. *Thalassemia* refers to DNA mutations resulting in normally structured globins but with reduced or negligible synthetic rates. Structural abnormalities may cause premature red cell destruction; easily denatured hemoglobins; hemoglobins with abnormal oxygen affinity; altered hemoglobin solubility; and, in a few instances, reduced globin synthesis. The heme moiety of hemoglobin is synthesized normally and is structurally normal. In this chapter only the few clinically significant hemoglobinopathies are discussed. The thalassemias are discussed in Chapter 3.

Structure and Function of Hemoglobin

The globin in hemoglobin consists of two pairs of identical polypeptide chains. In normal hemoglobin, hemoglobin A, one pair of polypeptide chains is designated α^A and the other pair is called β^A. Normal hemoglobin A is therefore written as $\alpha_2^A\beta_2^A$. A normal hemoglobin present in low concentration is hemoglobin A_2. It is made up of two α^A-chains and two δ^{A2}-chains. The major hemoglobin found in the fetus, so-called fetal or F hemoglobin, contains α^A-chains and, in place of β-chains, γ^F chains. Hemoglobin F is written as $\alpha_2^A\gamma_2^F$. The α-, β-, δ-, and γ-chains differ in their amino acid sequences. The structure of β-, δ-, and γ-chains is similar, whereas the amino acid sequence of α-chains differs considerably from these. α-Chain genes are carried on chromosome 16, and the β, γ, and δ structural genes are closely linked on chromosome 11. It is possible that the γ and δ structural genes resulted from reduplication of an original β-like gene.

Both the α- and the β-chains contain helical and nonhelical regions. The helices are labeled with capital letters, and an amino acid can be located in a helix by giving the letter corresponding to the helix and a number corresponding to the location of the amino acid in that helix. It is also possible to give the location of the amino acid by the number corresponding to the distance from the N-terminal amino acid. The N-terminal amino acid is assigned the number 1, and each succeeding amino acid is given the next higher number until the C-terminal end is reached. For example, the β-chain substitution in sickle cell hemoglobin is at a glutamic acid residue 6 places from the N-terminal end or at helix A3. To each of the four polypeptides is joined a heme group. The heme iron is covalently bonded with a histidine at F8. When hemoglobin is oxygenated, the oxygen covalently binds with heme and with globin at histidine E7. Bonds also exist between heme and other parts of the hemoglobin molecule. Interchain amino acid contacts of functional significance have been specified as $\alpha_1\beta_1$ and $\alpha_1\beta_2$.

The process of oxygenation of a hemoglobin molecule results in changes in the tertiary and quaternary structure of hemoglobin but leaves the primary amino acid and secondary helical structures unchanged. The tertiary structure, or the folding of the individual polypeptide chains, changes slightly with oxygenation, whereas the quaternary structure, or the manner in which the four polypeptide chains are joined to form a single molecule, changes significantly and accounts for the sigmoidal shape of the hemoglobin–oxygen dissociation curve. This change in oxygen affinity during oxygenation is called *heme–heme interaction*. The sequence of molecular changes on oxygenation occurs in the following manner: Oxygen is added first to the heme of an α-chain, then to a second α-chain, and finally to the two β-chains. After the second or third oxygen is added, the quaternary structure changes considerably. 2,3-DPG, which had stabilized the deoxygenated form of hemoglobin, is now expelled from the molecule. Movement occurs at the $\alpha_1\beta_1$ and $\alpha_1\beta_2$ contact points, particularly the $\alpha_1\beta_2$. Once the change from the deoxygenated to the oxygenated configuration is under way, oxygen affinity is greatly increased (accounting for the steep rise in the oxygen dissociation curve of hemoglobin), and oxygen is added to the hemes of the remaining β-chain or chains.

Details of the "respiration of hemoglobin" obviously have been omitted. The structure–function relationships of the hemoglobin molecule are interesting and important but will not be discussed further except as they relate to the pathogenesis of hemoglobin disorders.

Hemoglobin Nomenclature

Hemoglobins were first assigned a letter of the alphabet on the basis of their electrophoretic mobility. When the letters of the alphabet were used up, subsequent hemoglobins were named after the geographic location in which they were described. If the hemoglobin had characteristics of one of the letter hemoglobins, the geographic designation was used as a subscript, for example, hemoglobin $J_{Capetown}$. If the hemoglobin had been characterized as to the amino acid substitution, this was designated in a parenthesis after the globin chain involved: for example, hemoglobin S, $\beta6(A3)Glu \rightarrow Val$.

This means that there is a substitution 6 amino acids from the N-terminal end of the β-chain: glutamic acid is no longer present and valine has been substituted for it.

Pathogenesis of Hemoglobinopathies

Several different genetic mechanisms account for abnormal hemoglobin production:

1. Substitution of a DNA nucleotide for another *(point mutation)*. The hemoglobin product of this mutated DNA gene has a substitution of one amino acid for another. Almost always, only one of the three bases coding for the amino acid is changed. The location of an amino acid substitution will often determine the functional abnormality and the clinical findings. At least five different locations for substitutions have been described:
   a. Substitution at the surface of the hemoglobin molecule. Usually these are innocuous, since they do not affect tertiary structure, heme function, or subunit interaction. However, some surface substitutions as, for example, in hemoglobin S, result in a molecule with reduced solubility, and in stacking of hemoglobin chains to cause shape abnormalities and hemolytic anemia.
   b. Substitution in the internal nonpolar residues. This results in hemoglobin instability and in some cases hemolytic anemia (for example, hemoglobin$_{\text{Köln}}$).
   c. Substitution of tyrosine for histidine near the heme iron. The ionic bond between heme and tyrosine stabilizes the heme iron in the ferric state and leads to methemoglobinemia and cyanosis.
   d. Substitution at an $\alpha_1\beta_2$ contact point. This impairs heme–heme interaction and results in increased oxygen affinity and erythrocytosis (for example, hemoglobin$_{\text{Chesapeake}}$).
   e. Substitutions at an $\alpha_1\beta_2$ contact point and near the heme moiety. Decreased oxygen affinity and cyanosis result (for example, hemoglobin$_{\text{Kansas}}$).
2. Point mutation in a "stop" codon. Extra amino acids' residues are added to the normal hemoglobin chain (for example, hemoglobin$_{\text{Seal Rock}}$).
3. Mutation of a codon to a "stop" codon. A shortened chain results that can only be tolerated at its terminal amino acids (for example, hemoglobin$_{\text{McKees Rocks}}$).
4. Crossovers between chromosomal pairs, resulting in gene deletion or fusion of genes. Hemoglobins made up partially of β-chains and partially of Δ-chains may result from the latter (for example, Lepore hemoglobin).

5. "Frameshifts" in which a single DNA nucleotide is added or deleted. Codons further on in the chain will, therefore, be altered, usually in a nonsensical manner. These nonsense mutations can be tolerated only if the amino acids involved are at the end of a chain (for example, hemoglobin$_{Wayne}$).

Hemoglobin S

By far the most important hemoglobinopathies are those related to the presence of sickle hemoglobin (HbS). This hemoglobin is present in approximately 10 percent of blacks. Depending on many factors, which we will discuss, its presence may result in severe disease causing early death or in a clinically benign condition of importance only when the individual is stressed. Before detailing the clinical manifestations of the diseases related to sickle hemoglobin we shall discuss the pathogenesis of the anemia and the thrombotic tendency associated with it.

PATHOPHYSIOLOGY OF SICKLE HEMOGLOBIN

Sickle hemoglobin results from replacement of the sixth amino acid from the N-terminal end of the β-chain, glutamic acid, by valine. This replacement occurs because of the substitution in messenger RNA of uridine for adenine in the second nucleotide of the glutamic acid codon (adenine for thymidine in the DNA codon). As a result of the replacement of the hydrophilic amino acid, glutamic acid, by the hydrophobic amino acid, valine, cyclization of the N-terminal end of the β-chain of sickle hemoglobin takes place after deoxygenation. This is a valine–valine cyclization between the valine residues at the 1 and the 6 positions. The resulting structure interlocks with an adjacent normal or abnormal hemoglobin molecule in an oxygenated or deoxygenated state. This leads to the formation of hemoglobin polymers. When viewed from the side, the polymeric hemoglobin fibers have a helical structure. When viewed on end, each layer consists of 14 or 16 hemoglobin molecules (four chained tetramers) in each layer wound around a vertical axis. This polymeric structure is stabilized by noncovalent contacts between one of the cyclized valine residues in a hemoglobin S tetramer and an adjacent hemoglobin molecule. These polymers or gels can transform into true crystals. Intracellular gelation or polymerization is accompanied by deformation of the red cell into an elongated sickle form (Plate 37). These cells may revert to normal on exposure to oxygen, but some erythrocytes in the blood of patients with sickle cell anemia become irreversibly sickled. A noncovalent rearrangement of the submembrane spectrin-actin cytoskeleton during sickling may account for these irreversibly sickled cells.

It should be emphasized that two events must occur in order that polymers be formed: (1) the substitution of glutamic acid by valine and the formation of hydrophobic valine–valine bonds and (2) the deoxygenation of HbS to cause a configurational change in the hemoglobin that allows interlocking between the valine–valine ring structure and adjacent hemoglobin molecules. Once polymers have occurred in the red cells, deformability of the sickled cell decreases and blood viscosity increases. Sickled red cells flow poorly through small arterioles and may actually act as a plug. The interference with arteriolar blood flow results in infarction and death of tissues supplied by these arterioles. Enhanced adhesion of erythrocytes containing hemoglobin S to endothelial cells may help to initiate these microvascular occlusions.

Irreversibly sickled forms are also susceptible to fragmentation, loss of membrane, and hemolysis. They may be sequestered in the mononuclear phagocytic system, particularly in the liver, thereby causing hemolysis.

HEMOGLOBIN S CLINICAL SYNDROMES

Four important clinical syndromes are associated with sickle hemoglobins. In order to understand these syndromes, it is necessary to review the inheritance of sickle hemoglobin and the factors that moderate the formation of sickle cells.

Patients with a gene coding for hemoglobin S on one chromosome could have one of the following on the other chromosome that bears a β-chain locus:

1. Normal β-chain locus coding for hemoglobin A (HbAS)
2. Abnormal β-chain locus coding for hemoglobin S (HbSS)
3. Abnormal β-chain locus coding for hemoglobin C, β6(Glu → Lys) (HbSC), or other mutant hemoglobin
4. Gene that results in the continued production of hemoglobin F after infancy (hereditary persistence of fetal hemoglobin) (HbSF)
5. Thalassemia gene that suppresses normal production of hemoglobin A (HbS–thal)

The genes on both chromosomes are expressed and inherited as *autosomal codominants.*

Deoxyhemoglobin S molecules copolymerize most effectively with other hemoglobin S molecules, and in decreasing order, with hemoglobin C, D, O, Arab, A, and F. These in vitro observations parallel the clinical severity of disorders involving these mutant hemoglobins. The presence of α- or β-thalassemia genes may also ameliorate sickling, perhaps by decreasing intracellular hemoglobin concentration or increasing hemoglobin F.

The presence of hemoglobin A and F in cells with hemoglobin S will modify the severity of the sickling. This is particularly important in patients who are homozygous for hemoglobin S and have hereditary persistence of hemoglobin F, for in these individuals the presence of hemoglobin F markedly retards the sickling of the hemoglobin S. Similarly, patients with sickle cell trait with 50–55 percent A in each red cell (HbAS) have a benign clinical course.

Sickle Cell Trait (HbAS)

Sickle cell trait is an asymptomatic condition. However, some patients have diminished perfusion of the renal medulla, resulting in impairment of concentration of the urine. This hypoperfusion may also predispose to small medullary infarcts and hematuria. Before aircraft had pressurized cabins, patients with HbAS who flew in aircraft above 10,000 feet occasionally developed splenic infarcts due to hypoxia. Blood counts and peripheral smears are normal in patients with HbAS. Sickling tests (sodium metabisulfite) and solubility tests (dithionite) are positive in these patients. Hemoglobin electrophoresis shows somewhat more HbA than HbS.

Sickle Cell Anemia (HbSS)

Sickle cell anemia is the most serious of the sickling syndromes. Symptoms generally do not appear until the patient is about one year old, although hemolysis develops during the first 3 months and splenomegaly is detectable at about 6 months. By age 5 or 6 years, the spleen is no longer palpable since repeated occlusions by rigid sickled cells result in functional asplenia. The most prominent hematologic finding is chronic hemolytic anemia, with average hemoglobin concentrations of about 8 gm/dL. Irreversibly sickled cells as well as target cells and the polychromasia of stress reticulocytes are prominent on smear. After autosplenectomy, basophilic stippling, Pappenheimer bodies, and nucleated red blood cells are present as well. Bilirubin is chronically elevated and bilirubin stones often develop.

Various hematologic crises may intervene. As with other chronic hemolytic anemias, intercurrent infections may suppress marrow response to hemolysis, resulting in an erythropoietic arrest and worsened anemia. After resolution of the infection, augmented hematopoiesis is restored. A second hematologic complication is folate depletion, with a resultant megaloblastic picture. Patients with chronic hemolysis require chronic folate supplementation. Finally, patients with HbSS may develop splenic sequestration crisis. This sometimes fatal complication occurs in childhood when splenomegaly is present. For unclear reasons there is engorgement of splenic sinusoids with sickled cells and trapping of a large volume of blood in the spleen, which may result in hypovolemic shock and death.

Recurrent episodes of severe musculoskeletal pain account for the majority of hospital admissions for patients with HbSS. Painful crises may occur spontaneously or in association with infections. These episodes result from ischemia precipitated by plugging of arteriolar beds by sickled cells. Infarction may also occur in the mesentery, brain, liver, kidney, or lung. Other complications include leg ulcers, aseptic necrosis of the femoral or humeral heads, priapism, heart failure, and pregnancy-related problems, both for mother and child. Bacterial infection is a lifelong concern because the asplenic status of these patients impairs their immunologic response and because sites of infarction may predispose to infection. Infection is a leading cause of death in patients with HbSS.

Sickle Cell–β-Thalassemia (HbS–thal)

If a patient inherits two abnormal alleles, one for S hemoglobin and one for thalassemia, one of two different syndromes may result. In one, there may be 90 percent or more S hemoglobin and complete suppression of hemoglobin A synthesis. In the other, β-chain synthesis is not completely suppressed, and there may be 25 to 35 percent hemoglobin A. Because of the presence of hemoglobin A, the clinical course is much milder than when complete suppression of normal β-chain synthesis occurs. Patients with sickle cell–thalassemia have an extremely variable clinical picture ranging from mild to severe disease. The spleen may be enlarged. The severity of the disease seems to be correlated with the concentration of HbS present in the erythrocytes and with the amount of HbF, which is usually increased in this condition.

Sickle Cell–Hemoglobin C (HbSC) Disease

Individuals with *sickle cell–hemoglobin C disease* carry two abnormal β-alleles, those for hemoglobin S and hemoglobin C. These patients are sometimes severely affected but generally less so than with HbSS disease; this disorder is more likely to be compatible with long life. It includes many of the symptoms and signs described for HbSS disease. Unlike sickle cell anemia it may cause splenomegaly in adults. There are numerous reports of pregnancies with complications to the baby and mother. These patients are also predisposed to hemorrhages in the fundus of the eye. Corkscrew-shaped conjunctival capillaries are characteristically seen in this and other sickle hemoglobin syndromes.

Since patients with high concentrations of sickle hemoglobin in their erythrocytes often die prematurely, there must be some selective advantage to this hemoglobin in order to maintain its stability in African populations. Malaria is present in the populations affected by this disease, and it has been suggested that preferential sickling of parasitized cells containing hemoglobin S and their rapid removal from the circulation reduce the number of parasites and thereby ameliorate the malarial infection.

LABORATORY DIAGNOSIS OF THE SICKLE HEMOGLOBIN SYNDROMES

Irreversibly sickled cells are typically seen on Wright-stained peripheral blood smears from patients with HbSS disease and HbS–thalassemia. They may occasionally be present in HbSC disease but are not seen in smears from patients with sickle cell trait. Target cells (Plate 19) and poikilocytes are seen in the peripheral blood of all patients with hemoglobin S syndromes (except HbAS). The bone marrow is characterized by active erythropoiesis and investigation of the blood shows evidence of hemolytic anemia.

Hemoglobin molecules in alkaline solution have a net negative charge and therefore move toward the anode in an electrophoretic system. Routine hemoglobin electrophoresis is performed on cellulose acetate at pH 8.6 and separates HbA, HbF, HbS, and HbC. Since some hemoglobins comigrate under these conditions, for example, HbD with HbS and HbE with HbC, citrate agar electrophoresis at acid pH (pH 6.2) can be performed for further identification of mutant hemoglobins. In all sickle hemoglobin syndromes, sickling of red blood cells (Plate 37) can be demonstrated by sealing blood under a cover slip and adding 2% sodium metabisulfite. This agent chemically deoxygenates hemoglobin and thus induces sickling. This test is often used to screen for the presence of HbS. Solubility testing with dithionite can also be used for this purpose. In this test HbS is reduced by dithionite and the insoluble HbS opacifies the solution. Hemoglobin electrophoresis, however, is required for definitive diagnosis of the sickle hemoglobin disorders.

All hemoglobins that sickle are not necessarily hemoglobin S. Hemoglobin C_{Harlem}, hemoglobin $C_{Georgetown,}$ and the α-chain variant, hemoglobin I, sickle when deoxygenated. High concentrations of hemoglobin$_{Bart's}$ (γ_4) also sickle.

The clinical picture, hematocrit, hemoglobin electrophoresis, and assay for hemoglobin F, will usually enable us to distinguish among HbS syndromes. In a few cases special research techniques or a thorough study of the family may be required. Sickle cell trait (HbAS) is characterized by a normal hematocrit and blood smear. The sickle cell test is positive, and hemoglobin electrophoresis reveals almost equal quantities of HbA and S, but there is always a little more HbA than S. Sickle cell anemia (HbSS) is associated with anemia and severe clinical abnormalities, including painful crises. Hemoglobin electrophoresis reveals virtually all hemoglobin S, and the assay for fetal hemoglobin shows only moderate quantities. The only other diagnostic possibilities would be hemoglobin SD disease or another hemoglobin with the electrophoretic mobility of HbS. These can be distinguished by family studies, hemoglobin electrophoresis on acid–agar gel, or differential solubility studies. It is sometimes difficult to distinguish sickle cell anemia from sickle cell–thalassemia, particularly when hemoglobin A production is completely suppressed in the sickle cell–thalassemia patient. Sickle cell–thalassemia with complete suppression of hemoglobin A synthesis should be suspected if the patient has marked targeting and microcytosis. HbA_2 is usually significantly elevated and the patient often has splenomegaly. Family studies may help in the diagnosis. In some cases the differential diagnosis may require in vitro measurement of the biosynthesis of hemoglobin chains in the patient's reticulocytes.

Patients with hemoglobin S and hereditary persistence of fetal hemoglobin are characterized by the even distribution of fetal hemoglobin among all the red cells. When the Kleihauer technique is used, the presence of hemoglobin F is detected by acid elution of hemoglobin A from dried red cells. The remaining cytoplasmic hemoglobin F is stained pink, and under a microscope, hemoglobin F–containing cells are readily counted. Patients with sickle cell–thalassemia may have high hemoglobin F values, but the fetal hemoglobin will be seen in only a relatively small number of cells (heterogenous distribution). Patients with hemoglobin S and hereditary persistence of hemoglobin F will have similar quantities of hemoglobin F in many cells (homogenous distribution).

THERAPY FOR SICKLE HEMOGLOBIN SYNDROMES

Patients with mild HbS syndromes may require no therapy. Usually patients who require treatment have high concentrations of sickle hemoglobin and no ameliorating hemoglobins. Frequent, painful crises are the major problem with these patients. Hydration, treatment of any infections, and administration of oxygen and narcotics may be of palliative benefit in treating painful crises.

Much attention has been devoted to long-term solutions to this debilitating disease. Inhibition of HbS polymerization has been attempted by administration of sodium cyanate. Although red cell life span is increased with this technique, it is less clear that painful crises are suppressed. Moreover, cyanate is a toxic agent. Reduction of plasma osmolarity using arginine vasopressin (DDAVP) in an attempt to lower MCHC and prevent polymerization has also been tried. Success has been hampered by the complexity of the protocols involved. Since HbF inhibits HbS polymerization, antineoplastic agents that are capable of switching on HbF expression (e.g., hydroxyurea) hold promise. In initial studies this manipulation appears to decrease the rate of hemolysis as well as the number of irreversibly sickled cells. Although more difficult to ascertain, the number of painful crises may also be reduced.

In certain high-risk patients, partial exchange transfusion with normal blood can be performed in an attempt to minimize complications. Enough of the patient's blood is removed and replaced by normal blood to obtain a final hematocrit of between 0.30 and 0.35 with at least 50 percent hemoglobin A. This treatment has been used for life-threatening complications such as cerebrovascular accidents, as well as to prevent complications of pregnancy or surgery. The risks of transfusion-related infection, iron overload, and allosensitization to red cell antigens and the lack of controlled studies to demonstrate the effectiveness of transfusion present serious drawbacks to the routine use of this mode of therapy.

PRENATAL DETECTION

Prenatal diagnosis of sickle cell disease is now possible. Fetal cells are obtained by amniocentesis. Cellular DNA is treated with a "restriction" enzyme (Dde I or Mst II), which always cuts DNA in the same place (in this case a certain location on the β-chain locus). One site at which this enzyme cuts the normal β-globin gene is the place where the sickle mutation occurs. If the mutation is present, that cutting site is abolished, resulting in a DNA fragment (detected with a molecular probe and hybridization techniques) that is longer than normal. The genotype of the fetus is indicated by the length of the DNA fragments retrieved. A shorter fragment means the fetus is normal; a longer fragment means the fetus has sickle cell anemia; a mixture of long and short indicates sickle cell trait. Gene analysis of fetal DNA is now possible with chorionic villous biopsy at only 9 to 10 weeks of gestation.

Hemoglobin C Syndromes

Since hemoglobin C (HbC) is probably the second most common hemoglobinopathy (2–3% gene frequency in black populations), four important hemoglobin C syndromes will be discussed. HbC is caused by substitution of lysine for glutamic acid in the sixth position from the N-terminal end of the β-hemoglobin chain (same location as the substitution in HbS).

HEMOGLOBIN C TRAIT (HbAC)

Hemoglobin C trait is the most commonly encountered syndrome. Patients are asymptomatic and not anemic. The peripheral blood smear shows increased numbers of target cells (Plate 19), and hemoglobin electrophoresis reveals about 40 percent hemoglobin C migrating faster than HbS but slower than HbA.

HEMOGLOBIN C DISEASE (HbCC)

Hemoglobin C disease is characterized by a mild hemolytic anemia associated with splenomegaly and by a peripheral blood smear showing many target cells and some microspherocytes. Hemoglobin C crystals may appear after slow drying of a peripheral blood smear and may account for the marked targeting, with puddling and then crystallization of hemoglobin in the center of these cells. Occasionally these patients can have acute episodes of hemolysis when stressed, particularly by infections. In some cases they have gallstones. Since the prognosis is good, little is required in the way of therapy.

HEMOGLOBIN SC DISEASE (HbSC)

Hemoglobin SC disease is of intermediate severity between hemoglobin SS disease and hemoglobin CC disease. Patients may have a mild anemia, with hemoglobins ranging from 10 to 13 gm/dL and a reticulocytosis of 3 to 10 percent. In the peripheral smear, target cells are more prominent than sickled cells. The latter are often difficult to find. Hemoglobin electrophoresis shows equal amounts of hemoglobins S and C. The clinical course varies from asymptomatic to severe. The major vasoocclusive complications of HbSS, such as bone or joint crises, abdominal crises, pulmonary infarction, priapism, stroke, or gallstones, are generally uncommon. Interestingly, other complications of HbSS occur more frequently in patients with HbSC; these include aseptic necrosis of the femoral heads, renal papillary necrosis, proliferative retinopathy, and pregnancy-related problems. More than half of these patients have splenomegaly, but splenic hypofunction may sometimes be present, putting these patients at risk for sepsis.

HEMOGLOBIN C–β-THALASSEMIA (HbC–THAL)

HbC–thalassemia resembles HbCC disease clinically, but the concentration of HbC is greater than 50 percent. HbA may or may not be detectable. Occasionally, if HbA is absent, family studies are needed to distinguish HbC–thalassemia from HbCC. The disorder is usually symptomless; however, if a patient lacks HbA, moderate hemolysis may be present.

Hemoglobinopathies Associated with Cyanosis

Cyanosis can be caused either by increased levels of deoxyhemoglobin (> 5 gm/dL) or by the presence of methemoglobin. Methemoglobin is hemoglobin in which the iron moiety of heme is maintained in the ferric (Fe^{+++}) rather than the ferrous (Fe^{++}) state. Methemoglobinemia occurs if the enzyme systems of the red cell are unable, because of inherited defects or overwhelming oxidant stress, to maintain iron in the ferrous state. Toxic methemoglobinemia due to drugs has been reported with amyl nitrite (coronary artery vasodilator); acetanilid and phenacetin (analgesics); prilocaine (local anesthetic); dapsone; sulfonamide (sulfa antibiotic); menadione (vitamin K analogue); and naphthalene (moth balls). G-6-PD deficiency will enhance methemoglobin production.

Inherited abnormal hemoglobins with light absorption spectra somewhat different from those of normal methemoglobin arise from amino acid substitutions in the microenvironment surrounding the heme group. These *M hemoglobins* have substitutions in their α- or β-chains that fix the heme iron in a ferric state. The cyanotic or brownish color of an affected person's skin is secondary to the abnormal light absorption properties of the HbM hemes. They are detected by special electrophoretic techniques or by their spectroscopic characteristics. Other abnormal hemoglobins cause cyanosis because of their abnormally low affinity for oxygen (see p. 169) rather than by production of methemoglobin.

Patients with cyanosis or a purplish, brownish, or slate gray appearance to their skin since birth should be given a battery of tests: spectroscopic measurement of deoxyhemoglobin and methemoglobin concentrations, assay of the methemoglobin reduction enzyme systems, evaluation of oxygen affinity, and test for electrophoretically abnormal or unstable hemoglobins, and they should be asked about exposure to methemoglobin-producing drugs.

The cyanide moiety (CN) binds to heme and prevents normal oxygenation. Furthermore, normal respiration of the hemoglobin molecule is disturbed even if only one of the four heme groups is bound to CN. As a result of this abnormal heme—heme interaction, the oxygen dissociation curve becomes markedly abnormal and oxygen loading is markedly decreased at any given oxygen concentration. Death from cyanide poisoning actually results from the binding of CN to cytochrome oxidase, which inhibits this key enzyme in cellular respiration and causes cytotoxic hypoxia. In the presence of methemoglobin, which has a high affinity for CN, the formation of the cytochrome oxidase—CN complex is minimal. Therefore nitrites are administered to cyanide victims therapeutically in order to convert hemoglobin to methemoglobin.

Hemoglobinopathies Associated with Unstable Hemoglobins (Heinz Body Hemolytic Anemia)

Unstable, readily denaturable hemoglobins are the result of amino acid substitutions in areas critical to oxygen binding, at sites in the interior of the molecule, in helical regions, and at contacts between globin chains. Because the substitution often affects heme function, unstable hemoglobins may have increased or decreased oxygen affinity. These unstable hemoglobins are detected by the presence of a hemoglobin fraction that precipitates on incubation at 50°C or in buffered isopropanol at 37°C; by an abnormal electrophoretic band; or by the appearance of Heinz bodies, cytoplasmic inclusions made of denatured hemoglobin, in blood smears. These Heinz bodies can only be visualized with phase microscopy or supravital staining, and are seen particularly after splenectomy. Hemolytic anemia of varying severity is found in patients with unstable hemoglobins, and a hemolytic crisis may follow use of sulfa drugs. Interestingly, variability in the phenotypic expression of hemoglobin$_{Zürich}$ may be secondary to its high affinity for carbon monoxide and to stabilization of this unstable hemoglobin by carbon monoxide from cigarette smoking.

Hemoglobin$_{Köln}$ is probably the most commonly encountered example of an unstable hemoglobin. The anemia associated with it may be mild or severe and is not usually improved by splenectomy. Hemoglobin$_{Zürich}$ is expressed clinically only after exposure to sulfa drugs.

The sequence of events in the denaturation of unstable hemoglobins involves oxidation of heme iron, separation of unlike hemoglobin chains, formation of hemichromes (subunits with heme attached), heme–globin dissociation, and finally Heinz body formation. In some cases heme has been found in the Heinz bodies. Liberated heme is catabolized to dark brown dipyrroles (e.g., mesobilifuscin), which are excreted in the urine.

Normally in oxyhemoglobin there is polarization of the electron shared by the heme iron and bound oxygen. This shared electron is returned to the heme iron when oxygen is released from hemoglobin, and the iron therefore retains its ferrous (Fe^{++}) state. The return of the electron to iron is prevented if water enters the pocket in which heme sits. As a result superoxide (O_2^-) radicals (activated oxygen) are released. Methemoglobin production increases greatly if an amino acid substitution allows distortion of the heme pocket (e.g., hemoglobin$_{St. Louis}$), with increased entry of water or other small anions, increased production of superoxide, and oxidation of hemoglobin to methemoglobin. These changes also lead to denaturation and Heinz body formation.

Besides their appearance with unstable hemoglobins, Heinz bodies may be found in the blood or bone marrow of patients with thalassemia, HbH disease, or G-6-PD deficiency, or after ingestion of phenylhydrazine, phenacetin, naphthalene, nitrofurantoin, sulfasalazine, sulfa drugs, dapsone, or other oxidant drugs.

Hemoglobinopathies Associated with Abnormal Oxygen Affinity

Increased oxygen affinity (decreased P_{50}) is found not only with unstable hemoglobins such as Köln, Zürich, and Gun Hill but also with stable hemoglobins like Yakima, Rainer, and Bethesda. Tissue anoxia due to impaired release of oxygen initially stimulates erythropoietin production, sometimes resulting in erythrocytosis. Whether erythrocytosis develops depends on the concentration of the abnormal hemoglobin, its stability, and the nature of the mutation. Many of these hemoglobins have a defect at $\alpha_1\beta_2$ contact points or at the carboxyterminal end of the β-chain. These defects impair hemoglobin oxygenation, heme–heme interaction, or binding of 2,3-DPG to deoxyhemoglobin.

Decreased oxygen affinity (increased P_{50}) is found with the unstable hemoglobins Torino, Seattle, and others and with the stable hemoglobin Kansas. Either cyanosis due to increased concentration of deoxyhemoglobin or a lowered hematocrit due to decreased erythropoietin production may result from the decreased binding of oxygen to hemoglobin. The amino acid substitutions are near the heme group or the $\alpha_1\beta_2$ contact point.

Miscellaneous Types of Inherited Hemolytic Anemia

Patients with a blood type Rh_{null} have shortened red cell survival. Anemia is mild to moderate, but a characteristic stomatocytosis is seen on the blood smear. The etiology is believed to be a membrane abnormality associated with the absence of all Rh antigens on the red cell. Patients with Wilson's disease, an inherited disease associated with high serum copper levels, also suffer from hemolytic anemia. It is thought that hemolysis is due to increased oxidative stress on erythrocytes. About one third of patients with Gilbert's syndrome, an inherited disease associated with high levels of unconjugated bilirubin in an otherwise asymptomatic patient, have hemolytic anemia, which is often unexplained but may be due to a coexisting congenital hemolytic disease such as HS. These unusual causes of hemolytic anemia should not be considered until more common causes have been ruled out.

Approach to Patient with Hereditary Hemolytic Anemia

On the basis of the patient's history, physical examination, and blood smear, in particular the red cell morphology, a hereditary hemolytic anemia can usually be assigned to one of three categories. These are listed in Table 7-1 along with the associated erythrocyte abnormalities. Confirmatory tests are then performed to define the diagnosis further. For example, a finding of many target cells in a moderately anemic black patient with splenomegaly suggests the presence of a hemoglobinopathy. Hemoglobin electrophoresis may confirm the diagnosis of HbC disease. Indiscriminate laboratory screening without an adequate history, physical examination, or study of the peripheral blood smear is wasteful not only of laboratory resources but also of patients' money.

Approach to patient with hereditary hemolytic anemia

I. History
  A. Drug ingestion (oxidant drugs)
  B. Childhood anemia
  C. Gallstones
  D. Jaundice
  E. Family history of anemia, jaundice, splenomegaly, gallstones
II. Physical examination
  A. Pallor
  B. Jaundice
  C. Splenomegaly
  D. Skeletal and facial abnormalities suggestive of marrow expansion
III. Laboratory data
  A. Complete blood count
  B. Red cell morphology
  C. Reticulocyte count
  D. Haptoglobin, LDH, unconjugated bilirubin
IV. Tests to be considered after initial evaluation
  A. Family studies
  B. Hemoglobin electrophoresis
  C. Heinz body preparation
  D. Erythrocyte enzyme studies
  E. Osmotic fragility and autohemolysis
  F. Hemoglobin heat stability or isopropanol test
  G. X-rays of skull, hands, and long bones

Table 7-1. Morphologic red cell abnormalities with inherited hemolytic anemias

Anemia	Red cell abnormalities on blood smear
Membrane disorders	
Hereditary spherocytosis	Spherocytes
	Polychromasia
	Elevated MCHC
Hereditary elliptocytosis	Elliptocytes
	Poikilocytosis
Hereditary pyropoikilocytosis	Poikilocytosis
	Fragments
	Spherocytes
	Elliptocytes
	Depressed MCV
Enzyme disorders	
G-6-PD deficiency	Bite cells
	Heinz bodies (special stains required)
	Polychromasia
Pyruvate kinase deficiency	Acanthocytes
	Polychromasia
Pyrimidine-5'-nucleotidase deficiency	Basophilic stippling
Hemoglobinopathies	
HbS	Sickle cells
	Target cells
	Polychromasia
HbC	Target cells

Case Development Problems: Inherited Hemolytic Anemias

Each of the following patients has a hereditary hemolytic anemia. Indicate the mechanism(s) for the pathogenesis of the hemolytic anemia in each case.

1. An 18-year-old boy has a normal hemoglobin, many spherocytes in his peripheral blood, and Howell-Jolly bodies in his red cells.

   This patient may have been born with congenital spherocytosis. A splenectomy was done to cure his disease, but this left him with spherocytes in his peripheral blood and Howell-Jolly bodies in his red cells. The latter are remnants of DNA that are seen when the spleen has been removed.

2. A healthy 25-year-old black man with no history of anemia ingested primaquine as malarial prophylaxis. Within 3 days he had an episode of hemoglobinuria and was found to be anemic (hematocrit 30%) with a reticulocytosis of 8 percent. G-6-PD screen was reportedly normal at that time. By the time he was referred to you 2 weeks later, his hematocrit and reticulocyte count had normalized. His peripheral smear was notable only for occasional bite cells.

   This patient almost certainly has G-6-PD deficiency. Unlike other patients with congenital hemolytic anemias, he does not display hemolysis in the absence of a drug or metabolic stress. An acute hemolytic crisis was precipitated in this patient by primaquine ingestion. Older cells are destroyed, but younger ones with adequate G-6-PD levels are not lysed. Since the reticulocytes are rich in G-6-PD, the G-6-PD screening test done during a reticulocytosis is invalid. An ascorbate cyanide test would have reflected the G-6-PD deficiency during the reticulocytosis. After the reticulocytosis has resolved, a repeat G-6-PD test should demonstrate the deficiency. The persistence of bite cells is a clue that hemolysis has occurred. Bite cells result from the removal of red cell inclusions of denatured hemoglobin (Heinz bodies) and may persist for several days or weeks after the hemolytic episode.

3. A 10-year-old black girl was found to have splenomegaly on routine physical examination. Her health history was unremarkable. CBC showed a hematocrit of 33 percent with normal Wintrobe indices. Reticulocyte count was 3 percent. Peripheral smear showed many target cells, occasional sickle cells, and mild polychromasia. A sodium metabisulfite test was positive. Bilirubin was mildly elevated at 2.2 mg/dL, all indirect. Review of her parents' CBCs showed normal hematocrits and indices.

Her father's peripheral smear was normal, while her mother's smear showed frequent target cells.

Despite the positive sickle test, many features of this patient's presentation suggest that the diagnosis is not HbSS. Splenomegaly, while present in the first few years of life in patients with HbSS, should have disappeared before age 10 because of repeated splenic infarcts. In addition, patients with HbSS are usually more anemic and more symptomatic with painful crises by this age. This patient's picture is also inconsistent with HbAS, an asymptomatic condition, since the patient has evidence of mild hemolysis and has an abnormal smear. Additional clues to the diagnosis are the presence of target cells and sickle cells in her peripheral smear and target cells in her mother's smear. Hemoglobin electrophoresis showed this patient to have HbSC. These patients may be asymptomatic, like this girl, or may have a picture suggestive of mild to moderate HbSS. Splenomegaly is seen in more than 50 percent of patients with SC disease. The patient's mother has HbAC, and the patient's father has HbAS.

4. A 17-year-old black female with known HbSS presents with persistent fatigue and dyspnea on exertion after a recent viral infection. CBC shows a hematocrit of 15 percent with normal Wintrobe indices and a reticulocyte count of 1 percent. Her usual hematocrit is 25 percent. Mild leukopenia and thrombocytopenia are present as well. Peripheral smear is notable for sickled cells and the absence of polychromasia.

The patient's picture is suggestive of an aplastic crisis seen in HbSS. Intercurrent infections, bacterial or viral, are capable of suppressing the marrow's response to chronic hemolysis. Parvovirus, in particular, is implicated because of its predilection for immature erythroid cells. An alternative etiology to consider is folate depletion. Patients with chronic hemolysis require folate supplementation because of the high turnover of marrow cells. In the setting of folate deficiency, DNA synthesis is slowed and pancytopenia ensues.

5. A 25-year-old man of German ancestry is referred for evaluation of persistent jaundice despite splenectomy for a diagnosis of hereditary spherocytosis. He gives a history of lifelong scleral icterus and hyperbilirubinemia, although his hematocrits have always been normal. CBC shows a hematocrit of 40 percent with normal Wintrobe indices except for an MCV of 105fL. The reticulocyte count is 6 percent. Peripheral smear shows macrocytes, polychromasia, and Howell-Jolly bodies, but no spherocytes. Urine is mahogany colored. A Heinz body test is positive.

This patient has the unstable hemoglobin, $Hb_{Köln}$. More than 100 cases have been described, many of them in patients of Dutch or German ancestry. $Hb_{Köln}$ is characterized by well-compensated hemolysis and the findings in this case are characteristic. Heinz bodies are readily apparent after splenectomy. The dark urine is due to the pigment derived from degradation of heme released when Heinz bodies are metabolized. Pigmenturia does not correlate with the degree of hemolysis or jaundice. The absence of spherocytes in the smear and the lack of response to splenectomy demonstrate the error in the initial diagnosis of hereditary spherocytosis.

Topics for Discussion: Hereditary Hemolytic Anemias

Primary defect in hereditary spherocytosis
Relationship of congenital elliptocytosis to congenital spherocytosis
Red cell membrane sodium and potassium pumps
Structure and function relationships in G-6-PD variants
Abnormalities of glutathione and related enzymes in hemolytic anemia
Hemoglobin structure and the unstable hemoglobinopathies
Hemoglobins with abnormal oxygen affinity
Mild sickle cell syndromes
Hemoglobin F in thalassemia, sickle cell disease, and other hemoglobinopathies
Treatment of sickle cell disease
Molecular basis for sickle cell disease
Structure and function of spleen
Indications for and complications of splenectomy

Selected Readings

General Considerations

Dacie, J. V. *Haemolytic Anemias. Part I: The Congenital Anaemias* (2nd ed.). New York: Grune & Stratton, 1960.
Jacob, H. S. (ed.). Blood cell membranes I, II. *Semin. Hematol.* 16 : 1 : 95, 1979.
Jandl, J. H. *Blood: Textbook of Hematology.* Boston: Little, Brown, 1987.
Nathan, D. G., and Oski, F. A. *Hematology of Infancy and Childhood* (3rd ed.). Philadelphia: Saunders, 1987.
Rao, K. R. P. et al. Infection with parvovirus-like virus and aplastic crisis in chronic hemolytic anemia. *Ann. Intern. Med.* 98 : 930, 1983.

Hereditary Elliptocytosis/Spherocytosis

Agre, P., Orringer, E. P., and Bennett, V. Deficient red-cell spectrin in severe, recessively inherited spherocytosis. *N. Engl. J. Med.* 306 : 1155, 1982.

Becker, P. S., and Lux, S. E. Hereditary spherocytosis and related disorders. *Clin. Haematol.* 14 : 15, 1985.

Goodman, S. R. et al. Identification of the molecular defect in the erythrocyte membrane skeleton of some kindreds with hereditary spherocytosis. *Blood* 60 : 772, 1982.

Jandl, J. H. *Blood: Textbook of Hematology.* Section 7, Hemolytic Anemias Caused by Primary Defects of Red Cell Membranes. Boston: Little, Brown, 1987. pp. 237–257.

Knowles, W., Marchesi, S. L., and Marchesi, V. T. Spectrin: Structure, function and abnormalities. *Semin. Hematol.* 20 : 159, 1983.

Lux, S. E., and Wolfe, L. C. Inherited disorders of the red cell membrane skeleton. *Pediatr. Clin. N. Am.* 27 : 463, 1980.

Marchesi, V. T. The red cell membrane skeleton: Recent progress. *Blood* 61 : 1, 1983.

Palek, J. Hereditary elliptocytosis and related disorders. *Clin. Haematol.* 14 : 45, 1985.

Shohet, S. B. Spectrin and spherocytosis. *N. Engl. J. Med.* 306 : 1170, 1982.

Wintrobe, M. M. et al. Hereditary Spherocytosis and Other Hemolytic Anemias Associated with Abnormalities of the Red Cell Membrane. In M. M. Wintrobe et al. (eds.), *Clinical Hematology* (8th ed.). Philadelphia: Lea & Febiger, 1981.

Wolfe, L. C. et al. A genetic defect in the binding of protein 4.1 to spectrin in a kindred with hereditary spherocytosis. *N. Engl. J. Med.* 307 : 1367, 1982.

Erythrocyte Enzyme Deficiencies—
Congenital Nonspherocytic Hemolytic Anemias

Beutler, E. *Red Cell Metabolism: A Manual of Biochemical Methods* (2nd ed.). New York: Grune & Stratton, 1975.

Beutler, E. Red cell enzyme defects as nondiseases and as diseases. *Blood* 54 : 1, 1979.

Carrell, R. W., Winterbourn, C. C., and Rachmilewitz, E. A. Activated oxygen and haemolysis. *Br. J. Haematol.* 30 : 259, 1975.

Desforges, J. Genetic implications of G-6PD deficiency. *N. Engl. J. Med.* 294 : 1438, 1976.

Dreyfus, J. C., and Kahn, A. Red cell enzymopathies: Molecular mechanisms. *Clin. Biochem.* 17 : 331, 1984.

Jandl, J. H. *Blood: Textbook of Hematology.* Section 11, Heinz Body Hemolytic Anemia, and Section 12, Hemolytic Anemias Caused by Genetic Deficiencies in Glycolytic Enzymes. Boston: Little, Brown, 1987. pp. 335–360.

Mentzer, W. C. (ed.). Enzymopathies. *Clin. Haematol.* 10 : 3, 1981.

Miwa, S. et al. Four new pyruvate kinase (PK) variants and a classical deficiency. *Br. J. Haematol.* 29 : 157, 1975.

Valentine, W. N. Hemolytic anemia and inborn errors of metabolism. *Blood* 54 : 549, 1979.

Hemoglobinopathies

Alter, B. P. Advances in the prenatal diagnosis of hematologic diseases. *Blood* 64 : 329, 1984.

Bunn, F. H., and Forget, B. G. *Hemoglobin: Molecular, Genetic and Clinical Aspects.* Philadelphia: Saunders, 1986.

Dover, G. J. et al. Individual variation in the production and survival of F cells in sickle-cell disease. *N. Engl. J. Med.* 299 : 1428, 1978.

Hebbel, R. P., Moldow, C. F., and Steinberg, M. H. Modulation of erythrocyte-endothelial interactions and the vasoocclusive severity of sickling disorders. *Blood* 58 : 947, 1981.

Higgs, D. R. et al. The interaction of alpha-thalassemia and homozygous sickle-cell disease. *N. Engl. J. Med.* 306 : 1441, 1982.

Jandl, J. H. *Blood: Textbook of Hematology.* Section 13, Abnormal Hemoglobins and Hemoglobinopathies. Boston: Little, Brown, 1987. pp. 361–395.

Mears, J. G. et al. The sickle gene polymorphism in North Africa. *Blood* 58 : 599, 1981.

Murayama, M. Molecular mechanism of red cell sickling. *Science* 153 : 145, 1966.

Nathan, D. G., and Oski, F. A. *Hematology of Infancy and Childhood* (3rd ed.). Chapter 21, Methemoglobinemia. Philadelphia: Saunders, 1987. pp. 641–654.

Noguchi, C. T., and Schechter, A. N. The intracellular polymerization of sickle hemoglobin and its relevance to sickle cell disease. *Blood* 58 : 1057, 1981.

Orkin, S. H. Prenatal diagnosis of hemoglobin disorders by DNA analysis. *Blood* 63 : 249, 1984.

Schechter, A. N., and Bunn, H. F. What determines severity in sickle-cell disease? *N. Engl. J. Med.* 306 : 295, 1982.

Smith, R. P., and Olson, M. V. Drug-induced methemoglobinemia. *Semin. Hematol.* 10 : 253, 1973.

Steinberg, M. Review: The sickle hemoglobinopathies—genetic analyses of common phenocopies and new molecular approaches to treatment. *Am. J. Med. Sci.* 288 : 169, 1984.

Weatherall, D. J. (ed.). Haemoglobin: Structure, function and synthesis. *Br. Med. Bull.* 32 : 193, 1976.

8 Acquired Hemolytic Anemias: Immunohemolytic Anemias, Fragmentation Hemolysis, Hypersplenism, Chemicals and Toxins, PNH

Margot S. Kruskall

A variety of acquired clinical conditions result in shortened survival of previously normal red cells. These include immune-mediated destruction, red cell fragmentation disorders, acquired membrane defects, splenic effects, and the results of infections and environmental toxins. This chapter is subdivided according to the major types of acquired hemolytic anemia.

Immunohemolytic Anemias

Immunohemolytic anemias are the result of the binding of antibody, complement, or antibody plus complement to red cells. Antibodies formed against erythrocyte antigens may be either warm (active at 37°C) or cold (active at room temperature and below). In some cases, these antibodies activate a series of proteins, referred to collectively as complement; in others, the red cells are coated with antibody alone. As a result of complement activation by hemolytic antibodies, intravascular red cell lysis and release of hemoglobin may occur. Alternatively, and more frequently, immune lysis, due to either antibody or complement, is extravascular and happens slowly within cells of the macrophagic–phagocytic system (RES), particularly in the spleen.

Hemolytic Anemia, Antibodies, and Complement

Antibodies and complement play various roles in the pathogenesis of immunohemolytic anemias. The human complement system consists of many plasma protein components. A subunit of the first component of complement, C1, contains a combining site for the Fc portion of immunoglobulins and initiates the complement cascade. This C1 subunit reacts with IgG or IgM antibodies that have combined with their corresponding antigen. In the case of IgG antibodies, which are small in comparison to IgM, close proximity to one another is required to activate complement. Because red cell antigens are often widely separated, complement activation by IgG antibodies is uncommon. Hemolysis is typically "extravascular":

IgG-coated cells are destroyed within phagocytic cells. By contrast, two subunits of the same IgM molecule may serve to activate the first component of complement. As a result of the initial activation of C1 components, C4, C2, and then C3 are fixed and activated on the red cell. Complement components 5 through 9 may then be activated. This complete cascade leads to changes in the erythrocyte membrane, which, on electron microscopic examination, appear as transmembrane holes or pores. Hemoglobin leaks out, water is drawn in, and red cell lysis occurs. Thus, IgM antibodies can initiate severe "intravascular" hemolysis. In some instances complement is found on the red cell membrane without explanation. Both in these situations and in IgM-mediated hemolysis, the complement activation sequence frequently is not completed and hemolysis is extravascular.

Red Cell Destruction in Immunohemolytic Anemias

Antibody- and complement-coated red cells are generally sequestered and destroyed within mononuclear phagocytic cells, particularly in the spleen. If the spleen is removed, or the red cells are heavily coated with antibody, the liver may play a significant role in clearance of coated erythrocytes. In such situations, called *extravascular hemolysis*, hemoglobin is degraded to bilirubin, and the plasma level of unconjugated bilirubin is increased. In addition, bilirubin conjugated in the liver is excreted by the kidney and the intestines. In other cases, particularly where complement is strongly activated, such as paroxysmal nocturnal hemoglobinuria and ABO-incompatible transfusion reactions, destruction of red cells is largely *intravascular*. Plasma hemoglobin, hemoglobinuria, and urine hemosiderin are typical laboratory findings consistent with intravascular destruction. However, these laboratory findings may also be found in very severe cases of extravascular hemolysis. Serum haptoglobin is low in both extra- and intravascular hemolysis.

Classification of the Immunohemolytic Anemias

Immunohemolytic anemias fall into one of three major categories: autoimmune, in which the patient makes an autoantibody against his or her own red cells; alloimmune, where the patient's antibody is directed against foreign red cells; and drug-induced, where a drug-dependent or related antibody is responsible for hemolysis (Table 8-1).

Pathogenesis of Immunohemolytic Anemia

The surface of human red blood cells is covered with substances capable of provoking an immune reaction; these substances are

Table 8-1. Classification of immunohemolytic anemias

I. Autoimmune hemolytic anemia
  A. Warm autoimmune hemolytic anemia
  B. Cold agglutinin syndrome
  C. Paroxysmal cold hemoglobinuria
II. Drug-induced hemolytic anemias
III. Alloimmune hemolytic anemia
  A. Transfusion reactions
  B. Hemolytic anemia of the newborn

known as *blood group antigens*. The most important groups of red cell antigens are the ABO and Rh systems; in addition to these there are at least 400 other substances (see Chap. 9). Usually, the healthy immune system produces antibodies only to foreign antigens. Thus, for example, a membrane antigen on a transfused red cell may stimulate the production of antibodies in an individual if his or her own red cells lack that antigen. By contrast, in autoimmune hemolytic anemias, the immune system produces antibodies against the body's own red cell antigens. When this happens, red cells become coated with antibody, complement, or both.

There is no generally accepted explanation for why patients produce autoantibodies against their own red cells. Some investigators have suggested that minor damage to red cells leads a normal immune system to sense them as being foreign and therefore produce antibodies against them. However, it has not been demonstrated that the red cells of patients suffering from autoimmune hemolytic anemias actually have abnormal antigenic structures. Alternatively, the immune system may become deranged, falsely sensing normal red cell antigens as foreign, and producing autoantibodies in response. The cause of this derangement may be acquired, perhaps by infection with certain viruses. Animal models provide evidence that viruses can modify normal immune responses. Furthermore, inherited immune response genes may predispose certain individuals to autoimmune phenomena. Evidence for this exists in certain mouse strains, in which autoimmune hemolytic anemia is easily induced through the injection of autologous red cells mixed with an adjuvant. Family studies in humans also have yielded evidence suggesting genetic predispositions to autoimmune diseases. Finally, it is possible that a disorder of T cells, such as qualitatively or quantitatively abnormal T suppressor cells, may allow the development of otherwise forbidden autoantibodies.

Warm Antibody Autoimmune Hemolytic Anemia

This illness, more common than the two other autoimmune hemolytic anemias (cold agglutinin syndrome and paroxysmal cold hemoglobinuria), occurs in 1 to 3 individuals per 100,000 in the population. Approximately half of the cases are in patients already affected with other illness, such as lupus and chronic lymphocytic leukemia and lymphoma. This form of warm autoimmune hemolytic anemia (AIHA) is called "secondary." Other patients, with no associated diseases, are said to have "idiopathic" AIHA.

The initial presentation of warm AIHA is variable, depending on the rapidity of onset and severity of the anemia. In some patients, symptoms of anemia and signs of jaundice may predominate; more severe cases present with fever, abdominal or back pain, and red or dark brown urine. Mild to moderate splenomegaly is common.

The hematocrit may be nearly normal, or extremely low (<15%). The reticulocyte count is nearly always elevated, which helps compensate for the red cell destruction. However, 5 to 10 percent of cases may have reticulocytopenia. The white count may be elevated during active hemolysis. Occasional patients develop simultaneous thrombocytopenia, which also appears to have an autoimmune etiology; this combination of AIHA and thrombocytopenia is called "Evan's syndrome." The peripheral blood smear usually shows spherocytes, polychromatophils (when the reticulocyte count is increased) (Plate 25), and often some agglutination of red cells.

In general the rate of hemolysis is proportional to the concentration of cell-bound antibody. Some patients with relatively weak positive direct antiglobulin tests do not hemolyze at all. In others, hemolysis occurs so slowly that the bone marrow can increase erythrocyte production sufficiently to maintain a normal hematocrit, a *compensated autoimmune hemolytic anemia.*

LABORATORY TESTS

The hallmark of autoimmune hemolytic anemia is the presence of antibody or complement, or both, on the patient's own red cells. In the clinical blood bank laboratory, this is detected using the direct antiglobulin test (direct Coombs' test). Many blood bank tests (for example, ABO typing) depend on the ability of antibody-coated red cells to form agglutinates. However, red cells coated with IgG antibodies frequently will not agglutinate in a test tube. These antibodies are usually too small to span the distance between red cells, which are normally repelled from each other by their negative surface charges (ζ potential). In addition, cells coated only with complement will not agglutinate. However, the direct antiglobulin (Coombs) test solves this problem. Coombs reagent is an antiserum raised in rabbits against human γ-globulins and complement components. When added to IgG- or complement-sensitized red cells, these additional antibodies are able to bridge the gaps between red cells (Fig. 8-1). Agglutination indicates the presence of antibody or complement components, or both. Further information can be obtained from the strength of the reaction (1+ to 4+, where 4+ is

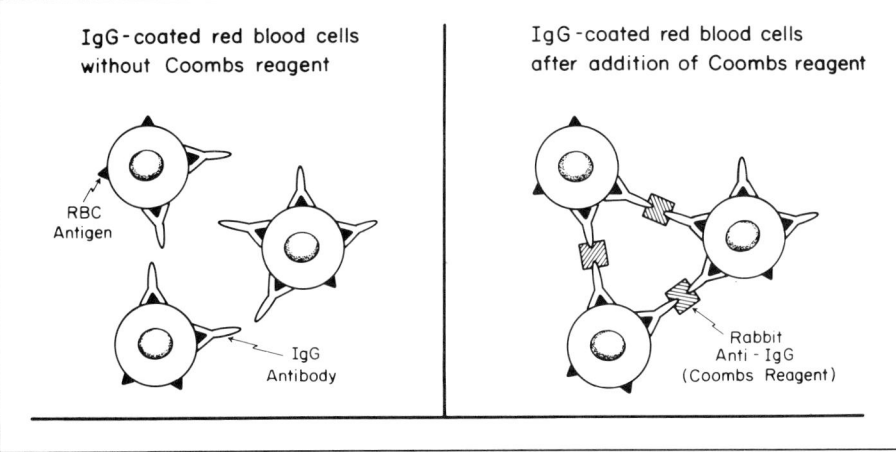

Fig. 8-1. The Coombs test: addition of Coombs reagent (antibody to human IgG, raised in rabbits) leads to agglutination of IgG-coated red cells. A similar reagent can be used to detect C3-coated cells. Usually a broad spectrum Coombs reagent containing both anti-IgG and anti-C3 is used first to look for either IgG or C3, or both proteins, on the red cell membrane. Then separate anti-IgG and anti-C3 reagents are used to determine the specificity of the reaction.

the strongest), and by using monospecific Coombs reagents (directed against γ-globulin only or complement only). When IgG is present on red cells, its specificity (the antigen it is directed against) can frequently be ascertained by stripping the antibody off the red cell and reacting this *eluate* with an assortment of other cells.

"Coombs tests" ("direct" and "indirect") are frequently confused and improperly ordered. The direct Coombs test, or direct antiglobulin test, is used to test a patient's red cells for antibody and complement components. The test is performed directly on the red cells, and on additional reagent red cells as needed. The phrase "indirect Coombs test" is a misnomer; what is actually performed is an "antibody screen." Here a patient's *serum* is tested for red cell antibodies. The serum is added to normal group O red cells; the cells are washed and Coombs reagent is added to enhance agglutination due to coating of the normal red cells with antibody in the patient's serum. The antibody screen is very useful in the diagnosis of immune hemolysis. It is also routinely performed during transfusion compatibility testing (the type and screen; see Chap. 9). The usual findings for the direct Coombs test and antibody screen in different disorders, which will be discussed in subsequent sections, are shown in Table 8-2.

In warm AIHA one may sometimes find both IgG and complement on the red cells, although in many cases only one is present. In a very small percentage of cases, the direct Coombs test is negative.

Table 8-2. Interpreting the direct Coombs test and antibody screen

Direct Coombs test	Antibody screen* (identification)	Interpretation
Positive	Negative	Autoimmune hemolytic anemia Drug-induced ABO-mediated acute hemolysis
Positive	Positive (Panagglutinin)	Autoimmune hemolytic anemia (high-titer antibody) α-Methyldopa (Aldomet)
	(Red cell specificity)	Non-ABO hemolytic transfusion reaction Paroxysmal cold hemoglobinuria
Negative	Positive (Red cell specificity)	Recent or distant allosensitization to red cell antigen

*Also known as the indirect Coombs test.

In such cases, an autoantibody is present, but in amounts too small to be detected by the standard Coombs test (threshold is 100 molecules of IgG), and specialized testing is required.

The specificity of the autoantibody causing warm AIHA has never been conclusively determined. As a rule, such antibodies are "panagglutinins," in that they can cause agglutination of many different types of cells in addition to the patient's own. Typically, the only cells with which warm autoantibodies do not react are those rare red cells that are missing some or all Rh antigens (Rh_{null} cells). It has been proposed that these autoantibodies recognize some feature common to all glycoprotein Rh antigens.

THERAPY

High-dose corticosteroids (60 mg per day or more) are typically the initial treatment for moderate or severe warm AIHA. Corticosteroids primarily affect the clearance of antibody-coated red cells and also reduce antibody synthesis and avidity of the antibody for red cells. Most patients respond within 2 weeks and some as quickly as a few days. Treatment is usually continued for many months. Relatively few patients achieve permanent cures using steroids. Some can be maintained for many years on low doses of steroids (<15 mg per day). However, because of the complications of long-term steroid use, patients who require higher doses should be considered for splenectomy.

Splenectomy is useful because it removes a major site of red cell destruction; in addition, antibody production is reduced. About 60 percent of patients are benefited by this operation. In others, although steroid dependence persists, the dose of drug can be reduced. Complications of splenectomy include perioperative infections, postsplenectomy thrombocytosis, thromboembolism, and death from overwhelming sepsis (more common in children). Although splenic sequestration studies using red cells radiolabeled with chromium 51 have been proposed as a test for predicting response to surgery (a high ratio of spleen to liver red cell uptake being associated with a good response), too many false positive and false negative results are obtained to justify their routine use.

Immunosuppressive drugs such as azathioprine (Imuran) and cyclophosphamide (Cytoxan) are usually reserved for patients in whom steroids and splenectomy have failed (or who have contraindications to the surgery). These drugs must be used with close attention to their side effects, including bone marrow suppression and its complications, such as infection and bleeding, sterilization and teratogenic effects, and later development of leukemia. Other recently reported therapies include high-dose intravenous γ-globulin, danazol, and plasmapheresis.

Blood transfusions carry special risks for patients with warm AIHA. Transfused red cells, like the patient's own red cells, will have a shortened survival because of hemolysis. This is usually of no serious consequence. More importantly, the autoantibody hinders the ability of the laboratory to identify red cell alloantibodies that the patient may have acquired as a result of previous exposure to red cells. Thus, if the patient also had an unrecognized alloantibody to the red cell antigen Jk^a, the transfusion of Jk^a-positive red cells could result in a severe transfusion reaction. Several techniques can be used to remove the patient's autoantibody from the serum, but there are many caveats to their use. Therefore, transfusions should be reserved for patients with severe, symptomatic anemia, after other measures, such as bed rest and oxygen, have already been tried.

Patients with chronic hemolytic anemias of any cause may become deficient in folic acid, which serves only to worsen the already present anemia. For this reason, folic acid, 1 mg per day, should be prescribed.

Cold Agglutinin Syndrome

This hemolytic anemia is less common than its warm counterpart. Cold agglutinin hemolysis occurs both as a self-limited syndrome in association with certain infectious diseases, such as infectious mononucleosis and *Mycoplasma* pneumonia, and as a chronic illness, often without cause, but sometimes accompanying lymphoma and other reticuloendothelial malignancies.

The laboratory features of the antibodies that cause cold agglutinin syndromes are important to the clinical presentation of the patient. These antibodies have specificity against antigens in the blood group system I-i. All human red cells have these antigens; fetal red cells have almost exclusively i, but over the first 18 months after birth, i is largely replaced by I. Cold autoagglutinins directed against I or residual i antigens are IgM pentamers that can agglutinate red cells, since the antibodies' large size enables them to bridge the distance between negatively charged red cells. This occurs predominantly at cold temperatures (4–20°C) but can also occur at body temperature. The patient with cold agglutinins is prone to the development of red cell agglutination in cooler parts of the microcirculation, leading to pain, blanching, and numbness in the toes and fingers, that is, Raynaud's phenomenon. IgM antibodies fix large amounts of complement on red cells, which may then be destroyed either extravascularly within mononuclear phagocytic cells or intravascularly, leading to hemoglobinemia and possibly hemoglobinuria.

The clinical findings in patients with cold agglutinin disease include cyanosis of extremities (acrocyanosis) and skin surfaces exposed to cold, mild jaundice, but usually no splenomegaly. Autoagglutination may interfere with results from automated cell counters and interpretation of blood smears unless care is taken to keep the specimen at 37°C. Spherocytes are not usually seen on blood smears. The direct Coombs test is positive due to the presence of complement; the IgM autoantibody is washed off during the test procedure and is not detected by the Coombs test. The antibody screen is positive, and anti-I is usually identified in high titer.

Chronic cold agglutinin syndromes are difficult to treat. Avoiding cold temperatures is of paramount importance; this step may be sufficient to alleviate hemolysis for patients with mild illness. Daily folic acid should be taken. Corticosteroids are far less effective than in warm AIHA. Immunosuppressive drugs such as chlorambucil have been useful in some patients. Other modalities, such as penicillamine and plasma exchange, are of little benefit except in isolated cases. A search for an underlying diagnosis, such as lymphoma, and treatment of the primary illness often result in amelioration of the hemolysis. Transfusions should be used cautiously. An in-line blood warmer should be used to prevent hemolysis of recently refrigerated red cells during transfusion.

Paroxysmal Cold Hemoglobinuria

This rare disease, characterized by hemoglobinuria following cold exposure, is caused by an IgG autoantibody to the red cell antigen P. This *Donath-Landsteiner autoantibody* is unique in that it binds to red cells at cold temperatures, in contrast to other IgG antibodies. Furthermore, it binds complement well, and brisk hemolysis results when the cells are warmed and the complement sequence proceeds to completion. In the past paroxysmal cold hemoglobinuria (PCH) was primarily a complication of tertiary syphilis, but now that advanced syphilis is less common, PCH is most likely to be associated with recent viral infections (measles, mumps, chickenpox, infectious mononucleosis). Hemolysis often occurs acutely, with the sudden onset of chills, fever, nausea, abdominal pain, and hemoglobinuria; the hemoglobin level falls rapidly. The direct antiglobulin test is positive, but usually only for C3 unless special attempts are made to perform the test at cold temperatures, when IgG may also be found. The Donath-Landsteiner test, which examines for hemolysis after the patient's serum and test red cells are incubated first at 4°C and then at 37°C, will demonstrate the presence of the Donath-Landsteiner autoantibody. Because nearly all cases are self-limited, the long-term prognosis for affected patients is good, and the mainstay of therapy is avoidance of cold temperatures.

Drug-induced Immunohemolytic Anemias

Four pathophysiologic mechanisms (Table 8-3) account for most cases of drug-induced red cell sensitization and positive direct Coombs tests. The drug-induced problem may result in serious hemolytic anemia on the one hand, or a laboratory abnormality without clinical sequelae on the other.

PENICILLIN: "HAPTEN" (DRUG ADSORPTION) MECHANISM

Pencillin binds strongly to the red cell membrane, and can be detected on red cells in many patients who are receiving high doses of this drug (10 million units or more) for conditions such as bacterial endocarditis. Although the drug coating by itself is not harmful, some patients develop high-titer antipenicillin IgG antibodies, which can react with the coated red cells. This may occur in as many as 3 percent of patients receiving high-dose penicillin, and by itself is not necessarily an indication to stop the antibiotic. A small proportion of these patients go on to develop hemolysis. The Coombs test is positive due to the presence of IgG; complement is not usually found. Antibodies can be detected only with penicillin-coated test cells. Cessation of the drug leads to quick amelioration of hemolysis.

QUINIDINE: "INNOCENT BYSTANDER" (IMMUNE COMPLEX) MECHANISM

In some patients previously sensitized to quinidine, and taking it again, the drug reacts with a quinidine antibody, often IgM, to form an immune complex. This complex is then adsorbed onto the red cell membrane; the red cell is considered an "innocent bystander" because it is not the direct target of the antibody. The immune complexes often activate complement, and an abrupt and life-threatening intravascular hemolytic anemia may develop. Sometimes, however,

Table 8-3. Drug-induced positive direct antiglobulin (Coombs) tests

Drug (example)	Mechanism	Coombs test		Eluate	Antibody screen
		IgG	C3		
Penicillin	Hapten	Pos	Neg	Positive with penicillin-treated red cells only	Positive with penicillin-treated red cells only
Quinidine	Innocent bystander (immune complex)	Neg	Pos	Usually negative	Positive only if drug added to test system
α-Methyldopa (Aldomet)	Unknown	Pos	Neg	Positive with all cells; no need for drug in test system	Positive with all cells; no need for drug in test system
Cephalosporins	Membrane modification	Pos	Pos	Neg	Neg

hemolysis is extravascular and of mild to moderate severity as in cold agglutinin disease. The Coombs test is positive for complement; the immune complexes themselves do not bind firmly to the cell. The serum antibody screen is negative unless quinidine is added to the test system. Hemolysis abates once the drug is discontinued. Many other drugs, including quinine, hydralazine, sulfonamides, phenacetin, isoniazid (INH), and rifampin, may occasionally cause hemolysis by this mechanism.

α-METHYLDOPA (ALDOMET): AUTOIMMUNE HEMOLYSIS BY UNKNOWN MECHANISM

In as many as one third of patients taking 2 gm α-methyldopa daily, a positive direct Coombs test develops after 3 to 6 months of use. Far fewer (between 1 and 5%) develop frank hemolysis. In patients taking lower doses of the drug, these serologic problems develop less frequently. The drug itself does not attach to red cells or antibodies, but somehow causes the development of red cell IgG autoantibodies, which closely resemble those found in warm AIHA. Many hypotheses have been put forth for the drug's action, including alteration of red cell antigens so that they appear foreign, or generation of abnormal clones of lymphocytes. The direct Coombs test is usually strongly positive with IgG; complement is rarely found. All patients with frank hemolysis have serum antibodies in addition to antibodies on the red cells. The hemolysis is gradual in onset, but may become quite severe. Levodopa (L-dopa) and mefenamic acid may also cause this type of hemolytic anemia.

Treatment of such patients includes discontinuing the drug, after which the hemolysis usually abates in days to weeks. The direct Coombs test, however, may remain positive for many months. In severe cases, steroids and other modalities used in the treatment of warm AIHA (which this drug-induced picture so closely resembles) can be employed. Blood transfusions should be administered only when absolutely necessary, and with the same precautions described for warm autoimmune hemolytic anemia.

CEPHALOSPORINS: MEMBRANE MODIFICATION

These drugs cause a positive direct Coombs test through a non-immunologic mechanism. Cephalothin and other cephalosporins are capable of altering the red cell membrane so that proteins, including complement and an assortment of γ-globulins, are nonspecifically adsorbed. As a result of the presence of these proteins, the direct antiglobulin test is positive. However, the red cell eluate does not react with any other cells, because the mixture of γ-globulins does not include any predominantly red cell antigen-specific antibody. The antibody screen is negative because no unusual drug-related antibodies are present. Hemolytic anemia does not occur in this situation.

Hemolytic Transfusion Reactions

The differential diagnosis of a positive direct antiglobulin test includes not just red cell autoantibodies but also alloantibodies—antibodies in the patient directed against foreign red cell antigens. These antibodies are either *"naturally occurring,"* in that individuals acquire them without specific exposure to the red cell antigen, or *"immune,"* from red cell transfusions (see Chap. 9).

ACUTE HEMOLYTIC TRANSFUSION REACTIONS

ABO antibodies are the most important example of naturally occurring red cell antibodies (so-called isoantibodies) that can cause severe, even fatal, hemolysis. For example, a patient whose red cells are group O has anti-A and anti-B in his or her serum. Like many other IgM antibodies, these isoagglutinins are potent complement fixers. If inadvertently transfused with group A red cells, this patient's anti-A would immediately react with the donor cells. Complement fixation and intravascular hemolysis would result. Signs and symptoms of acute hemolysis, including fever (the most common finding in such reactions), pain at the IV site, chest and back pain, hemoglobinemia, hemoglobinuria, renal failure, and disseminated intravascular coagulation, often follow. The direct Coombs test is positive due to complement fixation, but may become negative within hours to days, depending on how rapidly the group A cells are destroyed. The presence of urine hemosiderin beginning 3 to 5 days after the transfusion attests to the recent presence of hemoglobinemia. Mortality from ABO-incompatible transfusion reactions may approach 20 percent. Since the problem is almost always due to clerical rather than technical errors, including using for the crossmatch a blood specimen labeled with the wrong patient's name, or transfusing a unit of red cells intended for one patient into another, these reactions should be avoidable.

Most other red cell antibodies are due to sensitization to foreign red cell antigens. These so-called alloantibodies develop sometime after a patient is exposed to the antigen by transfusion. Thus, non-ABO antibodies such as anti-Kell cause red cell destruction only if a previously transfused patient in whom anti-Kell antibodies develop is given Kell-positive red cells again. This situation is uncommon, because an antibody screen is normally performed before every transfusion. However, it may occur if the pretransfusion antibody screen is improperly performed or interpreted, or if a patient requires emergency transfusion and there is insufficient time to perform the antibody screen. Most red cell antibodies that occur in response to immunization are IgG, and many fix complement poorly if at all. Thus, although antigen-positive cells immediately become coated with antibody, rapid intravascular hemolysis is uncommon; instead cells are slowly destroyed in the mononuclear phagocytic system. Symptoms and signs of hemolysis are usually present, as for ABO-mediated hemolysis, but the mortality rate is not as high. The direct Coombs test is positive, due to the presence of the IgG antibodies on the red cell, and becomes weaker and eventually negative as the transfused cells are eliminated. The serum antibody screen is positive both before and after the transfusion, due to the presence of the non-ABO antibody, and may persist indefinitely.

DELAYED HEMOLYTIC TRANSFUSION REACTIONS

In some patients, the titer of non-ABO antibodies after transfusion wanes, and the antibody becomes undetectable. If the patient then receives an antigen-positive unit, an anamnestic rise in antibody occurs over the next 3 to 21 days. This results in *delayed hemolysis.* Here, red cell destruction is usually leisurely, since the cells are eliminated only after they are coated with sufficient antibody, which depends on the rapidity with which it is produced. Often patients are completely asymptomatic, although in some, fever and mild jaundice develop. More serious complications, including renal failure, are rare. The direct Coombs test on a posttransfusion blood specimen is positive due to IgG-coated transfused red cells. The test becomes negative as the antibody-coated cells are removed from the circulation. The patient's antibody screen, negative before the transfusion, becomes positive shortly afterward. To avoid delayed hemolytic transfusion reactions, patients should receive red cells negative for antigens to which they have previously become sensitized for all future transfusions (even if the antibody screen once again becomes negative) and should carry a medical card with information about their antibody history.

Hemolytic Disease of the Newborn

This hemolytic process actually begins in utero to the baby of a mother with IgG red cell antibodies. IgG antibodies readily cross the placenta, as opposed to IgM antibodies, which cannot. In the past, many Rh(D)-negative women became sensitized to the red cell antigen D at the time of birth of a first Rh-positive child, because at birth it is common for a small volume of fetal cells to enter the maternal circulation. Today, Rh sensitization is much less common and largely preventable (see p. 190). Rh-positive fetuses carried by a sensitized Rh-negative mother can be severely affected by the IgG anti-D. Some babies develop profound in utero anemia with congestive heart failure (*hydrops fetalis*), leading to stillbirth. In others, with less severe anemia, rapidly rising serum bilirubin levels (indirect) develop after birth: In utero, the placenta handles bilirubin clearance, but newborns have limited ability to conjugate bilirubin. This leads in some cases to the clinical picture of *kernicterus*, an often irreversible encephalopathy due to accumulation of bilirubin in the brain.

Rh(D) sensitization of the Rh-negative mother is now almost completely preventable through the administration of a small dose of passive anti-D antibody (Rh immunoglobulin) after the birth of an Rh-positive child. In addition, Rh immunoglobulin is given at the beginning of the third trimester of pregnancy in Rh-negative women (because in some women fetal red cells begin to appear in the maternal circulation this early), as well as after miscarriages and abortions. IgG red cell antibodies to other antigens can also cause hemolytic disease of the newborn.

Approach to the Patient with a Coombs Test–positive Hemolytic Anemia

The Coombs test is frequently ordered in the initial evaluation of a patient with a hemolytic anemia. To determine the cause of the positive Coombs test, the approach outlined in Table 8-4 can be helpful.

The Role of the Spleen in Immune Red Cell Destruction

The normal spleen weighs 135 gm, and holds about 1 percent of the total blood volume. It contains T and B lymphocytes as well as elements of the mononuclear–phagocyte system. Abnormal or antibody-coated red cells, such as those found in hereditary spherocytosis, spur cell anemia, and immunohemolytic anemia, are often destroyed in the spleen. Normal red cells are able to traverse small holes in the basement membranes of the splenic sinuses and cords because of their relatively fluid membranes; abnormally rigid cells accumulate in the red pulp. Here they are exposed to the metabolic stresses of hemoconcentration and stagnation, with hypoglycemia and decreased pH. The cells gain Na^+, and lose K^+ and adenosine triphosphate (ATP). The end result of such stress and energy depletion is destruction by splenic phagocytes.

In immunohemolytic anemias, some abnormal cells are able to make a number of trips through the spleen before their demise, but they progressively lose red cell membrane to phagocytic cells, which have receptors for the Fc fragment of the IgG that coats these cells. This surface loss produces spherocytes. Because spherocytes have a decreased surface-to-volume ratio, their deformability is reduced, rendering them even more susceptible to trapping and lysis on subsequent passes through the spleen. Splenectomy may improve red cell survival in immunohemolytic anemias.

Table 8-4. Approach to the patient with a Coombs test–positive hemolytic anemia

Clinical data	Implications
I. History	
A. Cold intolerance	Cold antibodies
B. Medication use	Drug-induced problems
C. History of blood transfusions	Hemolytic transfusion reactions
D. Recent viral illness	In relation to PCH, *Mycoplasma* infection, infectious mononucleosis
E. Symptoms of anemia	May help in assessing chronicity
F. Jaundice, hemoglobinuria	Evidence of hemolysis, intravascular hemolysis
G. Weight loss and other constitutional symptoms	Illness associated with hemolysis such as lymphoma or SLE
II. Physical examination	
A. Jaundice	Consistent with hemolysis
B. Splenomegaly	Seen in most patients
C. Lymphadenopathy	Seen in some patients; look for underlying illness
III. Laboratory data	
A. Complete blood count and peripheral smear	Look for spherocytes, polychromatophilia; increased lymphocytes of CLL
B. Reticulocyte count	Usually high
C. LDH, fractionated bilirubin, haptoglobin	Evidence of hemolysis
D. As appropriate, bone marrow or lymph node biopsy, ANA, protein electropheresis	Looking for underlying illness
E. Blood bank tests: Broad-spectrum Coombs test IgG and C3 Coombs tests Red cell eluate Serum antibody screen and identification Cold agglutinin titer if appropriate	See text

PCH = paroxysmal cold hemoglobinuria; SLE = systemic lupus erythematosus; CLL = chronic lymphocytic leukemia; ANA = nuclear antibody; LDH = lactic dehydrogenase.

Acquired Coombs-negative Hemolytic Anemias

Spur Cell Anemia

Spur cell anemia occurs in approximately 5 to 10 percent of patients with severe liver disease. The red cells appear as spherocytes with numerous projections. In contrast to normal red cells, which contain equal amounts of cholesterol and phospholipid in the red cell membrane, these cells have acquired excess cholesterol from the patient's cholesterol-laden serum. The overloaded membrane becomes wrinkled and surplus membrane sticks out from the cell. Such cells are readily trapped by the spleen, with eventual red cell demise. The hemolytic rate may be severe in this condition, and is ameliorated only by splenectomy (often a high-risk procedure for patients with advanced liver disease) or, rarely, by improvement in the liver disease.

Heinz Body Hemolytic Anemias

Heinz body hemolytic anemias are a set of disorders resulting from oxidative damage to red cells. Although hemolysis is often precipitated by oxidant drugs or infection, there is usually an underlying metabolic defect in the red cells. These disorders are discussed in Chapter 7, describing the inherited forms of hemolytic anemia.

Hypersplenism

Any disease that causes an enlarged spleen can result in the syndrome of hypersplenism (Table 8-5). This problem is characterized by three features: (1) splenomegaly; (2) anemia, leukopenia, thrombocytopenia, or any combination of these cytopenias; and (3) bone marrow hyperplasia.

In performing its job as blood filter, the average red cell spends only about 20 seconds traversing the splenic cords and sinuses. However, in splenomegaly, these hemodynamic conditions are markedly altered. Red cells may spend as long as 2 hours in the spleen, and as much as 50 percent of the total red cell mass may be found in the splenic pool. This redistribution of red cells as well as plasma volume expansion (which occurs in splenomegaly for unknown reasons) contribute to a dilutional anemia. In addition, inherently healthy red cells may be hemolyzed during their overlong sojourn through the spleen. The net result is a mild to moderate anemia, with the hemoglobin rarely below 8 gm%, and a mild reticulocytosis.

The normal spleen houses approximately 30 percent of the body's platelets (called sequestration or "pooling"); these cells are in equi-

Table 8-5. Causes of hypersplenism in adults

Inflammation and infection
  Tuberculosis
  Subacute bacterial endocarditis
  Infectious mononucleosis
  Malaria
  Sarcoidosis
  Rheumatoid arthritis
Congestive splenomegaly
  Cirrhosis of the liver with portal hypertension
Hematologic disorders
  Congenital and acquired hemolytic disorders
  Chronic lymphocytic leukemia
  Chronic myelocytic leukemia
  Myelofibrosis and agnogenic myeloid metaplasia
  Lymphoma
Infiltrative splenomegaly
  Lipid storage diseases such as Gaucher's
Splenic cysts and tumors

librium with the circulating platelets and are not harmed by their spleen transit. With splenomegaly, as much as 90 percent of the platelet population may be found in the spleen, and peripheral thrombocytopenia results. These sequestered platelets may be available to the patient following stresses such as hemorrhage; thus, what may appear to be a dangerously low platelet count may not lead to serious bleeding. Granulocyte pooling and some granulocyte destruction also occur in very large spleens, but rarely is the granulocytopenia life-threatening. Felty syndrome is an exception; this triad of splenomegaly and leukopenia, in association with rheumatoid arthritis, may be associated with life-threatening infections. Here, in addition to hypersplenism, it is likely that marrow granulocyte development is inhibited by T suppressor cells.

The diagnosis of hypersplenism is usually easy once splenomegaly and cytopenias are discovered. More challenging is the investigation of an underlying illness to explain the splenomegaly. If the illness is treatable (for example, tuberculosis), the resulting resolution of splenomegaly usually resolves the hematologic problems. In other settings, splenectomy may be performed to reduce the pancytopenia. Splenectomized patients, especially children under the age of 5, are at increased risk of overwhelming sepsis due to encapsulated bacteria, particularly *Streptococcus pneumoniae, Haemophilus influenzae,* and *Neisseria meningitidis.* Prophylactic antibiotic therapy for young children, immunization against pneumococcal infections, and close observation and early treatment of infections are prudent steps in such patients.

HYPOSPLENISM

The surgical removal of the spleen, or loss of splenic function through autoinfarction, as occurs in sickle cell anemia, results in the syndrome of hyposplenism. The failure or loss of the spleen's filtering actions results in the appearance of a variety of morphologic changes in the peripheral blood (Table 8-6). For example, Howell-Jolly bodies, residual nuclear fragments in the red cell, appear as large (up to 1 μ), round, dark basophilic inclusion bodies (Plate 38). In individuals with normal spleens, such inclusions are "pitted" by the spleen and are not seen in the peripheral blood. Pappenheimer bodies (Plate 21), remnants of ferritin, may also be seen; they are clusters of small, dark inclusions with ragged edges. Also called siderocytes, they stain with Prussian blue because of their iron content (Plate 20). Acanthocytes and target cells may also be present. Finally, there are often scattered nucleated red cells and immature granulocyte precursors. The peripheral blood counts may also be altered, with either temporary or sometimes long-standing elevations of the platelet, granulocyte, and reticulocyte counts.

Table 8-6. Peripheral blood changes in patients with hyposplenism

Howell-Jolly bodies
Pappenheimer bodies (siderocytes)
Poikilocytosis (particularly targets and acanthocytes)
Macrocytosis
Nucleated red cells
Increased reticulocyte count
Increased Heinz bodies (requires supravital stains; seen only in patients with
   Heinz body hemolytic anemias and thalassemias)
Immature white cells
*Neutrophilia
*Increased platelet count (sometimes permanent)

*These changes are usually transient.

Microangiopathic Hemolytic Anemia

A variety of illnesses can lead to the presence of fragmented erythrocytes in the peripheral blood and a microangiopathic hemolytic
anemia. Helmet cells, triangles, and other fragments are prominent
and are called *schistocytes* (Plate 39). Microangiopathic hemolytic
anemia is typically associated with intravascular hemolysis, with
hemoglobinemia, possible hemoglobinuria, and hemosiderinuria
(see Chap. 6). Red cell fragmentation is seen in the following settings (see Table 8-7).

Disseminated intravascular coagulation (DIC) is a cause of red cell
fragmentation due to fibrin strand deposition within the microvasculature, as a result of unchecked activation of the coagulation
system (see Chap. 15). Over 50 causes for DIC have been identified;
the most common are sepsis, malignancy, and shock. The distorted
vessels of *massive cutaneous hemangiomas* (Kasabach-Merritt syndrome) can cause activation of coagulation factors and DIC. Surgery
is usually required to cure the hematologic problem.

Pathologic changes in the microvasculature occur in many autoimmune disorders, including *periarteritis nodosa* and *systemic lupus
erythematosus*. Changes in the vessel walls may directly cause
microangiopathic hemolysis or they may encourage local platelet
deposition and coagulation factor activation, which may lead to
fibrin deposition. The irregular arteriolar endothelium that develops
during *renal graft rejection* produces a similar picture. Similarly,
malignant hypertension may lead to red cell fragmentation, as cells are
forced through irregular, nonyielding vessels.

The terminal stage of *disseminated carcinoma* of the stomach,
breast, pancreas, or lung may be associated with a microangiopathic
hemolytic anemia, due to direct encroachment of tumor cells on
endothelial surfaces. In some instances, mucin from these adenocarcinomas may stimulate the coagulation system and cause the local
deposition of fibrin.

Table 8-7. Causes of microangiopathic hemolytic anemia

I. Fibrin deposition
  A. Disseminated intravascular coagulation
    1. Infections
    2. Malignancy
    3. Shock
    4. Obstetric complications (toxemia, abruptio placentae, amniotic
       fluid embolism)
    5. Snake bites
    6. Giant hemangioma (Kasabach-Merritt syndrome)
    7. Miscellaneous
II. Endothelial-platelet lesions
  A. Thrombotic thrombocytopenic purpura
  B. Hemolytic-uremic syndrome
III. Vascular abnormalities
  A. Vasculitis
    1. Systemic lupus erythematosus
    2. Periarteritis nodosa
    3. Renal graft rejection
  B. Disseminated carcinomatosis
  C. Malignant hypertension
  D. Malfunctioning cardiac prostheses; calcified or stenotic aortic valve
IV. Miscellaneous
  A. March hemoglobinuria

Following the insertion of a *prosthetic aortic valve,* a mild compensated hemolytic anemia is not uncommon, as red cells are now subject to more turbulence, pressure, and hammering on nonendothelial surfaces. Severe or worsening hemolysis after valve replacement suggests that the valve is functioning improperly. Calcified and stenotic abnormalities in native aortic valves can also cause mild fragmentation hemolysis. Prosthetic mitral valves cause hemolysis less frequently. Treatment of this hemolytic anemia often requires surgery to correct the valve problem.

Thrombotic thrombocytopenic purpura (TTP) is a very rare, potentially fatal cause of microangiopathic hemolytic anemia. The classic pentad of findings includes: (1) hemolytic anemia with many red cell fragments; (2) thrombocytopenia, sometimes with serious bleeding; (3) fever; (4) neurologic and psychiatric abnormalities, including convulsions, paralysis, hallucinations, or coma; and (5) renal abnormalities. Although the cause of this disease is not fully understood, immunologically mediated endothelial damage to vessels appears to be important. It has also been suggested that normal plasma contains a platelet aggregation–inhibiting factor that is absent in patients with TTP. Microthrombi are found in many small vessels. In contrast to DIC, coagulation factor depletion does not usually occur. The diagnosis is based primarily on clinical findings. Evaluation of small vessels on bone marrow, rectal, or gingival biopsies is sometimes helpful. Treatment is often life-saving, and the mainstays are plasma exchange or plasma infusion, often combined with use of platelet function–altering drugs such as aspirin and dipyridamole. Corticosteroids may also be helpful; heparin, dextran, and splenectomy are probably not effective. *Hemolytic–uremic syndrome* resembles TTP, but the kidney is affected earlier and more profoundly. This disease is more common in children than adults and often occurs after an infectious illness such as *Escherichia coli* gastroenteritis.

March hemoglobinuria has been reported in athletes after long-distance running and soldiers after long marches. Here red cells are mechanically destroyed by pressure within blood vessels of the soles of the feet. Anemia, if any, is mild, and the problem is self-limited.

Paroxysmal Nocturnal Hemoglobinuria

Paroxysmal nocturnal hemoglobulinuria (PNH) is a rare, acquired membrane disorder that results in red cells becoming unusually sensitive to the hemolytic action of complement. The susceptible red cells are *clonally derived*, meaning that all abnormal cells have descended from a single pluripotential stem cell with the PNH mutation. Recent research has identified as critical to the development of PNH the absence of a substance, "decay accelerating factor," that is present on the surface of normal red cells to speed the inactivation of complement. This defect is also present in granulocytes, platelets, and lymphocytes. It appears to be part of a more global defect in the membrane glycoproteins of these cells.

CLINICAL FINDINGS

Although specific predisposing factors have not been identified, many cases of PNH involve patients who have had or who eventually will develop marrow disorders, such as aplastic anemia, myelodysplastic or myeloproliferative disorders, or acute nonlymphocytic leukemia. Classically, the affected patient describes bouts of hemoglobinuria, usually worse on arising from sleep. The explanation for nocturnal hemolysis is unclear, although it has been attributed to the mild fall in pH that occurs during sleep; red cells are most sensitive to complement as the pH falls toward 7.0. Severe hemolytic attacks are accompanied by symptoms such as fever, back pain, and malaise.

LABORATORY ABNORMALITIES

Patients with PNH often have severe anemia, but in contrast to other acquired hemolytic anemias discussed in this chapter, no spherocytes or other morphologic abnormalities are seen on examination of the peripheral blood smear. The reticulocyte count is high. Over time, some patients develop hypochromic microcytic red cells due to progressive iron deficiency, resulting from hemoglobinuria and hemosiderinuria. Neutropenia and thrombocytopenia are common.

As in chronic myelogenous leukemia (CML), the leukocyte alkaline phosphatase (LAP) score is reduced in PNH granulocytes. Acetylcholinesterase levels in the erythrocytes are also decreased.

The biochemical hallmark of PNH is the ability to demonstrate hemolysis of the patient's red cells when the pH is dropped to between 6.5 and 7.0. The Ham test involves the addition of acidified serum from a normal volunteer to the patient's red cells. The normal serum provides complement, which may be depleted in patients with PNH. Lysis in this tube as compared to control tubes, in which the normal serum has been heated to destroy complement, is virtually diagnostic of PNH. The sucrose hemolysis ("sugar water") test can be used as a simple screening test. Here the patient's blood is added to isotonic sucrose, which is a low ionic strength solution. Complement is activated by the reduced ionic strength, and hemolysis occurs. Since occasional false positives occur, positive results require confirmation with the more complex and rigorous Ham test.

COURSE AND TREATMENT

A serious complication of PNH is an increased incidence of intravascular thromboses, possibly due to abnormal platelet function. Infections may also be a problem, because granulocytes, also affected by the PNH defect, function poorly. Renal failure due to hemoglobinuria and transformation to acute myelocytic leukemia or aplastic anemia are other complications.

There is no specific treatment for PNH. Some patients may benefit from prednisone, others possibly from androgens. Folic acid should be administered to counter the deficiency frequently seen in severe hemolytic anemias of any cause. Because the hemolysis results in hemosiderinuria, many patients become iron deficient. Paradoxically, iron administration may heighten hemolysis; this is because the red cells produced following iron repletion represent a new supply of complement-sensitive cells. Some reports suggest that red cell transfusions may also lead transiently to more severe hemolysis, because of complement components in the transfused plasma. Washed red cells are traditionally transfused to avoid this problem. Successful marrow transplantation has been reported; because of its risks, this option is currently reserved for patients with life-threatening disease.

Miscellaneous Causes of Acquired Hemolytic Anemia

In patients with extensive third-degree burns, hemolysis develops as a result of heat damage to red cells caught in the injured skin and tissues. Clostridial sepsis can result in rapid, massive hemolysis due to the action of a bacterial toxin that dissolves red cell membrane proteins and lipids. A variety of heavy metals may damage the red cell membrane. Thus, patients with Wilson's disease, an inherited disorder associated with high serum copper levels, often develop acute hemolysis early in their illnesses, when large amounts of unbound copper are suddenly released from the liver during infarctive episodes. Contamination of hemodialysis fluids by tap water with high copper concentrations has also been reported to cause hemolysis in patients undergoing dialysis. Exposure of red cells to water can produce hemolysis; for example, irrigation of the prostate bed with large amounts of water during surgery has caused acute severe hemolysis. This form of hemolysis is also seen in freshwater drowning victims. Hemolysis may also develop in patients with severe hypophosphatemia.

Approach to the Patient with Acquired Hemolytic Anemia

In addition to the acquired hemolytic anemias described in this chapter, congenital hemolytic disorders need to be considered even in the adult patient presenting for the first time with a picture of shortened red cell survival. On the basis of the patient's history, physical examination, and red cell morphology on a peripheral blood smear, hemolysis can usually be classified into one of the categories described in this chapter. Once this assignment has been made, confirmatory tests can be performed to define the diagnosis further. For example, the finding of many helmet cells and fragmented forms in an acutely ill patient is consistent with a microangiopathic hemolytic anemia; prolonged prothrombin time (PT), partial thromboplastin time (PTT), thrombocytopenia, and high levels of fibrin degradation products would confirm the diagnosis of DIC. A schematic for approaching patients with hemolysis is presented in Table 8-8.

Case Development Problems: Acquired Hemolytic Anemias

In each of the following cases, the patient has developed hemolysis. You are asked to determine the best diagnosis.

1. A 40-year-old woman with rheumatic valve disease (mitral and aortic stenosis) has been administered high-dose intravenous penicillin (20 million units per day) to treat subacute bacterial endocarditis for 3 weeks. Her hematocrit has fallen slowly during this treatment to 25 percent, and because of mild angina, she is transfused with a unit of packed red cells. One week later, you notice that she is jaundiced, and her hematocrit is still only 25 percent. In the process of crossmatching another unit, the laboratory reports these newly abnormal results to you:

Table 8-8. Approach to the patient with acquired hemolytic anemia

Clinical data	Implications
I. History	
A. Family history of anemia, jaundice, gallstones, splenomegaly	Congenital hemolysis such as spherocytosis
B. Cardiac valve disease or prosthesis	Microangiopathic hemolysis
C. Drug ingestion	G-6-PD, oxidant drugs, drug-induced immuno-hemolytic anemia
D. Infection	DIC, immunohemolytic anemia
E. Red or dark urine	Intravascular hemolysis or rapid hemolytic rate
F. Liver disease	Hypersplenism
G. Major burns	Thermal injury
H. Autoimmune disease, lymphoproliferative diseases	Immunohemolytic anemia, hypersplenism
II. Physical examination	
A. Jaundice	Confirms severity of hemolysis
B. Bleeding, purpura	DIC, TTP
C. Splenomegaly	Many causes of hemolysis
III. Laboratory data (initial)	
A. Complete blood count	To evaluate
B. Peripheral smear	extent and
C. Reticulocyte count	severity of
D. LDH, bilirubin, haptoglobin	hemolysis
E. Examine plasma, urine for hemoglobin	Intravascular or rapid extravascular hemolysis
IV. Tests to be considered after initial evaluation	
A. Coombs test	Immunohemolytic anemia
B. Urine hemosiderin	Intravascular hemolysis (microangiopathy, PCH, PNH)
C. Erythrocyte enzyme assays	G-6-PD
D. Sugar water/ Ham tests	PNH
E. Heinz body preparation	G-6-PD, oxidant drugs
F. DIC evaluation (PT, PTT, TT, FDPs)	DIC

G-6-PD = glucose-6-phosphate dehydrogenase; LDH = lactic dehydrogenase; TT = thrombin time; FDPs = fibrin degradation products.

Laboratory Data

Direct antiglobulin test	positive
IgG Coombs	positive
complement Coombs	negative
eluate	anti-c
Antibody screen	positive (without adding penicillin)
antibody identification	anti-c

This patient has a new positive direct Coombs test due to the presence of IgG antibodies. Furthermore, elution of the antibodies from the cells reveals that the IgG antibodies are specifically directed against the red cell antigen c. The same antibody is also found in the patient's serum. These results indicate a delayed hemolytic transfusion reaction. The patient must have been exposed to c-positive red cells through earlier transfusions or pregnancies, but the antibody titer had fallen to undetectable levels at the time of the crossmatch before the recent transfusion. The transfusion of c-positive cells resulted in an anamnestic rise in the patient's anti-c titer, and slow destruction of the transfused red cells without symptoms of acute hemolysis.

This patient is probably not going to have serious problems from the hemolysis. However, she should always receive c-negative red cells in the future, even if her antibody screen becomes negative again.

2. A 50-year-old woman with high blood pressure has been taking Aldomet (2 gm per day) for the past 2 years. Four years ago she was transfused with multiple units of blood following a car accident. She has received no blood since then. Now she is admitted for elective coronary artery surgery, and the blood bank cannot find compatible blood.

Laboratory Data

Direct antiglobulin in test (Coombs test)	positive (4+)
IgG Coombs	positive (3+)
C3 Coombs	negative
eluate	reacts with every cell— "panagglutinin"
Antibody screen	positive
antibody identification	reacts with every cell— "panagglution"

The positive direct antiglobulin test cannot be related to transfusion given 4 years ago, since transfused, antibody-coated cells should no longer be present. A panagglutinin is present both in the serum and on the red cells. Because the antibody is found on the patient's own cells, the antibody is by definition an autoantibody. The differential diagnosis includes warm AIHA and α-methyldopa–induced immune hemolytic anemia. There is no way to distinguish between these two problems based on the laboratory data. It is possible that other alloantibodies may be present in the serum in addition to the autoantibody, and special test procedures may be necessary to identify them in the process of finding blood.

It will not be possible to find "compatible" blood since the serum autoantibody will react with all donor cells. This patient's

Aldomet should be changed to another antihypertensive agent and surgery delayed if feasible. If the antibody is Aldomet-induced, the antibody should disappear from the serum over the next 6 months. If emergency transfusions are necessary in the interim, carefully chosen but incompatible units would have to be used.

3. A 65-year-old woman develops blue finger tips whenever she pulls food from her freezer; sometimes her urine becomes darker after these episodes. Her hematocrit is 23 percent, the reticulocyte count is 9 percent, lactic dehydrogenase (LDH) and bilirubin are elevated, and urine hemosiderin is present.

Laboratory Data

Direct antiglobulin test (Coombs test)	positive (4+)
IgG Coombs	negative
C3 Coombs	positive (4+)
eluate	not done
Antibody screen	positive
antibody identification	panagglutinin at cold temperatures (anti-I)
Cold agglutinin titer	1 : 1,000,000

The clinical story of sensitivity to cold is supported by the laboratory data, which demonstrate that the patient's cells have been strongly sensitized by complement. Note that an eluate has not been done—IgG is not present on the red cells (negative IgG Coombs test), and therefore there is no point in looking for antibody specificity. Furthermore, a cold-loving IgM panagglutinin (anti-I) is present in very high titers in the serum. This autoantibody has sensitized the patient's red cells with complement and is causing the cold agglutinin syndrome with intermittent intravascular hemolysis superimposed on chronic extravascular hemolysis.

4. A 29-year-old man of Italian extraction has a 10-year history of alcoholism. He now presents with jaundice and an enlarged spleen. Physical examination also reveals a slightly enlarged, nodular liver.

Laboratory Data

Hematocrit	30%
White blood count	3,000/cu mm
Platelet count	85,000/cu mm
Blood smear	hypochromia, target and tear-drop cells, polychromatophilia
Mean corpuscular volume (MCV)	80

Reticulocyte count	8%
Direct antiglobulin test (Coombs test)	negative
Bilirubin	increased (both direct and indirect)

On the basis of the information obtained thus far, the patient has a hemolytic anemia with microcytic red cells. The differential diagnosis for the hemolytic component includes hypersplenism; the target cells raise the possibility of a hemoglobinopathy or thalassemia. The microcytosis also supports thalassemia, as well as iron deficiency, the anemia of chronic disease, or lead poisoning.

Selective additional tests will be helpful, including:

Bone marrow examination: The patient has pancytopenia, and a careful examination of the marrow is warranted; the finding of hyperplasia of all three blood cell lines would be consistent with hypersplenism

Liver function studies, liver–spleen scan: To evaluate the degree of liver dysfunction and size of the spleen

Serum iron and total iron-binding capacity, and serum ferritin: To evaluate iron stores and the possibility of anemia of chronic disease

Hemoglobin electrophoresis, with A_2 and F levels: To confirm or eliminate the presence of β-thalassemia

5. A 28-year-old woman is acutely ill, with a fever (101°F), headaches, and confusion. In the last 3 days, her urine has turned dark. On examination she has petechiae.

Laboratory Data

Hematocrit	22%
Platelet count	5,000/cu mm
Reticulocyte count	10%
PT	normal
PTT	normal
Blood urea nitrogen (BUN)	55 mg%
Creatinine	4.5 mg%
LDH	2,300 IU
Haptoglobin	0
Direct antiglobulin test	negative
Antibody screen	negative

The patient has signs of a brisk hemolytic anemia that is Coombs negative. Associated with severe thrombocytopenia, renal failure, and neurologic signs and symptoms, the diagnosis is most likely TTP. This diagnosis would be supported by finding fragmented red blood cells in the blood smear. DIC appears unlikely because of the normal coagulation studies. The LDH and platelet count are the two earliest and best indicators of response to treatment, or relapse, in this condition.

6. A 24-year-old man with a microcytic anemia and low serum iron tells you that he has frequent headaches and abdominal pain, and that his urine seems very "concentrated" some mornings.

Consider the possibility of PNH. Red cells from such individuals are more readily sensitized to complement during sleep, and hemoglobinuria appears with the first morning's urine. Chronic hemoglobinuria and hemosiderinuria may lead to iron deficiency, which may compound the already present anemia due to hemolysis.

Selected Readings

Coombs test–positive Hemolytic Anemias

Bird, G. W. G. Paroxysmal cold hemoglobinuria. *Br. J. Haematol.* 37 : 167, 1977.

Bowman, J. W. The management of Rh-isoimmunization. *Obstet. Gynecol.* 52 : 1, 1978.

Frank, M. M. Complement in the pathophysiology of human disease. *N. Engl. J. Med.* 316 : 1525, 1987.

Griffin, J. P. Rapid screening for cold agglutinins in pneumonia. *Ann. Intern. Med.* 70 : 701, 1969.

Jones, S. Autoimmune disorders and malignant lymphoma. *Cancer* 31 : 1092, 1973.

Kirtland, H. H., Mohler, D. N., and Horwitz, D. A. Methyldopa inhibition of suppressor-lymphocyte function: A proposed cause of autoimmune hemolytic anemia. *N. Engl. J. Med.* 302 : 185, 1980.

NIH Conference. Pathophysiology of immune hemolytic anemia. *Ann. Intern. Med.* 87 : 210, 1977.

Petz, L. D. Transfusing the patient with autoimmune hemolytic anemia. *Clin. Lab. Med.* 2 : 193, 1982.

Petz, L. D. Drug-induced immune hemolysis. *N. Engl. J. Med.* 313 : 510, 1985.

Petz, L. D., and Garatty, G. *Autoimmune Hemolytic Anemias.* New York: Churchill Livingstone, 1980.

Pineda, A. A., Taswell, H. F., and Brzica, S. M., Jr. Delayed hemolytic transfusion reactions: An immunologic hazard of blood transfusions. *Transfusion* 18 : 1, 1978.

Worlledge, S. M. Immune drug-induced hemolytic anemias. *Semin. Hematol.* 10 : 327, 1973.

The Spleen and Hypersplenism

Aster, R. H. Platelet sequestration studies in man. *Br. J. Haematol.* 22 : 259, 1972.

Crosby, W. H. Splenic remodeling of red cell surfaces. *Blood* 50 : 643, 1977.

Diamond, L. K. The concept of functional asplenia. *N. Engl. J. Med.* 281 : 958, 1969.

Jacob, H. S. Hypersplenism: Mechanisms and management. *Br. J. Haematol.* 27 : 1, 1974.

Jandl, J. H., and Aster, R. H. Increased splenic pooling and the pathogenesis of hypersplenism. *Am. J. Med. Sci.* 253 : 383, 1967.

O'Neal, B. J., and McDonald, J. C. The risk of sepsis in the asplenic adult. *Ann. Surg.* 194 : 775, 1981.

Spivak, J. L. Felty's syndrome: An analytical review. *Johns Hopkins Med. J.* 141 : 156, 1977.

Microangiopathic Hemolytic Anemia

Antman, K. H. et al. Microangiopathic hemolytic anemia and cancer: A review. *Medicine* 58 : 377, 1979.

Bick, R. L. et al. Disseminated intravascular coagulation and blood component therapy. *Transfusion* 16 : 361, 1976.

Byrnes, J. J. Thrombotic thrombocytopenic purpura. *Adv. Intern. Med.* 26 : 131, 1980.

Drummond, K. N. Hemolytic–uremic syndrome—then and now. *N. Engl. J. Med.* 312 : 116, 1985.

Kelton, J. G., Moore, J. C., and Murphy, W. G. Studies investigating platelet aggregation and release inititated by sera from patients with thrombotic thrombocytopenic purpura. *Blood* 69 : 924, 1987.

Marsh, G. W., and Lewis, S. M. Cardiac hemolytic anemia. *Semin. Hematol.* 6 : 133, 1969.

Paroxysmal Nocturnal Hemoglobinuria

Nicholson-Weller, A., Spicer, D. B., and Austen, K. F. Deficiency of the complement regulatory protein, "decay accelerating factor," on membranes of granulocytes, monocytes, and platelets in paroxysmal nocturnal hemoglobinuria. *N. Engl. J. Med.* 312 : 1091, 1985.

Rosse, W. F. Treatment of paroxysmal nocturnal hemoglobinuria. *Blood* 60 : 20, 1982.

Miscellaneous Types of Hemolytic Anemia

Cooper, R. A. Hemolytic syndromes and red cell membrane abnormalities in liver disease. *Semin. Hematol.* 17 : 103, 1980.

Deiss, A., Lee, G. R., and Cartwright, G. E. Hemolytic anemia in Wilson's disease. *Ann. Intern. Med.* 73 : 413, 1970.

Jacob, H. S., and Amsden, T. Acute hemolytic anemia with rigid red cells in hypophosphatemia. *N. Engl. J. Med.* 285 : 1446, 1971.

Manzier, A. D., and Schreiner, A. W. Copper induced acute hemolytic anemia: A new complication of hemodialysis. *Ann. Intern. Med.* 73 : 409, 1970.

Sturgeon, P. Hematological observations of the anemia associated with blood type Rh_{null}. *Blood* 36 : 310, 1970.

9 Blood Transfusion

Margot S. Kruskall

In the early 20th century, transfusion therapy consisted of the use of freshly drawn whole blood to save the life of the exsanguinating patient. A number of important advances, including the ability to store red cells for many weeks, the development of techniques for blood component preparation, and recognition of the risks of transfusion-transmitted diseases, has led to the development of transfusion medicine as a medical specialty. Transfusion medicine specialists run blood collection facilities and hospital transfusion services, and are an important link between the blood bank laboratory and the patient and his or her physicians.

Blood Groups

The ABO System

The human red cell carries many antigens on its surface, but the first set discovered, the ABO system, remains the most important to transfusion therapy. Each ABO antigen, attached to membrane proteins, has a chain of sugars at its terminal (free) end. Group O red cells have large amounts of the antigen "H," which is the precursor of all ABO antigens. The addition of one sugar (N-acetylgalactosamine) to the end of the H sugar chain converts it to the antigen A; the addition of an alternate sugar (D-galactose) converts the H antigen to B. Group AB red cells contain a mixture of A and B antigens. ABO antigens are widely distributed on all tissues throughout the body, and are found as well in urine, saliva, and other fluids.

ABO antigen status is inherited (Table 9-1). More precisely, individuals inherit genes for transferases, the enzymes that attach the antigenic sugars to the ABO chains. Each person inherits two genes; alleles at each gene locus include the A transferase, the B transferase, or a null gene. Individuals homozygous for the null gene do not convert H substance to A or B; these individuals are group O. If both transferases are inherited, some H antigens are converted to A and others to B, and the red cells are AB. Individuals homozygous for one transferase (for example, A) convert more H substance to A than do individuals who are heterozygous for this transferase and the null gene, but both will have red cells that type as group A.

A curious and important phenomenon of the ABO system is the obligatory presence of ABO antibodies reciprocal to the missing ABO antigen. Thus, the individual whose red cells are group A will predictably have anti-B antibody in his or her serum; the individual whose red cells are group O will have both anti-A and anti-B, and the individual with group AB red cells will have neither. These immunoglobulin M (IgM) antibodies develop in all humans (except rare individuals with agammaglobulinemia) over the first 6 months after birth. They are called "naturally occurring," in that they develop without apparent exposure to transfusions of red cells; it has been shown that they occur in response to carbohydrate antigens in the environment (for example, antigens on bacteria) similar to A and B.

ABO IgM antibodies, being pentamers, are large enough and have enough binding sites to span the distance between corresponding antigens on two red cells. This is a boon to laboratory testing. The addition of anti-A to A red cells at room temperature results in visually apparent agglutination of the cells, without the addition of any other reagents. Thus, anti-A and anti-B typing sera are used to identify ABO antigens on the patient's red cells (*forward-typing*). Furthermore, the patient's serum can be checked for the presence of the predicted ABO antibodies, by adding it to red cells of known ABO type (*back-typing*) (Table 9-1). Any results that are discrepant must be carefully evaluated before the patient is assigned an ABO type, since an error can have lethal consequences.

ABO antibodies are termed *clinically significant* because of their ability to cause hemolysis of red cells bearing the corresponding antigens. These antibodies fix complement very efficiently and red cell destruction is usually rapid and intravascular. Thus, the transfusion of group A red cells into a group O individual (who has

Table 9-1. ABO blood groups: genotypes and phenotypes

Phenotype	Genotype	Serum antibody	Forward type Patient cells with:		Back type Patient serum with:	
			Anti-A	Anti-B	A cells	B cells
A	A O A A	Anti-B	+	−	−	+
B	B O B B	Anti-A	−	+	+	−
AB	A B	None	+	+	−	−
O	O O	Anti-A and -B	−	−	+	+

+ = positive; − = negative.

anti-A and -B antibodies) will result in acute destruction of the cells. For this reason, patients must be transfused with ABO-compatible red cells, and, as a rule, ABO-identical donors are chosen. When the identical type is not available, compatible blood donors can be used (Table 9-2). Thus, a group A individual (with anti-B in his or her serum) can be transfused with group O, as well as group A, donor cells. Since type O cells are not affected by any ABO antibodies, and are compatible with recipient plasma of any ABO type, group O individuals are referred to as *universal donors.* Conversely, group AB patients, who lack anti-A and -B antibodies, can receive any ABO type of blood (*universal recipients*).

In looking for compatibility one must be concerned with antibodies in the recipient's, but not the donor's, serum. The recipient has a large volume of plasma containing ABO antibodies. By contrast, although the group O donor has anti-A and anti-B in the accompanying plasma in the bag, the total volume is small, these antibodies are rapidly diluted in the recipient's blood volume, and they do not cause hemolysis of the recipient's cells.

Other Blood Groups

Many other blood group systems have been discovered. Typically, such systems have come to light when serum from a previously transfused patient reacts with one or more of a set (*panel*) of human red cells in a previously unknown pattern. Alternatively, the birth of a baby with a Coombs-positive hemolytic anemia (hemolytic disease of the newborn; see Chap. 8) may lead to the discovery that the mother's serum has a new, previously undescribed antibody to an antigen on the baby's and father's red cells. In many cases, other patients' sera can be used to identify additional alleles within the newly discovered system.

Antibodies to most of these antigens occur only after a patient has been exposed through transfusion (*immune antibodies*). Fortunately, most blood group antigens are not very immunogenic. Furthermore, only some antibodies are clinically significant; others cause problems only in the test tube.

Table 9-2. Choosing ABO-compatible red cells for transfusion

Patient blood type	Safe donor types			
	A	B	AB	O
A	Yes	No	No	Yes
B	No	Yes	No	Yes
O	No	No	No	Yes
AB	Yes	Yes	Yes	Yes

Rh System

The Rh system is important both because the antigens are relatively good immunogens compared to other blood group systems and the antibodies are clinically significant. The system consists of three closely related genes and many alleles, but the most important antigen is *D*. Individuals who have this antigen on their red cells are called *Rh-positive;* individuals who lack the Rh antigen are Rh-negative. Among whites, 85 percent are Rh-positive and 15 percent are Rh-negative; a smaller proportion of blacks are Rh-negative. Despite years of search, no alternative allele to D has been found in Rh-negative individuals. Conceptually, however, it is useful to use the notation "d" to denote the absence of D. Thus, Rh-positive individuals are either DD or Dd and Rh-negative individuals are dd. Two other allelic pairs of antigens are also important: C and c, and E and e. Patients inherit one antigen from each parent. Thus, red cells are either C-positive (CC), c-positive (cc), or express both antigens (Cc), and are also either E-positive (EE), e-positive (ee), or express both antigens (Ee).

Because the genes for these alleles are so closely linked, it is the rule that parental combinations of Rh antigens are inherited almost as one gene. Thus, for example, if an individual has the alleles CDe on one haplotype, and cde on the other, children get either one allele combination or the other (but not, for example, Cde). This phenomenon is helpful in predicting the Rh type of a fetus carried by an Rh-negative mother, and in paternity testing.

In contrast to the ABO system, relatively little is known about the biochemistry of Rh antigens, although it is likely that they are proteins, and integrally important to the stability of the red cell membrane. This comes from observations that Rh_{null} red cells (found in rare families; all Rh antigens are missing) are spherocytic and associated with a chronic hemolytic picture.

Also in contrast to the ABO system, antibodies to Rh antigens occur only after a person has been sensitized to the antigen through transfusion or pregnancy. Thus, an Rh-negative individual transfused with Rh-positive red cells may develop anti-D. Because the D antigen is the strongest immunogen of all red cell antigens, this may occur in up to 70 percent of such individuals. Sensitization may also occur in an Rh-negative mother carrying an Rh-positive fetus, most commonly at the time of birth, when fetal red cells routinely escape into the maternal circulation. Antibodies to other Rh antigens (C, c, E, and e) can also be made in response to transfusion or pregnancy. All of these immune antibodies are IgG. Serious hemolytic transfusion reactions can result when a previously sensitized patient is transfused with red cells bearing the corresponding Rh antigen. Fortunately, because these antibodies do not fix complement well, and because red cell destruction is largely mild and extravascular, mortality from such reactions is lower than with ABO incompatibilities.

Because the D antigen is so immunogenic, it is standard practice to type all patients' red cells for the presence of the D antigen, and to give Rh-negative individuals Rh-negative blood to prevent the formation of anti-D.

Kell, Duffy, and Kidd Blood Group Systems

Antigens in the Kell system (important alleles K and k), Duffy system (Fy^a, Fy^b), and Kidd system (Jk^a, Jk^b) may each lead to the development of immune antibodies after an antigen-negative individual is exposed through transfusion or pregnancy. Fortunately, the immunogenic potential of these antigens is much less than that of the antigen D. However, these antibodies can cause clinically significant, at times severe, hemolysis. Patients with such antibodies must receive antigen-negative blood for transfusion.

The I-i Blood Group System

This set of carbohydrate antigens has several unusual features. First, the two most important antigens, I and i, are (with very rare exception) universally present on human red cells. Neonatal red cells contain predominantly i antigen. However, over the first 18 months of life, the number of I antigen sites increases, and i decreases, so that red cells have predominantly I.

Curiously, the antibodies inspired by these antigens are all IgM cold-loving *autoantibodies* (*cold agglutinins*). Many otherwise normal individuals have some anti-I in their serum, demonstrable when testing is performed at 4°C. This antibody is usually present at titers of less than 1 : 64 and does not cause hemolysis. Higher titers of the cold agglutinin anti-I sometimes appear during infection with *Mycoplasma pneumoniae*, because the I antigen is similar to a *Mycoplasma* lipopolysaccharide. Very high titers of anti-I cause the hemolysis seen with cold agglutinin disease (see Chap. 8). Anti-i have been found following infectious mononucleosis and in rare individuals has caused transient hemolysis.

The MNSs Blood Group System

These glycoprotein antigens are associated with red cell membrane proteins: the M and N antigens with glycophorin A, and S and s with glycophorin B. Anti-S can cause clinically significant hemolysis; the other antibodies are only rarely clinically important.

The P Blood Group System

Alloantibodies to these carbohydrate antigens do not cause significant hemolysis. The IgG autoantibody to P, also called the Donath-Landsteiner antibody, is unusual in favoring cold temperatures. It causes the hemolysis of paroxysmal cold hemoglobinuria (see Chap. 8).

The Lewis Blood Group System

In contrast to all the antigens previously described, Lewis antigens (Le^a and Le^b) are not integral to the red cell membrane. Instead, they are soluble substances in the plasma that adsorb to red cells. Although IgM antibodies to Le^a and Le^b are common, they are typically of no clinical significance.

Compatibility Testing

Because most patients have naturally occurring antibodies that can cause hemolysis (the ABO antibodies, anti-A and anti-B) and some patients develop immune antibodies in other blood group systems that are clinically significant, the choice of red cells for transfusion must be made carefully to avoid life-threatening hemolytic transfusion reactions. The process by which donor red cell components are chosen for transfusion to a patient is called *compatibility testing,* and includes the following steps.

Red Cell Typing

The patient's *ABO type* is determined from both forward- and back-typing (see Table 9-1). Typically this and all blood bank testing are done in small test tubes, mixing one or two drops of patient cells with each of two reagent antibodies, anti-A and anti-B (forward type), plus two drops of patient serum with one drop each of A and B cells (back type). Agglutination, if present, is enhanced by spinning the tubes in small centrifuges for 15 to 30 seconds. The Rh type is also determined using patient cells and anti-D reagent. No back type is performed here, because very few Rh-negative patients actually have anti-D.

Antibody Screen

The patient's serum is tested for "unexpected" (i.e., non-ABO) antibodies. To do this, two drops of the patient's serum are mixed with each of two or three specially chosen reagent red cells. Each red cell must be group O (so that the expected ABO antibodies will not cause agglutination). Furthermore, all the major alleles of the clinically important blood group systems must be present on one or more of these cells. Thus, one or more cells must be Rh-positive, at least one must be C-positive, at least one must have c, and so forth. Each tube is examined for agglutination at room temperature (to look for IgM antibodies), as well as at 37°C (IgG antibodies). Many IgG antibodies can coat red cells, but because of their 7S size are unable to bridge the gap between neighboring cells to agglutinate them. As a last step, therefore, Coombs reagent is added. This rabbit antiserum to human IgG facilitates agglutination of IgG-coated red cells. The antibody screen is sometimes called the "indirect Coombs test" because of the use of the Coombs antiserum, but the term *antibody screen* is more accurate and less confusing. Any agglutination, at any phase of testing, is interpreted as a positive antibody screen, and additional testing must usually be done with other reagent red cells to figure out the precise identity of the antibody or antibodies (*antibody identification*).

Crossmatch

Potential donor components are chosen to match the patient's red cell type (ABO and Rh). In addition, if any other clinically important antibodies have been identified, the donor red cells must be negative for the corresponding antigens. Finally, to be sure that the selected donor blood is compatible with that of the recipient, two drops of the donor's red cells are mixed with the patient's serum and studied at room temperature, at 37°C, and after the addition of the Coombs reagent. The absence of agglutination is required for a compatible crossmatch.

Blood Component Therapy

Modern-day transfusion therapy relies on the use of blood components rather than whole blood for the treatment of hematologic diseases. Component preparation allows better storage of individual components. For example, red cells survive best at 1 to 6°C while platelets require room temperature. In addition, factors from plasma can be optimally concentrated (for example, pooled factor VIII can be prepared in a highly concentrated lyophilized form). Also, several patients can be treated with different components from the same unit of blood.

Whole Blood

Each unit consists of 450 ± 50 mL blood collected from a donor, and mixed with 63 mL anticoagulant and red cell preservative solution such as CPDA-1. Such anticoagulant preservative solutions typically include citrate, which binds calcium, and phosphate, dextrose, and adenine, to improve red cell survival. Typically, platelets and plasma are separated from the red cells shortly after donation, and plasma may be further fractionated.

Packed Red Cells

Although whole blood is still used in some situations of massive hemorrhage, most anemic patients do not require plasma and platelets, and thus should be transfused with packed red cells. Preparation of packed red cells from whole blood involves the removal of approximately 80 percent of the plasma, so that the volume of the component is about 250 mL. One unit of packed red cells typically raises a recipient's hematocrit by 3 percent. Because of the risks and complications of blood transfusions (see later in text), red cells should only be transfused to treat symptomatic anemia, or to prevent symptoms of imminent hypoxia. Furthermore, nontransfusion alternatives should always be attempted first (for example, iron therapy for iron deficiency anemia).

White-cell–poor Red Cells

Packed red cells still contain white blood cells. Some recipients who have developed HLA antibodies in response to previous transfusions or pregnancies may have febrile transfusion reactions because of the presence of donor white cells. White cells can be largely removed by centrifugation, or, as of more recently, with the use of filters specifically designed for this purpose.

Washed Red Cells

Components that are essentially devoid of plasma can be prepared using continuous-flow centrifugation instruments that flush the cells with isotonic saline. Such preparations are needed for rare individuals who are IgA-deficient and have had life-threatening reactions to plasma containing IgA. In addition, the washing procedure removes white cells, and washed red cells are sometimes used for individuals who continue to have reactions to white-cell–poor red cells prepared by filtration. Washing is time-consuming and expensive. Furthermore, because the procedure involves reentering the plastic bag that contains the red cells, washed red cells must be used within 24 hours to avoid possible growth of contaminating bacteria.

Frozen Red Cells

Packed red cells can only be stored at refrigerator temperatures for 42 days. Membrane and metabolic changes occur to the red cells during this 1 to 6°C storage. The effect of such changes (the *storage lesion*) is such that, if transfused after longer periods of storage, fewer than 80 percent of red cells survive even 24 hours in the recipient. However, it is possible to freeze cells within a short period of time after collection, and maintain them at −70°C for as long as 10 years. Freezing requires the addition of glycerol, a *cryoprotectant* that enters the red cells and limits the formation of intracellular ice crystals, which are lethal to the cell. Glycerol must be removed before transfusion, since excess glycerol in thawed red cells may lead to hemolysis. This is done using a series of wash solutions in a continuous-flow centrifugation instrument. As with washed cells, the technique is labor-intensive and costly, and the thawed cells outdate within 24 hours. At present, uses for frozen red cells are limited: Rare red cell types are often frozen and autologous blood can be frozen (although this is not often necessary). In addition, frozen red cells have lower numbers of white cells than washed red cells, and may be useful for the rare individual who continues to have febrile reactions to filtered or washed components.

Platelets

Two methods of platelet preparation are now commonly used. Slow centrifugation of an individual whole blood unit separates platelet-rich plasma, and the platelets can then be further concentrated by additional centrifugation. Typically, six to ten of these *platelet concentrates* are pooled so that there are sufficient platelets for an effective transfusion. The phrase "random donor" is also often applied to these platelets, because multiple unselected individuals' components are used. Alternatively, platelets can be prepared using *plateletpheresis* techniques. Here, blood drawn from a single donor is anticoagulated and passed through a centrifuge, where platelet separation takes place; red cells and plasma are returned to the donor. The number of platelets in each pheresis product is counted and converted to "units," where each unit (5.5×10^{10} platelets) is roughly equivalent to a random-donor concentrate. One pheresis donor typically can give the equivalent of six or seven units of platelets. The attribute "single donor" is usually applied to pheresis platelets to distinguish them from pooled platelet concentrates. Advantages to using single-donor platelets include a reduction in the number of donor exposures for the recipient; this is particularly important for the individual who is likely to receive few transfusions overall. In addition, selected HLA-compatible donors can be chosen for recipients refractory to random, unselected donors (see below). The possibility that exposure to platelets from fewer donors may reduce or delay platelet refractoriness is controversial at this time.

Platelets must be stored at room temperatures (20–24°C), since refrigeration quickly destroys their ability to aggregate. Storage for up to 5 days is currently allowed. With longer intervals, progressively lower pHs in the bag lead to reduced survival of the transfused platelets in recipients. In addition, the incidence of bacterial contamination within the bag increases; this blood component is a good culture medium because it is stored at room temperature rather than in the cold. One or two bacteria accidentally introduced, through breaks in sterile technique at the time of collection, can multiply to clinically significant levels over 5 to 7 days.

Platelets are indicated for the correction of severe thrombocytopenia—for example, to a patient with a platelet count of less than 50×10^9 who is bleeding. In addition, platelets are commonly used prophylactically in patients with platelet counts less than 20×10^9 per liter, to prevent hemorrhage. However, there is little clinical evidence that prophylactic transfusions at this level of platelets are necessary, and some evidence that platelet counts above 10×10^9 may not require transfusions in the absence of serious bleeding.

Typically, transfusion of one random concentrate or one single-donor "unit" raises the platelet count in the recipient by between 6 and 12×10^9/cu mm. This increment is affected by a number of factors. For example, it may be less than expected if the recipient is febrile, because fever reduces the platelets' half-life; if the recipient has a big spleen, because a large proportion of transfused platelets may be sequestered in that organ; or because of rapid platelet destruction due to idiopathic thrombocytopenic purpura (ITP) or alloimmunization. Therefore, a platelet count should always be checked one hour after the transfusion to ensure that the expected increment has been achieved.

Approximately 25 percent of patients treated with repeated platelet transfusions eventually become *refractory*, in that posttransfusion increments become very poor or absent. This dangerous situation is often due to the development of antibodies directed against HLA antigens on the platelets. Such patients can sometimes be treated with platelets from HLA-compatible donors.

Granulocytes

Pheresis techniques can also be used to obtain concentrates of white cells from normal donors. Such components have been used successfully to treat severely neutropenic patients with bacterial infections unresponsive to appropriate antibiotics. However, the granulocytes must be transfused as soon as collected, since it is not possible to preserve their function by storage at any temperature. It is also difficult to obtain adequate numbers of granulocytes from an individual donor. Furthermore, granulocyte transfusions are frequently accompanied by fever and respiratory symptoms in the recipient; these reactions have occasionally proved fatal. Recent improvements in antibiotic regimens allow most neutropenic patients to be treated without resort to granulocyte transfusions.

Fresh Frozen Plasma

When a unit of whole blood is stored at refrigerator temperatures, the activity of many of the plasma coagulation factors deteriorates. This is particularly true of the labile coagulation factors, V and VIII. Fresh frozen plasma (FFP), prepared by separating donor plasma from red cells at the time of donation and freezing it immediately, results in a product that maintains good levels of all coagulation factors. FFP is typically used to correct severe coagulopathies due to multiple factor deficiencies, as with warfarin (Coumadin) overdose or liver disease. It is also indicated for the treatment of factor deficiencies where relatively low levels of the factor are needed to prevent or stop bleeding (for example, factor XI). It is not practical as treatment for hemophilia A, because of the large volumes of FFP that would be required to bring factor VIII activity in the patient to adequate levels.

Cryoprecipitate

One approach that concentrates factor VIII in plasma is the preparation of cryoprecipitate. Here, a unit of frozen plasma is allowed to thaw in a refrigerator. Factors that are cold-precipitable (including factor VIII and fibrinogen) do not go back into solution during thawing, and can be concentrated by centrifugation, and then refrozen. A typical bag of cryoprecipitate contains 100 units of factor VIII (the amount normally present in 100 mL plasma) in a 20-mL volume. Cryoprecipitate can be used to treat hemophilia A and is particularly useful for von Willebrand's disease. Although the half-life of transfused factor VIII is usually 8 to 12 hours, for unexplained reasons transfusion can correct the factor VIII level and bleeding time for as long as 48 hours in von Willebrand's disease. Cryoprecipitate also appears to correct bleeding in uremia; the typical dose is 10 bags, pooled.

Clotting Factor Concentrates

A series of precipitation steps, performed on large volumes of plasma pooled from thousands of donors, can further concentrate specific factors such as factor VIII. Such concentrates are usually lyophilized, so that as many as 1,000 units can be reconstituted in only 50 mL saline. Until recently, concentrates caused a high incidence of non-A, non-B hepatitis and human immunodeficiency virus (HIV) infection. Modifications in the preparation, including heat treatment and purification using mouse monoclonal antibodies, have significantly reduced this problem. A recombinant factor VIII product is currently being tested as well.

In addition to factor VIII concentrate, factor IX preparations (which also contain factors II, VII, and X) are available for treatment of hemophilia B. Factor IX concentrate may also be useful in patients with hemophilia A and factor VIII antibodies, since these concentrates have "factor VIII bypassing activity" (probably due to activated clotting factors that therefore no longer need factor VIII). However, factor IX concentrate has also caused thromboses and DIC, presumably for the same reason, and should be used cautiously.

Immunoglobulin

A variety of immunoglobulins for intramuscular injection can be prepared from plasma, including hepatitis B immunoglobulin (HBIG) and Rh immunoglobulin (see Chap. 8). Preparation of γ-globulin can now be accomplished so as to minimize microaggregates of protein, making the globulin safe for intravenous injection. Intravenous immunoglobulin (IVIG) is now used to treat congenitally hypo- and agammaglobulinemic patients. In addition, high-dose IVIG (400 mg/kg) has been shown to temporarily increase the platelet count in ITP, possibly because excess IgG blocks the receptors on mononuclear phagocytes that take up IgG-coated platelets. The fractionation techniques involved in the preparation of all immunoglobulins appear to completely eliminate infectious viruses.

Albumin

The preparation of albumin involves long periods of heating plasma at 60°C, which renders it completely free of risk of infectious disease. Indications for the use of albumin are limited. It has traditionally been used as a volume expander, although salt solutions probably work as well and are much less expensive. It is also used as a replacement fluid during plasma exchange.

Transfusion Reactions and Complications

Many different reactions to blood components can occur (Table 9-3). However, the most serious, and paradoxically often the most preventable, is the acute hemolytic transfusion reaction due to the transfusion of incompatible red cells.

Table 9-3. Transfusion reactions

Transfusion reaction	Signs and symptoms	Useful laboratory findings	Treatment	Prevention
Acute hemolysis	Fever Pain at IV site Back pain Jaundice Hypotension	Positive DAT (Coombs) Hemoglobinemia Hemoglobinuria Elevated LDH, bilirubin Absent haptoglobin Elevated BUN, creatinine DIC	Support blood pressure Maintain urine output Dialysis for renal failure	Avoid clerical errors
Delayed hemolysis	Fever Jaundice	Positive DAT (Coombs) Positive antibody screen Fall in hematocrit	None	Antigen-negative blood
Febrile nonhemolytic	Fever	None	None	White-cell–poor red cells (filtered or washed) if reactions are recurrent
"Noncardiogenic" pulmonary edema	Dyspnea	Anti-HLA antibodies	Respiratory support	White-cell–poor red cells
Allergic	Urticaria	None	Antihistamines	Plasma-free components (washed red cells) if reactions are recurrent
IgA deficiency	Flushing Dyspnea Hypotension	Absent IgA Anti-IgA antibodies	Epinepherine Blood pressure support	IgA-deficient or plasma-free components
Bacterial contamination	Fever Shock	Positive blood culture Positive bag culture	Blood pressure support Antibiotics	Report to blood collection facility
Graft-versus-host disease	Aplastic anemia Mucositis Skin rash Liver disease	Identification of donor T cells (difficult) Skin biopsy	Unknown (?anti–T cell antibodies, immuno-suppressive drugs)	Irradiated blood components for immuno-compromised patients

BUN = blood urea nitrogen; DIC = disseminated intravascular coagulation.

Acute Hemolysis

The most common symptom of abrupt hemolysis due to incompatible blood is fever, but any untoward sign or symptom in a transfusion recipient should prompt suspicion of a hemolytic transfusion reaction. Red cell hemolysis may occur briskly, with intravascular hemolysis, particularly when the antibodies fix complement efficiently (as do ABO antibodies). This results in hemoglobinemia and hemoglobinuria within hours after the transfusion; serum haptoglobin disappears and urine hemosiderin appears 3 to 5 days after the event. Complement by-products released during complement fixation, including the anaphylotoxins C3a and C5a, cause symptoms such as pain at the IV site and cardiovascular shock. Back pain is related to the development of oliguria and renal failure, and is thought to be the result of antigen–antibody complexes rather than free hemoglobin directly. Non-ABO antibodies, such as those to the blood group systems Rh, Kell, Duffy, and Kidd, can also cause acute hemolytic transfusion reactions, but these are often less severe because red cell destruction is primarily extravascular. Although free hemoglobin may be seen with marked extravascular destruction, elevations in just bilirubin and lactic dehydrogenase (LDH) are more common. With all acute hemolytic transfusion reactions, the post-transfusion direct Coombs test becomes positive because of coating of the transfused cells with antibodies.

The mortality associated with ABO incompatibilities is close to 20 percent and is correlated with the volume of incompatible blood transfused. Therefore, it is important to recognize acute hemolysis early and discontinue the transfusion. As with all reactions, the blood bank should be notified; posttransfusion specimens should be sent for a direct antiglobulin test (DAT or Coombs test), visual inspection of the plasma for free hemoglobin, and other markers of hemolysis (LDH, bilirubin, haptoglobin). Treatment should include close observation, blood pressure support if needed with fluids and pressors, and dialysis if needed for renal failure.

Clerical errors are the most frequent cause of ABO incompatibility, and usually occur when a specimen for testing is mislabeled with another patient's name, or when blood crossmatched for one patient is given to another.

Delayed Hemolysis

Delayed hemolysis occurs only with non-ABO antibodies and is an infrequent but largely unavoidable complication. Usually the primary exposure to a foreign red cell antigen (through transfusion or pregnancy) results in only a transient rise in antibody. Subsequently, antibody screens become negative, until the patient is exposed to the same antigen again with a new transfusion. Now a secondary, anamnestic antibody response occurs, typically beginning over the next 3 to 10 days. Hemolysis is often leisurely because it depends on the rate of antibody production. Fever and jaundice develop in some affected patients during this period. Just as often, the patient is entirely asymptomatic, in which case proof of the reaction can be assembled only some time later, when the hematocrit is lower than expected and a new positive direct Coombs test and antibody screen are noted. No treatment is necessary. Future transfusions must be with antigen-negative blood, even if the antibody once again becomes unmeasurably low.

Febrile Transfusion Reactions

The most common reaction to the transfusion of blood, particularly red cells and platelets, is fever, sometimes accompanied by chills or rigors. HLA antibodies in the recipient directed at antigens on white cells in the donor component are responsible for this picture. Unfortunately, fever is also the most common early symptom of acute hemolysis, and it is not possible to distinguish between the febrile, nonhemolytic reaction and acute hemolysis at the bedside. *Therefore, every transfusion-related fever should be evaluated and the transfusion should be discontinued.* Usually the febrile reaction is mild and happens only once to a patient. However, some patients have recurrent febrile reactions, or develop severe symptoms, including respiratory distress due to pulmonary leukoagglutination. Such patients should receive white-cell–poor components for future transfusions.

Noncardiogenic Pulmonary Edema (Transfusion-associated Acute Lung Injury)

This uncommon problem is also due to HLA leukoagglutinating antibodies. Often the offending antibodies are in the donor rather than the recipient. The transfusion of red cells or plasma results in acute respiratory distress. The clinical picture resembles that of acute pulmonary edema, but cardiac filling pressures are normal. The patient usually improves in 12 to 24 hours. If due to a donor's HLA antibodies, the reaction is unlikely to occur in the same patient again. Recurrent reactions should be assumed to be due to recipient antibodies, and such patients should receive white-cell–poor components.

Allergic Reactions

Urticaria may sometimes be seen in response to the transfusion of foreign plasma proteins. Since hives do not occur in acute hemolytic reactions, it is not necessary to stop the transfusion unless the patient is very uncomfortable. Antihistamines and a slower transfusion rate are often sufficient treatment for this problem.

IgA Deficiency

A life-threatening reaction to plasma may occur in the rare individual who is IgA deficient and has IgG anti-IgA antibodies. The infusion of very small amounts of plasma causes wheezing, facial flushing, and cardiovascular collapse, resembling anaphylaxis. Treatment includes discontinuation of the transfusion and administration of epinephrine. Future transfusions must be either plasma-free (for example, washed or frozen red cells) or from IgA-deficient donors.

Bacterial Contamination

Despite the best blood collection techniques, it is possible to inadvertently introduce bacteria during the phlebotomy. These organisms may survive and grow even in refrigerated red cells, but do particularly well in platelet concentrates because they are stored at room temperature. The recipient of a contaminated component is made acutely ill, with fever and possibly shock, and must be treated for sepsis. This complication is fortunately uncommon.

Graft-versus-host Disease

The immunocompromised patient is at risk for the transfusion complication of graft-versus-host disease (GVH). Viable donor lymphocytes cause symptoms of GVH similar to those seen in bone marrow transplant recipients as a result of transplanted lymphocytes; these symptoms include skin rash, mucositis, and liver dysfunction. In addition, however, transfused donor lymphocytes attack the transfusion recipient's marrow, causing profound and often fatal aplastic anemia. (Aplastic anemia does not develop in the bone marrow transplant recipient because his or her marrow is also of donor origin.) Irradiation of blood components with 1,500 rad kills viable lymphocytes. Such treated components should be given when transfusion is required in patients with congenital or acquired immunodeficiencies, including bone marrow transplant recipients, premature newborns, and patients with Hodgkin's disease. Recently, cases of fatal GVH have been observed in immunologically normal recipients following transfusion of blood from first-degree relatives (so-called directed or patient-orchestrated donations). Blood components from family members offer no medical advantages over routine blood bank components, but, if used, should also be irradiated.

Hepatitis

Transfusion-transmitted diseases remain an important risk to blood transfusion therapy today. It is possible to screen for some infections, such as hepatitis B, and as a result this virus is an uncommon cause of posttransfusion hepatitis. The likelihood of posttransfusion hepatitis due to so-called non-A, non-B hepatitis virus after transfusion of blood has been estimated to be anywhere between 2 and 12 percent. Although many infections are asymptomatic, some progress to chronic hepatitis and cirrhosis. To reduce this incidence, blood collection facilities currently draw blood from volunteer, as opposed to paid, donors, because studies have shown that the latter group transmits a sevenfold increased incidence of hepatitis. Furthermore, donors are excluded not only if they relate a history of hepatitis or exposure to the virus, but also if their blood has anti-HBc or elevated levels of the liver enzyme ALT ("surrogate" or nonspecific tests that identify some carriers of non-A, non-B hepatitis). Recently, a specific hepatitis C virus has been found to account for most cases of non-A, non-B hepatitis. Now that the hepatitis C virus has been cloned, a specific antibody test has been added to the donor screening procedure and the incidence of this complication has fallen substantially.

Acquired Immunodeficiency Syndrome

The recognition that HIV could be transmitted by blood transfusion led to the rapid development of tests to identify infected donors by the presence of serum HIV antibodies. These tests [the enzyme-linked immunosorbent assay (ELISA) screening test and confirmatory Western blot], which were added to donor-screening procedures in mid-1985, have helped to eliminate virtually all cases of transfusion-transmitted AIDS except from the rare donor who has been recently infected and in whom antibodies have not yet developed. The risk of AIDS from blood is now somewhere between 1 in 40,000 and 1 in 250,000. The number of transfusion-transmitted AIDS cases continues to rise, however, as individuals exposed before 1985 become symptomatic; the incubation period between transfusion and disease may be as long as 13 years.

Other Infectious Diseases

Blood transfusions can also transmit cytomegalovirus (CMV). The disease is asymptomatic or mild in otherwise healthy individuals. Blood components from documented CMV-negative donors are given to immunocompromised patients, such as bone marrow transplant recipients, who are at risk from clinically important CMV infection. Malaria, babesiosis, Epstein-Barr virus, and toxoplasmosis have also been transmitted by blood. A newly recognized virus, HTLV-1, which causes T cell lymphoma, has also been shown to be transmitted by blood. This disorder is rare in the United States but endemic in Japan. It is expected that blood donors will soon be tested for antibodies to this virus.

Miscellaneous

The rare syndrome, *posttransfusion purpura,* presents as sudden, extreme thrombocytopenia in a patient transfused with red cells 7 to 10 days earlier. Although incompletely understood, the syndrome occurs only in patients whose platelets are Pl^{A1}-negative (2% of the population), and who have made anti-Pl^{A1} antibodies. These antibodies destroy Pl^{A1} platelets from the transfused component, and for unclear reasons, the patient's own Pl^{A1}-negative platelets also disappear. The syndrome is self-limited, provided the patient survives a 4- to 6-week period of profound thrombocytopenia. Plasmapheresis may be helpful in removing the antibodies.

It has been suggested that blood transfusions may alter the immune system of recipients, so as to increase the risk of metastases in cancer patients, for example. This hypothesis is controversial, and requires further analysis.

Alternatives to Traditional Transfusion Therapy

The risks of transfusion therapy suggest that nontransfusion therapeutic alternatives be tried first when possible. For example:

DDAVP, a synthetic vasopressin derivative, has been shown to cause release of endothelial stores of factor VIII. It is useful for many forms of von Willebrand's disease and for mild factor VIII deficiency before surgical procedures. In addition, it may be useful in correcting the bleeding diathesis associated with uremia.

Vitamin K is an effective and rapid treatment for Coumadin overdose; the prothrombin time begins to correct 8 to 12 hours after injection. Only life-threatening hypoprothrombinemia should be treated with fresh frozen plasma instead of vitamin K.

Nutritional anemias (due to iron, vitamin B_{12}, or folate deficiency) should be treated with the appropriate hematinic. Transfusions may even be dangerous for the severely anemic patient with a high cardiac output because of the risk of sudden congestive heart failure.

Erythropoietin therapy with recombinant human erythropoietin has virtually replaced red cell transfusions for patients with anemia due to renal insufficiency. There is evidence that erythropoietin can also ameliorate anemia in patients with AIDS receiving anti-HIV therapy and in patients with chronic diseases, such as cancer. Treatment with erythropoietin is expensive but may well become a safe alternative to red cell transfusion in many anemic states.

Autologous Blood Transfusion

Many patients undergoing surgical procedures can avoid homologous blood transfusions through techniques that allow the collection and retransfusion of their own blood, including:

Preoperative autologous blood donation. Most patients are able to donate one unit a week of their own blood, particularly if iron is taken to prevent iron deficiency. Autologous units can be stored liquid (for up to 6 weeks) or frozen for later use during surgery.

Intraoperative and postoperative blood salvage. Blood suctioned from the surgical field, once discarded, is now often collected, washed (to remove surgical field debris), concentrated, and transfused back to the patient. Red cells from postoperative mediastinal chest tube drainage can also be returned to the patient.

Intraoperative hemodilution. The patient is made intentionally anemic at the start of surgery by withdrawing two or more units of blood, which are kept in the operating room for transfusion back at the end of the procedure. Proponents of this technique point to the savings in red cells for any given surgical blood loss.

Blood Substitutes

Research into oxygen-carrying alternatives to blood has been directed at either avoiding the use of blood entirely or circumventing the use of red cells, with their crossmatch and storage requirements. Solutions of the synthetic compounds called *fluorocarbons* (similar to organic compounds, with a carbon backbone, but with fluorine instead of hydrogen) can carry oxygen in amounts equivalent to those in human blood, provided that the oxygen tension is close to 100 percent. A trial of the fluorocarbon mixture Fluosol-DA 20% in severely anemic Jehovah's Witnesses, who refuse blood for religious reasons, was recently completed. Unfortunately, the results showed no superiority of Fluosol over nonblood fluids, and licensure of this product by the Food and Drug Administration was denied. Other fluorocarbons and synthetic compounds are under development but not ready for human trials.

Hemoglobin in solution can carry oxygen, and can be prepared from outdated blood. Its circulation time is short, and interference with renal function occurs. However, removal of most of the red cell membrane debris (*stroma-free hemoglobin*) reduces the incidence and severity of renal failure. Additional modifications have also been necessary, including polymerization of hemoglobin monomers to increase the circulation time and addition of pyridoxal phosphate to reduce the very high P_{50} of free hemoglobin. Clinical trials with stroma-free hemoglobin are just beginning.

Therapeutic Pheresis

The selective removal of a component of the blood such as plasma can be accomplished relatively efficiently with the use of automated centrifugation devices called cell separators. In addition to donor pheresis for products such as single-donor platelets, some therapeutic indications for such techniques have emerged. *Plasmapheresis* (also called *plasma exchange*) was originally used to treat the hyperviscosity of Waldenström's macroglobulinemia. In the last two decades, plasmapheresis has also been tried, with varying degrees of success, in a variety of diseases with a known or hypothesized abnormal plasma constituent, such as an antibody. For example, plasmapheresis is often helpful in myasthenia gravis, where an IgG antibody against acetylcholinesterase receptors causes the muscle weakness. Plamapheresis is also beneficial in Goodpasture's syndrome (with IgG antibodies against renal and pulmonary basement membrane) and familial hypercholesterolemia (with high concentrations of cholesterol and low-density lipoproteins). In thrombotic thrombocytopenic purpura, plasma exchange often appears to be lifesaving, but the factor that causes this illness has not been identified. The effect of plasma exchange in other autoimmune diseases, such as systemic lupus, rheumatoid arthritis, and ITP, and a variety of neurologic disorders, including multiple sclerosis, Guillain-Barré syndrome, and chronic demyelinating disorders, is more variable. Plasmapheresis has potential risks: Rare patients have died from thromboemboli of unclear etiology both during and after the procedure, and cases suggesting that extensive plasma removal predisposes to serious infections have been reported. Furthermore, the procedure is very expensive to perform. Controlled randomized trials are needed to clearly establish the indications for this controversial form of therapy.

Therapeutic plateletpheresis has been employed in essential thrombocythemia to rapidly reduce platelet counts of greater than 1,000,000/cu mm in symptomatic patients. Similarly, leukapheresis has been advocated as initial treatment of leukemia when the blast count exceeds 100,000, to treat or prevent leukostasis. Leukapheresis is now also being used to collect lymphocytes from patients with advanced cancers. The cells are cultured with interleukin-2 to generate lymphokine-activated killer cells (LAK cells), and then injected back into the patient along with interleukin-2. This protocol has resulted in a small but definite number of partial or complete remissions, particularly with renal cancer and melanoma.

Case Development Problems: Blood Transfusion

1. The red cells from a 59-year-old man with chronic lymphocytic leukemia are agglutinated with reagent anti-A (forward type), but his serum does not react with either A cells or B cells. Explain.

   This patient may have become severely hypogammaglobuline-mic from his leukemia. As a result antibodies, including the anti-B he would have been predicted to have, may have fallen to undetectable levels. An explanation for any ABO-type discrepancies must be uncovered, and the ABO type firmly established, to prevent transfusion with the wrong blood type and subsequent hemolysis.

2. A newborn baby's red cells type as group O. The mother is group A and her husband is group B. Can the husband really be the father of the child?

   Yes, if the mother's genotype is AO and the father's is BO, one in four children can be expected to be OO.

3. A 45-year-old woman who needs red cell transfusions has a positive antibody screen, and the following antibodies are identified: anti-Kell, anti-I (low-titer), and anti-P_1 (room temperature reactions only). What blood should be crossmatched?

   Although some red cell alloantibodies cause significant hemolysis, many others are harmless in vivo, and are only a problem in the test tube. Anti-Kell can cause significant hemolysis, and therefore Kell-negative red cells must be chosen for the crossmatch. This is relatively easy, as only 10 percent of donors are Kell-positive. Neither the low-titer anti-I nor the room temperature anti-P_1 causes clinically significant hemolysis of transfused red cells, and no special search for antigen-negative units is necessary.

4. Major unexpected bleeding occurs during an exploratory laparotomy on a 54-year-old man. The blood bank had performed a type (group A–positive) and antibody screen (negative) before surgery, but no blood had been crossmatched. Can this patient be transfused emergently?

   If no unexpected antibodies were found using an antibody screen, the likelihood of any crossmatches being incompatible is extremely small (<1 in 50,000). Group A, Rh-positive packed red cells could be issued immediately, following a rapid room temperature mix of the patient's serum and donor red cells to ensure ABO compatibility. A complete crossmatch would be done in retrospect to confirm the absence of problems.

5. A patient who is being transfused with red cells complains of chills shortly after the transfusion begins; his temperature is 101°F. What is the appropriate course of action?

   The transfusion should be discontinued immediately, so that an investigation to rule out acute hemolysis can be conducted. This includes checking for clerical errors, both at the bedside and in the blood bank. The blood bag and posttransfusion specimens should be sent to the laboratory so that additional testing, including the patient's direct Coombs test and inspection for free hemoglobin, can be done. No new transfusions should be given to the patient until this evaluation is completed, so as to avoid compounding an error (for example, giving additional ABO-incompatible units).

6. A 45-year-old woman with chronic myelocytic leukemia has been transfused with platelets because of chemotherapy-induced thrombocytopenia. The pretransfusion count was 8,000/cu mm; the 1-hour posttransfusion count is 16,000/cu mm. What could have caused the poor increment?

   Possible explanations include splenomegaly, which accompanies chronic myelocytic leukemia (CML) and could result in the sequestration of the majority of transfused platelets; fever, which reduces the half-life of platelets in vivo; bleeding, which consumes platelets; and platelet refractoriness due to alloimmunization to HLA antibodies. Determining the etiology of the poor response is essential to planning future platelet transfusions; for example, larger-volume platelet transfusions can result in satisfactory increments in patients with splenomegaly, while HLA-matched components may be needed to counter refractoriness to randomly selected platelet donors.

7. A 64-year-old man who had coronary artery bypass surgery 6 years ago presents to you with weight loss, diarrhea, and easy bruising. His past medical history is significant for two units of blood transfused during the surgery. On examination he has diffuse lymphadenopathy and oral thrush. His platelet count is 15,000/cu mm. What is the probable diagnosis?

   Consider the diagnosis of transfusion-transmitted AIDS. The adenopathy and weight loss are consistent with HIV infection, the diarrhea suggests an opportunistic gastrointestinal pathogen, and immune thrombocytopenia is a frequent concomitant to AIDS. Although antibody conversion occurs relatively quickly after transfusion, the incubation period before symptomatic illness from HIV may be quite long. It is likely that cases of transfusion-associated AIDS related to pre-1985 transfusions will continue to be diagnosed over the next decade. It is vital that such cases be reported to the center that collected the blood for transfusion, so that the involved donors can be tested, the implicated donor identified, and other recipients of blood from the same donor contacted.

8. Which blood component would be most suitable for each of the following patients?

A 75-year-old man with transfusion-dependent aplastic anemia.

Packed red cells.

A 60-year-old woman with a negative antibody screen but recurrent febrile reactions to packed red cells.

White-cell–poor red cells.

A severely anemic 35-year-old patient with alloantibodies to Kell, S, E, and Kidd (Jk^b).

Red cells from a rare donor registry, probably frozen.

A 27-year-old woman with Stage IV Hodgkin's disease, for postoperative anemia.

Packed red cells, irradiated.

A 43-year-old man who had a life-threatening anaphylactoid reaction to a previous transfusion of plasma because of IgA deficiency.

Washed red cells (and FFP from an IgA-deficient donor, if needed).

Selected Readings

General

Huestis, D. W., Bove, J. R., and Busch, S. *Practical Blood Transfusion* (3rd ed.). Boston: Little, Brown, 1981.

Klein, H. G. Transfusion medicine: The evolution of a new discipline. *J.A.M.A.* 258 : 2108, 1987.

Mollison, P. L. *Blood Transfusion in Clinical Medicine* (7th ed.). Oxford: Blackwell Scientific Publications, 1983.

Widmann, F. K. (ed.) *Technical Manual* (9th ed.). Arlington, VA: American Association of Blood Banks, 1985.

Blood Groups

Issitt, P. D. *Applied Blood Group Serology* (3rd ed.). Miami: Montgomery Scientific Publications, 1985.

Marcus, D. M. (ed.). Blood group immunochemistry and genetics. *Semin. Hematol.* 18 : 1, 1981.

Components

Consensus Development Conference. Fresh-frozen plasma: Indications and risks. *J.A.M.A.* 253 : 551, 1985.

Daly, P. A. et al. Platelet transfusion therapy—one hour post-transfusion increments are valuable in predicting the need for HLA-matched preparations. *J.A.M.A.* 243 : 435, 1980.

Higby, D. J., and Burnett, D. Granulocyte transfusions: Current status. *Blood* 55 : 2, 1980.

Howard, J. E., and Perkins, H. A. The natural history of alloimmunization to platelets. *Transfusion* 18 : 469, 1978.

Janson, P. A. et al. Treatment of bleeding tendency in uremia with cryoprecipitate. *N. Engl. J. Med.* 303 : 1318, 1980.

Kruskall, M. S. et al. Transfusion therapy in emergency medicine. *Ann. Emerg. Med.* 17 : 327, 1988.

Oberman, H. A., Barnes, B. A., and Friedman, B. A. The risk of abbreviating the crossmatch in urgent or massive transfusion. *Transfusion* 18 : 137, 1978.

Synder, E. L. (ed.). *Blood transfusion therapy: A physician's handbook* (3rd ed.). Arlington, VA: American Association of Blood Banks, 1987.

Complications of Blood Transfusion

Bove, J. R. Transfusion-associated hepatitis and AIDS: What is the risk? *N. Engl. J. Med.* 317 : 242, 1987.

Heal, J. M. et al. Fatal *Salmonella* septicemia after platelet transfusion. *Transfusion* 27 : 2, 1987.

Leitman, S. F., and Holland, P. V. Irradiation of blood products: Indications and guidelines. *Transfusion* 25 : 293, 1985.

Pineda, A. A., Brzica, S. M., and Taswell, H. F. Hemolytic transfusion reaction: Recent experience in a large blood bank. *Mayo Clin. Proc.* 53 : 378, 1978.

Walker, R. H. Special report: Transfusion risks. *Am. J. Clin. Pathol.* 88 : 374, 1987.

Alternatives to Blood Transfusion

Gould, S. A. et al. Fluosol-DA as a red cell substitute in acute anemia. *N. Engl. J. Med.* 314 : 1653, 1986.

Kruskall, M. S. et al. Utilization and effectiveness of a hospital autologous preoperative blood donor program. *Transfusion* 314 : 1233, 1986.

Popovsky, M. A., Devine, P. A., and Taswell, II. F. Intraoperative autologous transfusion. *Mayo Clin. Proc.* 60 : 125, 1985.

Sehgal, L. R. et al. Polymerized pyridoxylated hemoglobin: A red cell substitute with normal oxygen-carrying capacity. *Surgery* 95 : 433, 1984.

Warrier, A. I., and Lusher, J. M. DDAVP: A useful alternative to blood components in moderate hemophilia-A and von Willebrand's disease. *J. Pediatr.* 12 : 228, 1983.

Pheresis

Fauci, A. S. et al. Immunomodulators in clinical medicine. *Ann. Intern. Med.* 106 : 421, 1987.

Shumak, K. H., and Rock, G. A. Therapeutic plasma exchange. *N. Engl. J. Med.* 310 : 762, 1984.

Paul R. Reich
Marshall E. Kadin
Peter F. Weller

Leukocytes prevent and fight infections: Granulocytes do this by their ability to phagocytize bacteria, and lymphocytes by their role in cell-mediated immunity and antibody production. Qualitative and quantitative disorders of granulocytes and lymphocytes are discussed in this chapter; proliferative and malignant diseases of leukocytes are discussed in Chapters 12 and 13. For each of the cells classified as leukocytes—neutrophilic granulocytes, basophils, eosinophils, lymphocytes, and monocytes—a description of known origin, morphology, function, and cell kinetics, and the differential diagnosis of quantitative abnormalities, such as leukopenia or leukocytosis, are given. Only a small number of laboratory procedures useful for diagnosing abnormalities of leukocytes are available: total white blood cell count, white blood cell differential, and peripheral blood and marrow morphology.

Several of the diseases that cause anemia also affect leukocytes. For example, in megaloblastic anemia there is frequently an associated depression of the total white blood cell count and in particular the granulocyte count. Once the diagnosis of megaloblastic anemia is made and treatment instituted, the white blood cell count returns to normal.

Table 10-1 summarizes leukocyte abnormalities found in peripheral blood.

Quantitation of Leukocytes

The total *white blood cell* or *leukocyte count* in the peripheral blood is usually determined by an electronic, automatic counter. The Coulter counter enumerates white cells as they pass between electrodes and creates a pulse due to displacement of electrolytic solution. A lysing agent is required to rupture the red cell membranes, so that red cells will not be counted. The total leukocyte or white blood cell count is normally 4.5 to 11.0×10^9 per liter. Another electronic counter, the Technicon H1, works somewhat differently, and also differentiates among the various types of leukocytes. An optical system uses light scattering to assay size of the white cells. Leukocytes are stained for

Table 10-1. Abnormalities of leukocytes and diseases associated with these abnormalities

Abnormality	Description	Associated diseases
Leukocytosis	White blood cell count > 11.0 × 10^9/L	Any physiologic or pathologic stress, corticosteroids, leukemia, etc.
Neutrophilic leukocytosis (granulocytosis)	Neutrophilic leukocyte count > 7.5 × 10^9/L	Infection, intoxication, tissue necrosis, myeloproliferative syndromes, leukemia (e.g., chronic myelocytic), hemorrhage, hemolysis
Neutropenia or granulocytopenia	Neutrophilic count < 1.5 × 10^9/L	Drugs, infection, congenital, megaloblastic anemia, aplastic anemia, acute leukemia, lupus erythematosus, rheumatoid arthritis, postirradiation, autoantibodies, hypersplenism, myelophthisis
Toxic granulation (Plate 43)	Distinct small black or purple cytoplasmic granules	Infections, inflammatory diseases, burns
Döhle bodies (Plate 40)	Small (1–2 µg) blue cytoplasmic inclusions in neutrophils	Infections, inflammatory diseases, burns
Pelger-Huët anomalies (Plates 41 and 42)	Neutrophil with bilobed nucleus or no segmentation of nucleus. Chromatin is coarse.	Hereditary acute or chronic myelocytic leukemias, myelodysplastic syndromes
May-Hegglin anomaly	Basophilic cytoplasmic inclusions of leukocytes, similar to Döhle bodies.	May-Hegglin syndrome (hereditary) includes thrombocytopenia and giant platelets
Alder's anomaly	Prominent azurophilic granulation in leukocytes, similar to toxic granulation. Granulation is seen better with Giemsa's stain.	Gargoylism and associated hereditary mucopolysaccharidoses
Chédiak-Higashi anomaly	Gray-green, large cytoplasmic inclusions	Chédiak-Higashi syndrome
Eosinophilia	Eosinophil count > 0.6 × 10^9/L	Allergic disorders, collagen diseases, parasitic infections, Hodgkin's disease, chronic myelocytic leukemia, pernicious anemia, tissue necrosis (e.g., postirradiation), sarcoid, malignancies, chronic skin diseases, hypereosinophilic syndromes
Basophilic leukocytosis	Basophil count > 0.05 × 10^9/L	Chronic myelocytic leukemia, other myeloproliferative syndromes
Myeloid "shift-to-the-left"	Presence of bands, metamyelocytes, and perhaps some earlier forms in peripheral blood	Infections, tissue necrosis, myeloproliferative syndromes, leukemia (chronic myelocytic), leukemoid reaction

Table 10-1 (continued)

Abnormality	Description	Associated diseases
Hypersegmented neutrophil (Plate 27)	Mature neutrophil with more than 5 distinct lobes	Megaloblastic anemia, hereditary constitutional hypersegmentation of neutrophils, iron deficiency anemia
Lymphocytosis	Lymphocytes $> 9.0 \times 10^9$/L in young children, 7.0×10^9/L in older children, and 5.0×10^9/L in adults	Infectious mononucleosis, viral infections, chronic lymphocytic leukemia, lymphomas
Atypical lymphocytes (Plates 49–51)	Lymphocytes with excessive, vacuolated cytoplasm. May contain lobulated (monocytoid) nucleus and sometimes nucleoli.	Infectious mononucleosis, viral hepatitis, and other viral infections; drug sensitivity
Monocytosis	Monocyte count $> 1.0 \times 10^9$/L	Chronic infectious and inflammatory diseases, e.g., tuberculosis or bacterial endocarditis; recovery from bone marrow suppression, lymphomas, solid tumors, myelodysplastic syndromes
Plasmacytosis (Plate 52)	Plasma cells present (none are normally seen) in peripheral blood	Multiple myeloma, plasma cell leukemia, viral illnesses, serum sickness
Leukemic cells (lymphoblasts, myeloblasts, etc.)	Presence of lymphoblasts, myeloblasts, monoblasts, promyelocytes (none normally present in peripheral blood)	Leukemia (acute or chronic), leukemoid reaction (rarely), myeloproliferative syndromes, recovery from bone marrow suppression, myelophthisis
Auer rods (Plate 62)	Rodlike, 1–6 μg long, red-purple, refractile inclusions in primitive neutrophils	Acute nonlymphocytic leukemia
Histiocytosis	Presence of phagocytic cells (none normally seen in peripheral blood)	Chronic infectious disease (e.g., subacute bacterial endocarditis), malignant histiocytosis, certain viral illnesses

the enzyme peroxidase, and can therefore be characterized by both size and peroxidase content. Eosinophils and neutrophils stain strongly with peroxidase and can be separated by their different size and intensity of staining (eosinophils are smaller and stain more intensely with peroxidase). Neutrophils have intermediate levels of peroxidase and monocytes only little of this enzyme. Lymphocytes are smaller than eosinophils and neutrophils, and do not stain with peroxidase. Although all leukocytes, especially immature neutrophils, cannot be differentiated by this machine, the instrument alerts the operator to the presence of abnormal or atypical cells, which must then be identified under the microscope.

Table 10-2. Normal human peripheral blood white cell differential count

Cells	Ranges (%)	Cells ($\times 10^9$/L)
Total WBC	—	4.5–11.0
Neutrophils	40–75	1.50–7.50
Lymphocytes	15–45	0.60–5.00
Monocytes	1–10	0.00–0.80
Eosinophils	1–7	0.05–0.60
Basophils	0–2	0.02–0.05

White cell differential counts are commonly still performed by microscopic examination. A drop of blood is placed on a slide or cover slip and smeared into a thin film. This film is stained with Wright's or Giemsa's stain. At least 100 cells are identified under the microscope and classified as neutrophils, bands, lymphocytes, monocytes, eosinophils, or basophils. Any cells that are not usually seen in the peripheral blood and that are therefore abnormal, such as nucleated reds or "blast" cells, are also classified and counted. The results are expressed as percentages. Table 10-2 shows the upper and lower limits of normal for each cell type.

Nucleated red cells are counted as white cells by both manual and electronic methods. The WBC can be corrected for the presence of nucleated reds by using the nucleated red cell differential count, for example,

$$\text{Total WBC} = 6.0 \times 10^9 \text{ per liter}$$
$$\text{nucleated reds} = 10 \text{ per 100 WBC}$$
$$\text{then } (6.0 \times 10^9) - (0.1 \times 6.0 \times 10^9) = \text{corrected WBC}$$
$$= 5.4 \times 10^9 \text{ per liter}$$

Granulocytes

The term *granulocytes* comprises neutrophils, eosinophils, and basophils. Neutrophils are the most common and important of these cell types, and will be discussed first. It should be pointed out that, although technically incorrect, the word granulocyte is often used synonymously with *neutrophil.* Another, more appropriate synonym for neutrophil is polymorphonuclear leukocyte, often abbreviated to *poly* or *polymorph.*

Neutrophils

Peripheral blood granulocytes are predominantly segmented neutrophils (polymorphonuclear leukocytes), although some nonsegmented, less mature neutrophils are also found in normal blood. Morphologic characteristics of neutrophil precursors in the bone marrow are described in the chapter on hematopoiesis (Chap. 1).

ABNORMAL NEUTROPHIL MORPHOLOGY

Döhle bodies (Plate 40) are pale blue, single or multiple, cytoplasmic inclusions about 0.5 μg in diameter. They are seen in patients with bacterial infections and burns, and following the administration of anticancer agents such as cyclophosphamide. Döhle bodies consist of residual ribonuclear proteins. Similar blue cytoplasmic inclusion bodies in neutrophils are seen in an inherited disorder called *May-Hegglin anomaly*, in which the patients have low white blood cell and platelet counts and giant platelets. The acquired Döhle bodies seen in infections are different ultrastructurally from the inclusion bodies in the May-Hegglin anomaly.

The Pelger-Hüet anomaly takes two forms, acquired and inherited. In the heterozygous inherited condition (Plate 41), the mature neutrophil is characterized by two nuclear lobes, both of which are round and connected by a thin strand of chromatin, giving a dumbbell or *pince-nez* appearance. These cells function normally. In the homozygous inherited form (Plate 42), the nucleus is round rather than segmented. Both these anomalies, the dumbbell-shaped and the round, nonsegmented nucleus, may be seen in acquired conditions such as the myelocytic leukemias, and particularly the myelodysplastic syndromes. Occasionally such *Pelgeroid anomalies* are found in patients with infections or drug reactions. In these cases the acquired changes may be reversible.

Toxic granulations (Plates 40 and 43)—distinct dark, black, or purple cytoplasmic granules—are often seen in polys from patients with infections. They are fused primary and secondary granules loaded with alkaline phosphatase and lytic enzymes, and they are often found in association with Döhle bodies and sometimes cytoplasmic vacuolization.

In *Alder's anomaly*, a rare abnormality, cytoplasmic inclusions resembling toxic granules are found in the granulocytes, monocytes, and lymphocytes of children with familial disorders called the *mucopolysaccharidoses*. Hypersegmentation of the *neutrophil nucleus* may be inherited, but is more commonly seen in megaloblastic anemias. Sepsis can cause vacuolization of granulocytes, nuclear pyknosis (shrinkage), and loss of normal neutrophilic granules. Hypogranularity of neutrophils is often observed in the myelodysplastic disorders and acute nonlymphocytic leukemia. The very rarely encountered *Chédiak-Higashi anomaly* is a familial disorder characterized by abnormally large primary granules in the cytoplasm of mature granulocytes and lymphocytes. Affected patients have partial albinism, susceptibility to bacterial infections, and photophobia, and usually die of a lymphomalike illness. The function of their lymphocytes, especially *natural killer (NK) cells* (see Lymphocyte section), is abnormal and probably contributes to their susceptibility to pyogenic infections and neoplasia. Treatment with interferon and bone marrow transplantation have helped patients with this disease.

NEUTROPHIL POOLS AND KINETICS

Granulopoiesis has been investigated by labeling leukocytes with radioactive (tritiated) thymidine, chromium 51, or diisopropylfluorophosphate 32 (^{32}DFP). From these and other studies, the functioning of the committed granulocytic stem cell and the organization of maturing granulocytes into functional pools have been deduced. Pluripotential stem cells with ability to replicate themselves and to differentiate into committed stem cells are described in Chapter 1. Cells derived from pluripotential stem cells serve as committed stem cells for the granulocytic series. The first recognizable member of the granulocyte series to develop from the granulocytic progenitor cell is the myeloblast. Myeloblasts, promyelocytes, and myelocytes retain the ability to divide. More differentiated cells, metamyelocytes, bands, and polys, mature but do not undergo mitosis.

Once the mature granulocyte (poly) is in the bloodstream, it may exist in one of two pools, the circulating granulocyte pool (CGP) or the marginal granulocyte pool (MGP). Cells in these pools are constantly interchanging, and equilibration between pools occurs rapidly. The CGP is quantified by the routine white blood cell count. Granulocytes in the marginal pool are not counted, since they remain in the intravascular space close to the endothelium but outside the mainstream of the circulation. Equal numbers of granulocytes are present in each of these pools, so shifting from the MGP to the CGP can approximately double blood neutrophil counts. Such shifting has been seen after stress or corticosteroid or epinephrine administration. In inflammatory disease it is possible for the MGP to increase while the CGP remains stable. This is sometimes referred to as *masked granulocytosis*. A shift of cells from the MGP to the CGP is sometimes referred to as *pseudoneutrophilia*.

In the marrow there are also two granulocyte pools: the mitotic pool, consisting of dividing cells, myeloblasts through myelocytes; and the maturation-storage pool, consisting of late myelocytes, metamyelocytes, bands, and segmented neutrophils. Marrow neutrophil differential counts are obtained by counting at least 200, and preferably 500, cells in Wright-stained smears of bone marrow specimens. Normal percentages of each cell type are given in Table 10-3.

The cells in the mitotic pool divide by going through a cell cycle consisting of the following phases: G_1 (postmitotic rest period), S (DNA-synthetic phase in which chromosomes replicate from diploid to tetraploid number), G_2 (premitotic rest period), and M (period of mitosis). The so-called generation time for cells capable of successive divisions is the time from one mitosis to the next. As we will see,

Table 10-3. Normal marrow granulocyte differential count

Cell type	Range (%)*
Myeloblast	1–2
Promyelocyte	2–4
Myelocyte	8–16
Metamyelocyte	10–15
Band forms	15–20
Mature granulocytes	10–20
Eosinophils	1–5

*Erythroid and other cell lines make up the difference from 100%.

knowledge about cell cycles both for normal granulocytes and in pathologic states such as leukemia is important in planning rational chemotherapy.

The normal human marrow contains 18.0×10^9 nucleated marrow cells per kilogram of body weight. Of this number, 11.4×10^9 per kilogram are in the granulocytic series. The marrow granulocyte reserve (MGR), consisting of bands and mature granulocytes, is put at 8.8×10^9 cells per kilogram. There is disagreement about this number, but it is considerably larger than the number of mature neutrophils in the peripheral blood. The bone marrow releases into the bloodstream 1.6×10^9 (another estimate is 0.7×10^9) cells per kilogram per day of mature granulocytes. There are 0.39 cells $\times 10^9$ per kilogram in the marginal granulocytic pool and 0.31×10^9 cells per kilogram in the circulating granulocyte pool. The total blood granulocyte pool is 0.7 cells $\times 10^9$ per kilogram of body weight.

The average life span of the granulocyte in the peripheral blood is 10 to 14 hours. It survives in tissues for only a short time. Thus, it spends most of its time in the bone marrow, a relatively short time in the peripheral blood, and, once it has entered the tissues, it does not return, but dies performing its phagocytic function.

Mobilization of granulocytes into the tissues can be studied by abrading a section of the skin and, at different intervals, placing a glass slide over the injured area *(Rebuck skin window)*. By allowing the leukocytes to stick to the glass and then staining them with Wright's stain, an estimate of the number of cells available for mobilization to inflamed sites and their differential counts can be obtained. Normally cells appear in 2 to 4 hours. Initially the responding cells are mainly granulocytes, but at 24 hours monocytes predominate. The neutrophil response is impaired in patients who receive steroids or ethanol and in individuals with acute leukemia, diabetes mellitus, and some forms of neutropenia. Some leukopenic patients have normal skin window responses despite a low CGP, their MGP and MGR being normal or near-normal.

Neutrophil kinetic studies employing tritiated thymidine, ^{32}DFP, or radiochromium can be used to determine the relative contributions of defects in granulocyte production, survival, or margination to abnormal granulocyte counts found in patients.

Epinephrine causes a neutrophilic leukocytosis by mobilizing granulocytes from the marginal pool. Etiocholanolone or endotoxin increases release of stored marrow neutrophils. Endotoxin also causes increased margination of neutrophils. Thus, patients with gram-negative sepsis and endotoxemia typically have initial neutropenia followed by neutrophilic leukocytosis. The rise in neutrophil count seen immediately after the administration of adrenal corticosteroids is due to release of marrow neutrophils and to delayed migration from the blood, that is, demargination. Transient neutropenia in hemodialysis patients is caused by intravascular margination of neutrophils in the lungs.

Patients with severe neutropenia ("agranulocytosis") due to accelerated peripheral blood loss of granulocytes may show "maturation arrest" of their marrow granulocyte precursor cells. Most of the granulocyte precursors present are immature. There is, however, no functional block or "arrest" in the maturation of the myelocytes; rather, there is depletion of the MGR by greatly increased peripheral demand and perhaps by the antibodies that are mediating destruction of neutrophils in the peripheral blood. The marrow may actually be producing normal or increased amounts of granulocytes, yet only immature cells will be seen. In such a case a misdiagnosis of acute leukemia should be avoided. Similarly, during recovery from drug-induced agranulocytosis due to marrow suppression there may be transient marrow hyperplasia and an increased number of immature forms. This can be severe enough to be mistaken for myelocytic leukemia. The reason for the shift is not peripheral demand, but rather the starting up of granulocyte production from the stem cell level.

NEUTROPHIL PRODUCTION CONTROL MECHANISMS

The control mechanisms by which a normal blood neutrophil level is maintained are not completely known. It is believed that when the peripheral blood granulocyte count falls, stimulatory factors come into play that lead to increased production of blood granulocytes and release of granulocytes from the marrow granulocyte reserve. GM-CSF and G-CSF clearly play a role in these processes but other factors may also be of importance. If the marrow granulocyte reserve is reduced, as occurs in cyclic neutropenia and following subtotal marrow suppression by cyclophosphamide, the normal, stable blood leukocyte count will be altered, and oscillations may occur in the leukocyte count. Such oscillations have been seen in some patients with marrow damage, chronic granulocytic leukemia, and cyclic neutropenia.

The marrow granulocyte mitotic pool is clearly under humoral control. Factors such as GM-CSF and G-CSF stimulate committed granulocyte progenitor cells to increase neutrophil production. The colony-stimulating factors (CSFs) and other hematopoietic growth factors are discussed more fully in the chapter on hematopoiesis (see Chap. 1).

NEUTROPHILIC LEUKOCYTOSIS

Neutrophilia ($> 7.5 \times 10^9$ neutrophils per liter) is far more common than neutropenia. Infections and inflammatory diseases cause neutrophilia more commonly than do neoplastic conditions such as leukemia. Almost any stress to the human body can result in leukocytosis with increased granulocyte counts. Even pregnant women and cigarette smokers can have elevated white cell counts. Because the causes of neutrophilia are so numerous, a rational approach to diagnosis is difficult. Luckily the patient's history usually suggests a primary cause, often a nonhematologic disease. Examination of the peripheral blood and bone marrow will usually reveal any primary blood disorder. Therapy for granulocytosis is essentially treatment of the underlying disease.

NEUTROPENIA

Leukopenia means a *total* white blood cell count of less than 4.0×10^9 per liter. *Granulocytopenia,* or *neutropenia,* is present when the "absolute" granulocyte count (WBC × neutrophil fraction) is less than 1.5×10^9 granulocytes per liter, counting only neutrophilic granulocytes at the band or mature cell (poly) maturation level. Severe and frequent infections usually do not appear until the "absolute" granulocyte count falls to 0.5×10^9 per liter or less. Some increase in infections may be seen in the range of 0.5 to 1.0×10^9 granulocytes per liter. As will be seen, granulocytopenia may be caused by a large variety of disorders.

The term *agranulocytosis* refers to a syndrome consisting of the abrupt disappearance of virtually all circulating granulocytes, usually accompanied by fever, sore throat, and necrosis of oral mucus membranes. If the granulocytopenia is not corrected, sepsis may occur. Although agranulocytosis may be caused by a variety of disorders, it is usually associated with drugs.

One may wish to assess the bone marrow reserves of neutrophils in patients with neutropenia. Examination of a bone marrow specimen suggests normal reserves if normal numbers of bands and mature neutrophils are present. Functional tests are also available. For example, 40 mg prednisone, a synthetic adrenal steroid, will normally increase the peripheral blood granulocyte count by about 4 to 5×10^9 per liter 5 hours after its administration. Similar tests may be done with bacterial endotoxin or etiocholanolone. The problem with corticosteroids is that they not only promote release of granulocytes from the marrow but also interfere with normal egress of granulocytes from blood vessels into tissues, thereby complicating the interpretation of any increment in circulating granulocytes.

Pathophysiology

Granulocytopenia is caused primarily by either decreased production of granulocytes in the marrow or increased destruction of circulating neutrophils (see p. 239).

Decreased production of neutrophils. Drugs and ionizing radiation are common causes of decreased marrow production of granulocytes. Examination of a marrow specimen shows absent or decreased neutrophil precursor cells.

Damage to stem cells, interference with normal DNA metabolism, and destruction of the marrow stroma and microcirculation are possible causes of drug-induced marrow aplasia. Study of the phenothiazine drugs indicates that they cause myeloid hypoplasia or aplasia by interfering with DNA synthesis. Unexplained host factors affect susceptibility to the marrow-damaging effects of the phenothiazines. Many patients receiving these drugs develop neutropenia but only a few develop agranulocytosis. Several other classes of drugs also produce mild suppression of neutrophil production commonly and granulocytosis rarely; examples include the antithyroid drugs, sulfa drugs, and semisynthetic penicillins. Cessation of drug therapy usually results in recovery after 1 to 2 weeks. Ionizing radiation probably owes its effect on granulocyte production to its DNA-damaging ability. Hematopoietic stem cells are destroyed by low to moderate radiation doses. Very high doses may inflict irreversible damage on the marrow stroma or microcirculation, preventing regeneration. Fortunately, the damage done by carefully planned radiotherapy is reversible, with leukocyte, red cell, and platelet counts returning to normal in a few weeks following cessation of therapy. Similarly, chemotherapeutic drugs used for treatment of cancer patients often suppress hematopoietic stem cells, with temporary decreases in the leukocyte, red cell, and platelet counts. Some chemotherapeutic drugs may also damage the marrow stroma.

Some inherited and cyclic neutropenias are also associated with myeloid hypoplasia. Rare familial diseases, such as Kostmann's syndrome and cyclic neutropenia, may be caused by hypoplasia or aplasia of granulocyte precursors. Cyclic neutropenic patients usually have leukocyte counts that oscillate at intervals of 15 to 35 days. At the nadir of the leukocyte count, their marrows are devoid of granulocytic precursors, and infections may develop. Between attacks the bone marrow appears normal. There is evidence that cyclic neutropenia is due to damage to pluripotential marrow stem cells, the cycling being an expression of deranged control mechanisms. Indeed, the blood levels of reticulocytes and platelets also

---

> **Causes of neutropenia***
>
> **I.** Decreased production of granulocytes
>   A. Congenital hypoplasia (Kostmann's syndrome)
>   B. Drugs, including anticancer agents
>   C. X-irradiation
>   D. Inherited and cyclic neutropenias
>   E. Chronic benign neutropenia
>   F. Myelophthisis (marrow replacement, e.g., by leukemia or lymphoma)
>   G. Megaloblastic anemia (ineffective granulocytopoiesis)
>   H. Myelodysplastic syndromes (abnormal differentiation with ineffective granulocytopoiesis)
>   I. Acute leukemia, lymphocytic or myelogenous
>   J. Aplastic anemia
> **II.** Increased destruction of circulating granulocytes
>   A. Hypersplenism
>   B. Viral and bacterial infections
>   C. Leukocyte antigen–antibody reactions, including autoimmune neutropenia and drug-induced antibody-mediated destruction

*Many of the above conditions are associated with a decreased hematocrit and platelet count as well as a reduced number of neutrophils.

vary cyclically. Further support for the defective stem cell hypothesis comes from a report of a patient who, while undergoing bone marrow transplantation as treatment for leukemia, acquired cyclic neutropenia from her histocompatible sibling donor.

Chronic benign neutropenia is a fairly common disorder that is due to impaired granulocyte release from the bone marrow. Only rarely is the defect severe enough to predispose to infections.

Myelophthisic anemia with replacement of the bone marrow by lymphoma, myeloma, carcinoma, granuloma, or fibrosis is another not uncommon cause of granulocytopenia, particularly in older patients. The red cell and platelet counts are usually also affected.

Ineffective myelopoiesis (production of abnormal granulocytes, which die before their release from the marrow) occurs in patients with megaloblastic anemia or myelodysplastic disorders and is characterized by hypercellularity of the marrow but decreased numbers of granulocytes in the peripheral blood. This is usually accompanied by anemia and thrombocytopenia. Some patients with acute lymphocytic or myelogenous leukemia present with low total leukocyte counts. However, the differential count usually demonstrates blast cells, and the hematocrit and platelet count are typically decreased. Finally, aplastic anemia is associated with a decrease in the leukocyte, red cell and platelet counts in the peripheral blood.

Increased destruction of neutrophils. Three general types of neutropenia due to increased leukocyte destruction are discussed here. The first is caused by hypersplenism and is usually corrected by splenectomy. Almost any disease that enlarges the spleen can lead to hypersplenism and increased sequestration and destruction of mature neutrophils. Hypersplenism also leads to increased destruction and sequestration of red cells and increased sequestration of platelets. It is often seen in association with cirrhosis of the liver, congestive or infiltrative splenomegaly, and *Felty's syndrome* (rheumatoid arthritis with high latex fixation titers and splenomegaly). Felty's syndrome is complex and may also include a marrow production defect for granulocytes, neutrophil dysfunction, increased immunoglobulin G on granulocyte surfaces, and a clinical course characterized by infections sometimes not ameliorated by splenectomy.

The second type is related to infections. Although the mechanism is unclear, viral and bacterial infections can be associated with neutropenia. In many cases not only is increased peripheral destruction or utilization of leukocytes present, but there is decreased production and sometimes increased margination of polys as well.

A third type is due to immunologic mechanisms. In a few neonates maternal isoimmunization and transplacental passage of leukoagglutinins from the mother to the fetus result in destruction of fetal neutrophils. In such cases the mother has been sensitized during previous pregnancies by fetal leukocytes carrying the father's antigenic determinants or by prior transfusion therapy. The antibodies may be directly cytotoxic or cause leukocyte agglutination and subsequent destruction or removal from the circulation. In adults similar white cell antibodies are a common cause of febrile transfusion reactions but seldom are associated with sustained neutropenia.

Autoantibodies directed against a patient's own leukocyte antigens may produce "autoimmune" neutropenia in patients with diseases such as systemic lupus erythematosus, rheumatoid arthritis, and leukemia/lymphocytosis of large granular lymphocytes (LGL syndrome). This mechanism may account for the mild neutropenia often seen in patients with disorders such as systemic lupus. Autoimmune neutropenia may also be idiopathic, that is, without apparent cause or association with other diseases.

Drugs such as aminopyrine can act as haptens against which antibodies are developed. When these antibodies and the drug are present together, an immediate reaction takes place, characterized by fever, chills, and destruction of peripheral blood neutrophils. All the complications of agranulocytosis then occur. The bone marrow appears hyperplastic with only immature granulocyte precursors present, giving rise to the misnamed "maturation arrest" phenomenon (see p. 236). Agranulocytosis subsides 1 to 3 weeks after discontinuation of the drug. Presumably the reaction between drug and antibody causes granulocyte destruction either by agglutination of granulocytes; by coating neutrophils with antibody, which causes their subsequent destruction in the reticuloendothelial system (RES); or by a complement-mediated cytotoxic effect of the antigen–

Common drugs that cause neutropenia
Alcohol
Allopurinol
Aminopyrine*
Antibiotics: chloramphenicol, furadantin, sulfa drugs,* ampicillin and other penicillins,* cephalosporins, gentamicin, metronidazole, griseofulvin, pyrimethamine
Anticonvulsants: diphenylhydantoin, phenobarbital, carbamazepine (Tegretol)
Antithyroid compounds*: thiouracils, methimazole, carbimazole
Benzene
Cancer chemotherapy agents: methotrexate, vincristine, vinblastine, procarbazine, hydroxyurea, cytosine arabinoside, daunomycin, 5-fluorouracil, 6-mercaptopurine, 6-thioguanine, azathioprine, alkylating agents, etc.
Cimetidine
Cinchona alkaloids: quinine, quinidine
Diazepam
Gold salts*
Imipramine and other tricyclic and tetracyclic antidepressants
Indomethacin and other nonsteroidal antiinflammatory agents
Phenothiazines
Phenylbutazone*
Tolbutamide

*Antibody-mediated in at least some patients.

antibody reaction on the cell membrane. This drug–antibody mechanism must be distinguished from granulocytopenia due to drug-induced leukocyte antibodies that do not require presence of the drug for their action and that are directed against leukocyte antigens and not against the drug itself. Possibly the drug combines with or alters the granulocyte membrane, so that the host reacts against a non–self-antigen by forming a leukocyte antibody. (Drugs suspected of causing neutropenia by an antibody-mediated mechanism are marked with an asterisk in the list above.)

Tests for antibody-mediated neutropenia are generally of two types. In the first, leukoagglutination is used as an endpoint after mixing normal granulocytes, patient's serum, and, in possible drug reactions, the suspected agent. Unfortunately, leukocytes tend to agglutinate under all conditions in vitro, and this test is not in common use. More recently developed tests detect the presence of IgG on granulocyte surfaces. Using the latter method antineutrophil antibodies have been described on granulocytes and in serum of patients with autoimmune disease and drug-induced agranulocytosis. The IgG is detected on cell surfaces by standard immunologic methods for the detection of γ-globulin and by several recently developed techniques. Fluoresceinated antibodies raised against IgG are used in conjunction with a fluorescence microscope or a cell sorter to detect white cell antibodies. A cell–cell recognition assay detects IgG on the surface of a granulocyte by observing the biochemical reaction of normal granulocytes to opsonized, that is, antibody-coated, cells. The oxidation of glucose increases in granulocytes exposed to IgG-coated neutrophils. A staphylococcal slide assay detects cells with surface IgG antineutrophil antibody by their ability to bind staphylococci rich in a substance called "protein A." All of these tests can be adapted to detect antibody in serum or on granulocyte surfaces.

Although the detection of leukoagglutinins and antineutrophil IgG is possible, and drugs can be added to reaction mixtures to see whether they promote agglutination or IgG deposition, the assessment of results in suspected cases of autoimmune or drug-induced granulocytopenia is complicated by several factors. Prior pregnancy or transfusions can evoke antibodies that cause incorrect interpretation of assay results. Furthermore, the antibodies detected may not be cytotoxic and, therefore, are less likely implicated as a cause for agranulocytosis in vivo.

Approach to the Patient with Neutropenia

The patient's history, with particular emphasis on ingestion of drugs, exposure to radiation, and cytotoxic cancer chemotherapy, is very important in evaluating possible marrow damage. The physical examination, with attention to signs of cancer, leukemia, lymphoma (for example, lymphadenopathy or splenomegaly), bleeding, or infection, is helpful in determining whether the marrow is possibly infiltrated, as in leukemias, or whether granulocytes are being excessively used or destroyed, as with hypersplenism or infection.

The hematocrit, platelet count, and reticulocyte count give some indication of the overall status of the marrow. Examination of the peripheral blood smear may suggest acute leukemia, megaloblastic anemia, aplastic anemia, or other primary diseases as the underlying cause for granulocytopenia. Occasionally study of the cyclic pattern of the white cell count or investigation of family members may be helpful.

The bone marrow examination is often helpful. If there is complete or partial absence of myeloid precursors, a production deficit is likely. "Maturation arrest," a "shift-to-the-left" with mainly immature granulocytic precursors present, suggests increased neutrophil destruction in both blood and marrow, with exhaustion of the marrow granulocytic reserve. A more severe shift-to-the-left, with presence of only blast cells and perhaps promyelocytes, is usually diagnostic of acute leukemia. Splenomegaly accompanied by a hypercellular bone marrow with normal proportions of granulocyte precursors is usually all that is needed to suggest hypersplenism as the cause of the granulocytopenia.

> **Approach to patient with neutropenia**
>
> **I.** History
>   A. Drugs
>   B. Anticancer therapy
>   C. Radiation exposure
>   D. Family history
>   E. Other diseases (cancer, lupus)
> **II.** Physical examination
>   A. Cancer signs
>   B. Lymphadenopathy
>   C. Splenomegaly
>   D. Signs of bleeding or infection
> **III.** Laboratory tests
>   A. Blood counts, including red cells, platelets
>   B. White cell differential
>   C. Peripheral blood smear for red and white cell morphology
>   D. Bone marrow examination
> **IV.** Other procedures to consider when relevant
>   A. Test for marrow reserves with etiocholanolone, endotoxin, or
>   corticosteroids
>   B. Marrow cytogenetics (myelodysplasia, leukemia)
>   C. Tests for leukocyte antibodies
>   D. ANA, rheumatoid factor to check for disorders often
>   associated with neutropenia, such as systemic lupus
>   erythematosus or rheumatoid arthritis

Therapy for Neutropenia

Rapidly progressive and overwhelming infection remains the most serious complication of severe granulocytopenia. Patients with neutropenia and febrile illnesses must be treated with antibiotics immediately after appropriate cultures are obtained. Prophylactic antibiotics are not indicated in afebrile, granulocytopenic patients, because superinfection with resistant organisms becomes a distinct possibility.

Adrenal corticosteroids are of no value unless an autoimmune mechanism is identified, and actually inhibit margination and phagocytic functions of the few remaining neutrophils. New preparations of γ-globulin that permit intravenous administration are being employed for the treatment of autoimmune neutropenias, perhaps working by inhibiting clearance of antibody-coated neutrophils. Certainly, any suspected drugs or toxic agents should be stopped or removed. Patients who are acutely ill with granulocytopenia and sepsis may rarely benefit from granulocyte transfusion (see Chap. 9).

Lithium carbonate has been used to treat neutropenia associated with Felty's syndrome, cyclical neutropenia, aplastic anemia, and cancer chemotherapy. Lithium appears to increase colony-stimulating activity from monocytes. It is probably of limited clinical value. More promising are GM-CSF and G-CSF. In clinical trials these hematopoietic growth factors have been shown to increase granulocyte production in many conditions. They are now used commonly to hasten recovery of neutrophil levels after cancer chemotherapy and bone marrow transplantation. They may also increase the neutrophil count and help control infection in some patients with aplastic anemia, myelodysplasia, and some forms of congenital and drug-induced neutropenia.

NEUTROPHIL FUNCTION—PHAGOCYTOSIS

The prime function of neutrophils is ingestion of bacteria, or phagocytosis, through which they play a major role in combating pyogenic infection. The monocyte and the macrophage, which also phagocytize bacteria, are discussed later (p. 250).

Chemotaxis, or the attraction of leukocytes toward sites of infection, injury, or inflammation, is mediated by substances in serum called *chemotaxins,* which are released by bacteria or tissues. Antibody–antigen reactions with activation of complement components also play a role in the release of chemotactic substances that attract leukocytes. The complement system, as well as the blood coagulation system including agents such as kallikrein and plasminogen activator, may react and interact to cause chemotaxis. Neutrophils themselves may release chemotactic substances, and lymphocytes have been found to elaborate lymphokines that have chemotactic activity.

Neutrophils adhere preferentially to vascular endothelium adjacent to a site of inflammation. This directed adherence requires that chemotactic peptides formed as by-products of inflammation modify the granulocyte so that it will adhere. Once it is attached to vascular endothelium, the neutrophil attenuates and squeezes through junctions between endothelial cells (diapedesis). Leukemic myeloblasts are not able to attenuate normally.

The capacity of corticosteroids to diminish the accumulation of neutrophils in inflamed sites may be due to their ability to reduce cell adherence to endothelium.

As a result of chemotaxis, phagocytes crawl toward inflamed sites. This leukocyte migration is characterized by the throwing out of pseudopods. The pseudopods are quite filmy and thin, and, as they stream forward, the granules in the main body of the leukocyte move with them, followed last by the cell's nucleus.

The locomotor apparatus of neutrophils consists of a contractile system, not unlike that in muscle, which includes actin and myosin. Actin filaments interact with the contractile protein myosin to produce movement. The reaction is energized by the enzymatic splitting of adenosine triphosphate (ATP). It is modulated by *actin-binding protein,* which arranges actin fibers into a three-dimensional, branching network with actin fibers at right angles to each other;

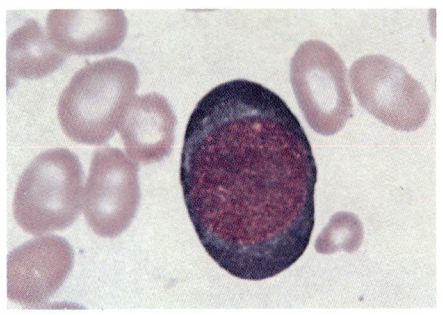

1. Pronormoblast (erythroblast)

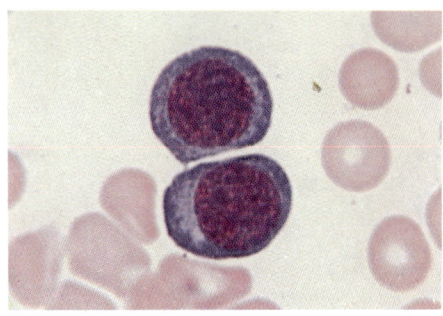

2. Basophilic normoblasts

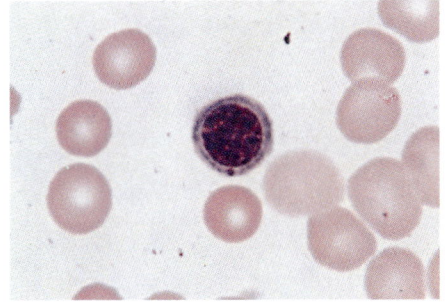

3. Polychromatophilic normoblast

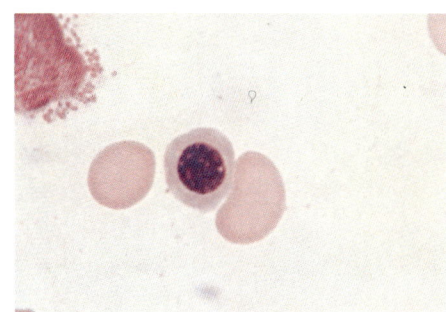

4. Orthochromatophilic normoblast

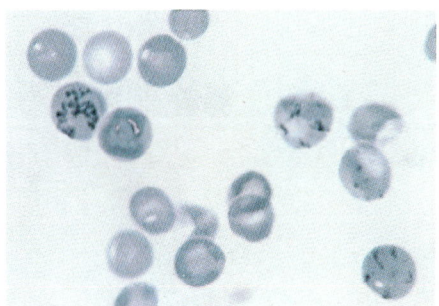

5. Reticulocytes—new methylene blue stain

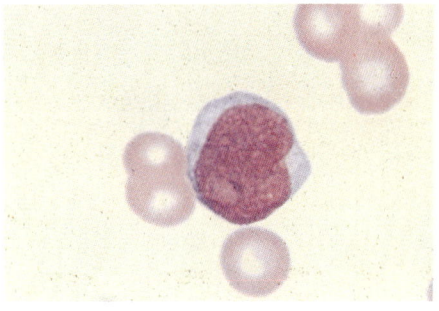

6. Myeloblast

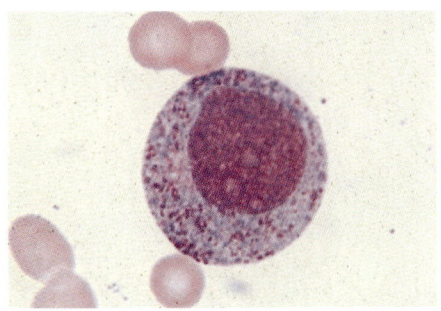

7. Promyelocyte

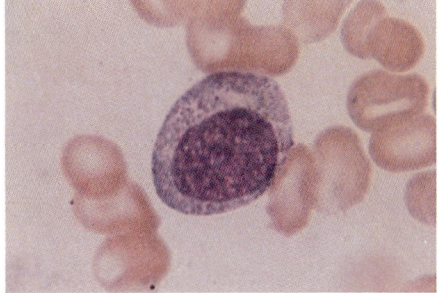

8. Myelocyte

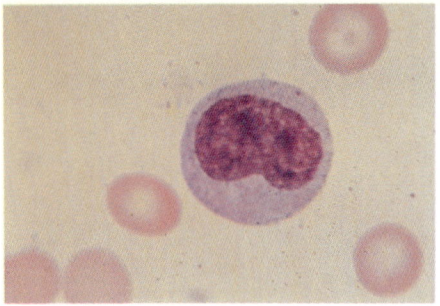

9. Metamyelocyte

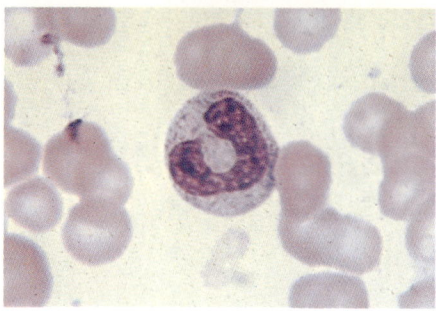

10. "Band" or "stab" form

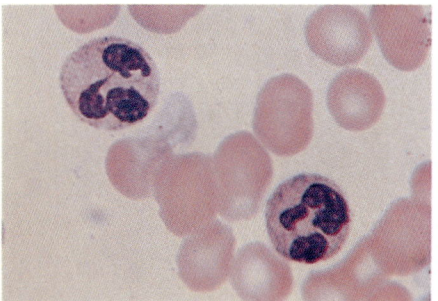

11. Neutrophil (poly)

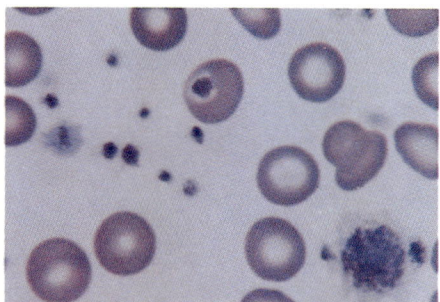

12. Platelets (note giant platelet at bottom, right)

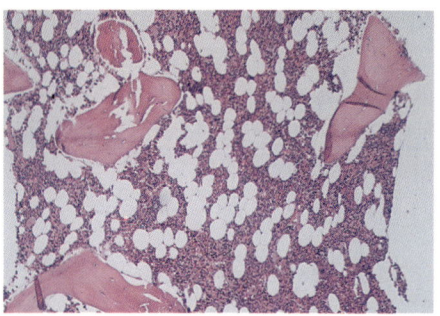

13. Normal bone marrow biopsy, H&E

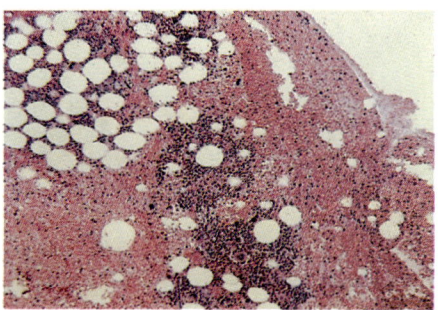

14. Normal clot section of bone marrow, H&E

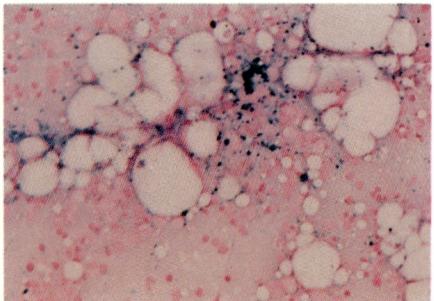

15. Normal bone marrow aspirate stained with Prussian blue, showing storage iron (low power 160×)

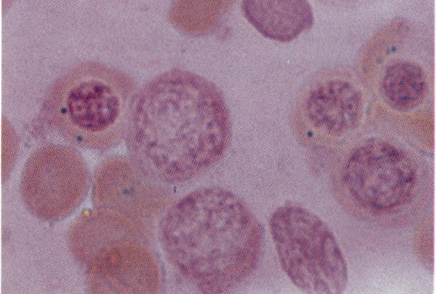

16. Normal bone marrow aspirate stained with Prussian blue, showing iron granules within normoblasts; such cells are called sideroblasts, H&E (oil immersion power 1000×)

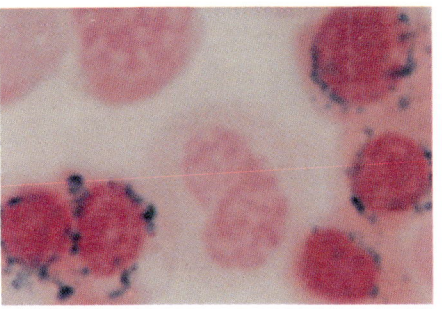

17. Bone marrow from patient with sideroblastic anemia, showing ringed sideroblasts

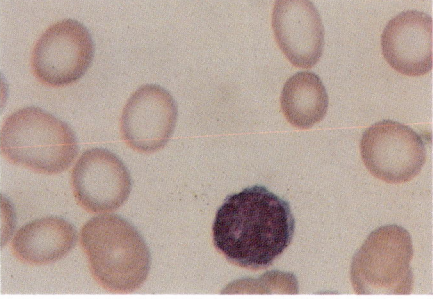

18. Microcytosis and hypochromia (diameter of many red cells is smaller than that of small lymphocyte nucleus)

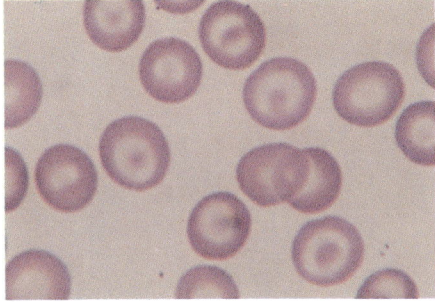

19. Target cells

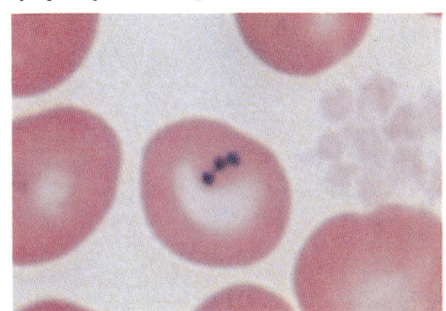

20. Pappenheimer bodies—iron stain

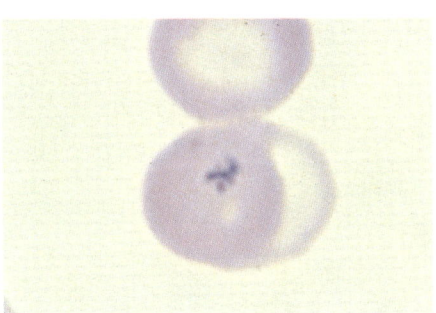

21. Pappenheimer bodies—Wright stain

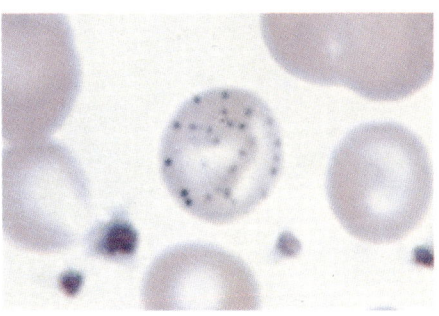

22. Coarsely stippled red cell

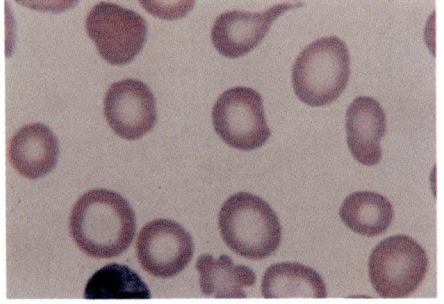

23. Thalassemia minor

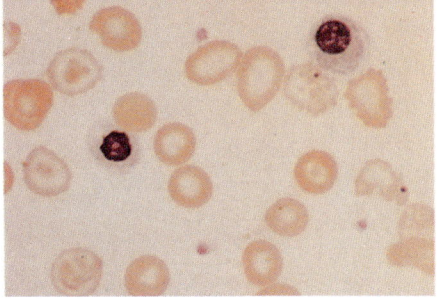

24. Thalassemia major

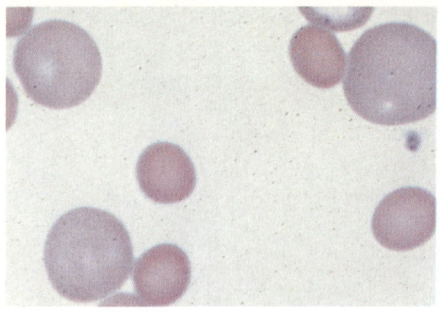

25. Polychromatophils and spherocytes

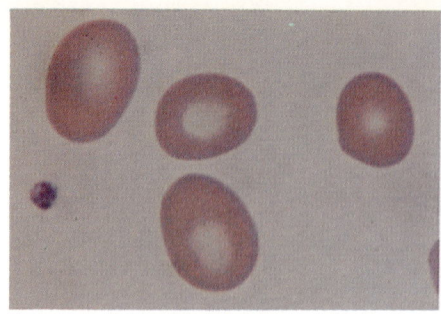

26. Macroovalocytes (megaloblastic anemia)

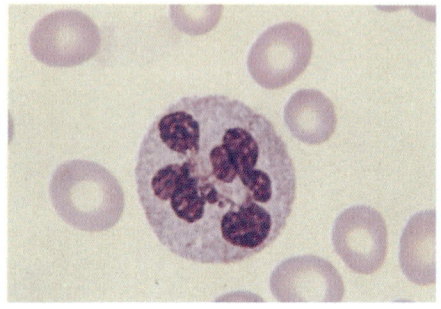

27. Hypersegmented poly (megaloblastic anemia)

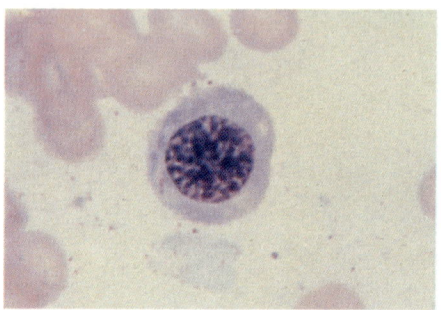

28. Megaloblast—bone marrow aspirate in megaloblastic anemia (note immature nuclear chromatin pattern)

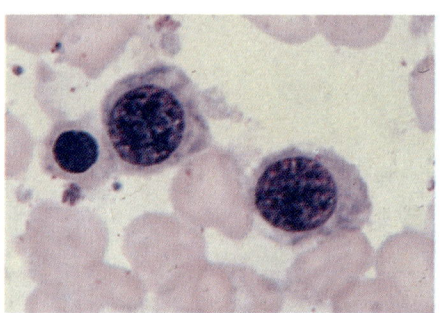

29. Megaloblasts (bone marrow aspirate in megaloblastic anemia)

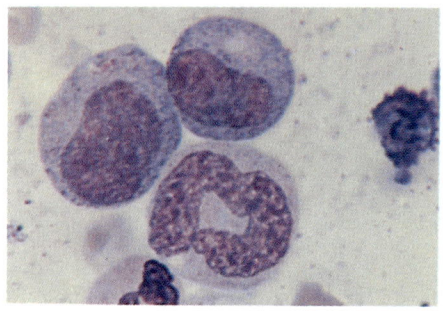

30. Giant band or metamyelocyte (bone marrow aspirate in megaloblastic anemia)

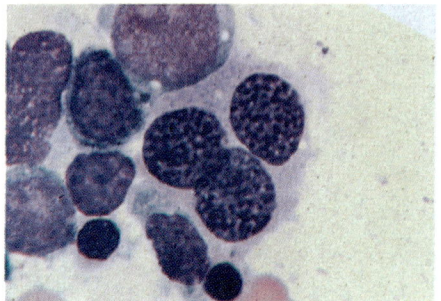

31. Multinucleated erythroid precursor, as seen in congenital dyserythropoietic anemia or sometimes in acute erythroleukemia (bone marrow aspirate)

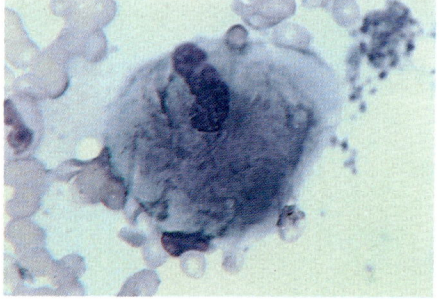

32. Gaucher cell, bone marrow aspirate

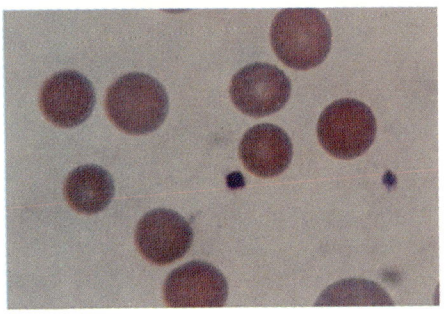

33. Spherocytes

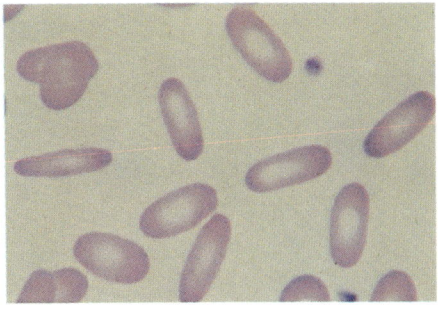

34. Elliptocytes (hereditary elliptocytosis)

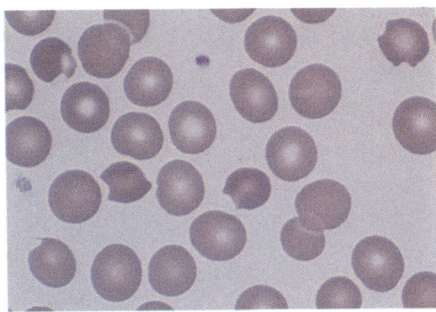

35. Bite cells (G-6-PD deficiency or other form of oxidant hemolysis)

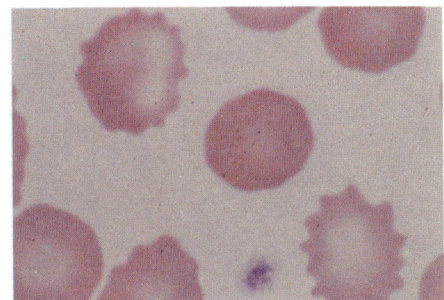

36. Burr cells

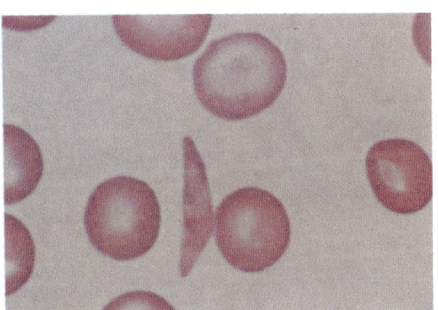

37. Sickle cells

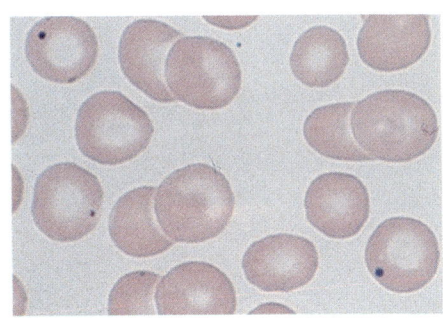

38. Howell-Jolly bodies

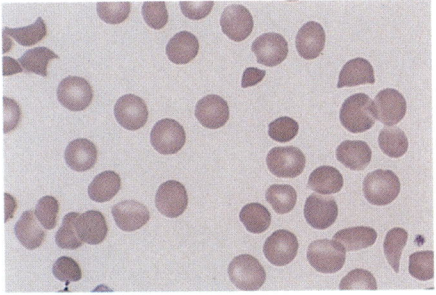

39. Schistocytes (red cell fragments, helmet cells)

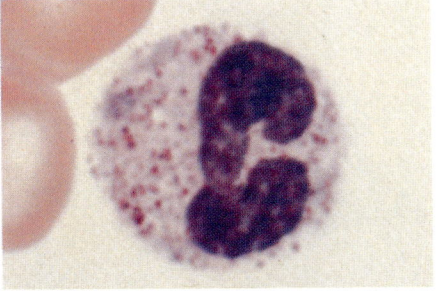

40. Döhle bodies (top, left, in cytoplasm) and toxic granulation in neutrophil

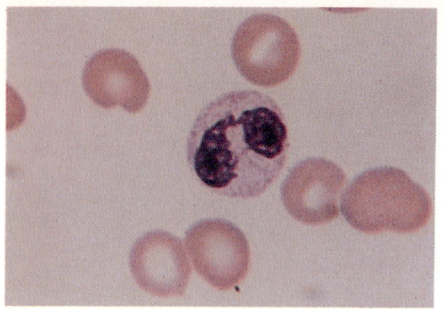

41. Pelger-Huët anomaly—heterozygous

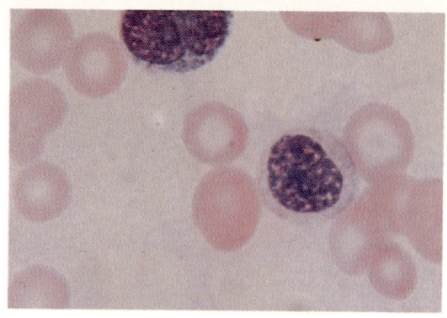

42. Pelger-Huët anomaly—homozygous

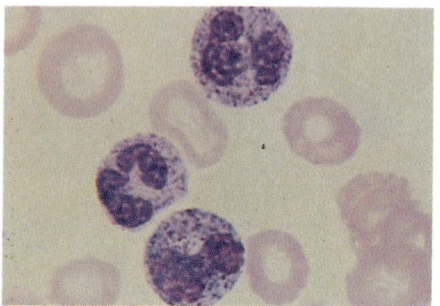

43. Toxic granulation in neutrophils

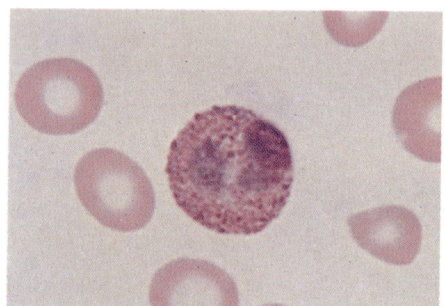

44. Eosinophil

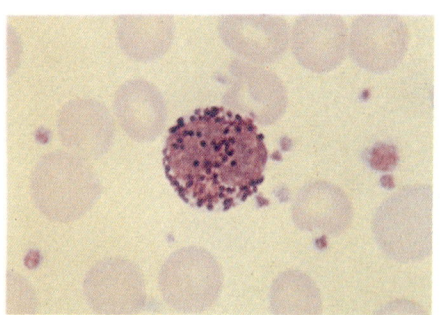

45. Basophil

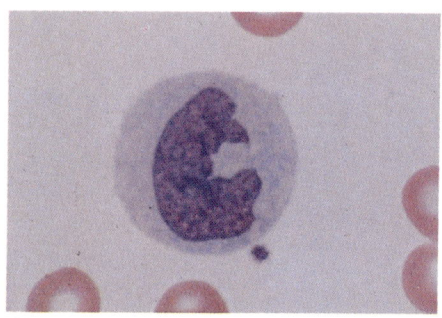

46. Monocyte

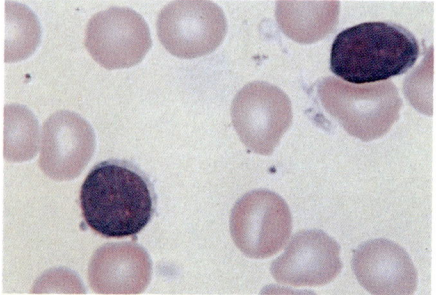

47. Lymphocyte, small

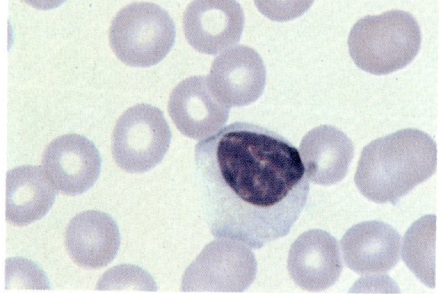

48. Lymphocyte, large

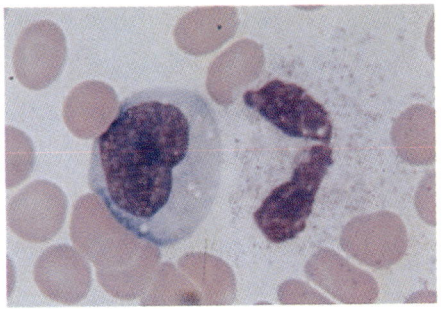

49. Atypical lymphocyte

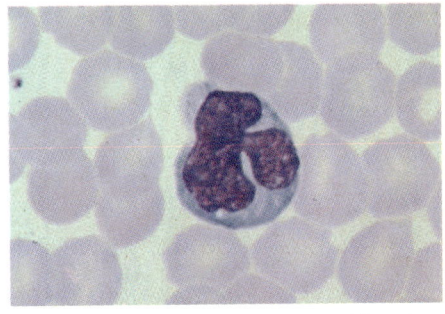

50. Atypical lymphocyte—monocytoid nucleus

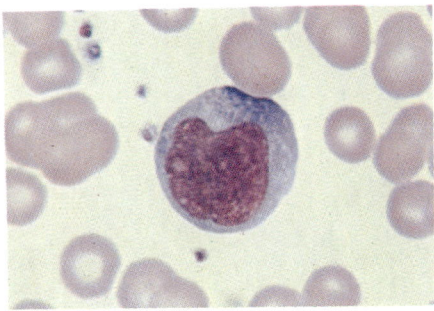

51. Atypical lymphocyte—containing one or more nucleoli

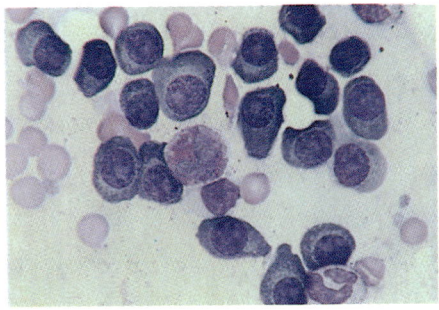

52. Multiple myeloma, bone marrow aspirate (plasma cell neoplasm)

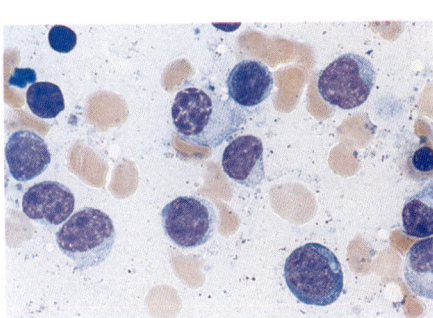

53. Plasmacytoid lymphocytes (plymphocytes) in macroglobulinemia, bone marrow aspirate

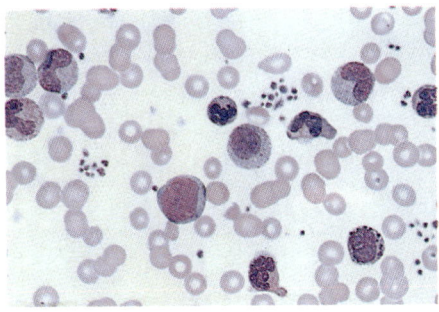

54. Chronic myelogenous leukemia, peripheral blood

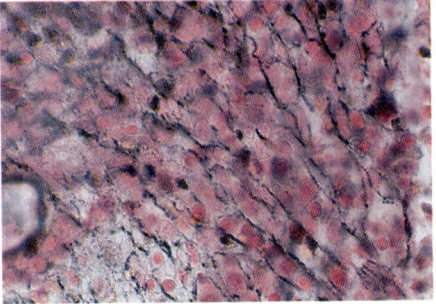

55. Myelofibrosis, bone marrow biopsy, reticulin stain

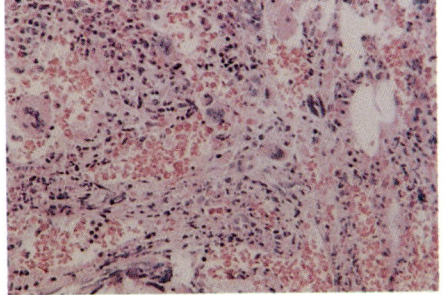

56. Myelofibrosis, bone marrow biopsy, H&E stain

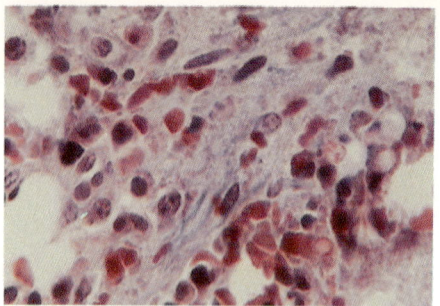

57. Myelofibrosis, bone marrow biopsy, Masson trichrome stain (collagen fibers stain green or blue)

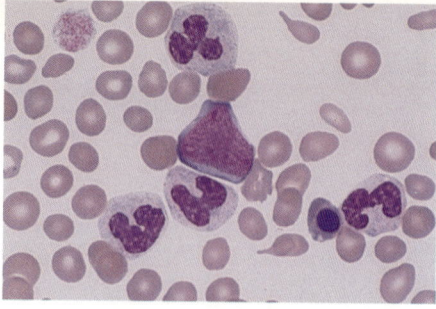

58. Leukoerythroblastic (myelophthisic) blood picture, peripheral blood (note teardrop red cells; also giant platelet, left, upper corner)

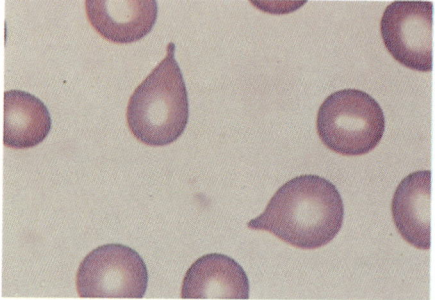

59. Teardrop cells

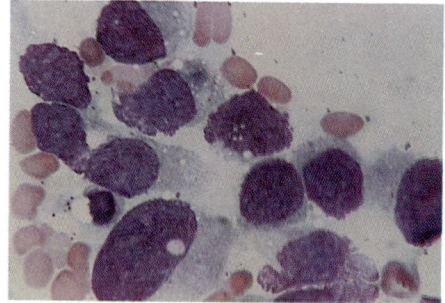

60. Tumor cells in bone marrow aspirate

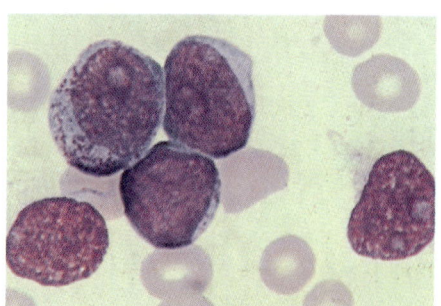

61. Acute myelogenous leukemia, M2 type. Two myeloblasts, one promyelocyte in marrow aspirate (note granules in the lower blast)

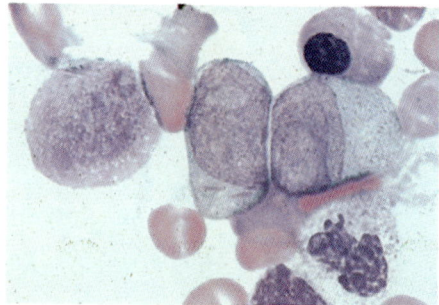

62. Auer rods in acute myelogenous leukemic cell, bone marrow aspirate

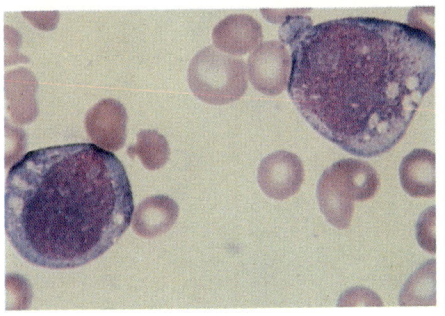

63. Acute promyelocytic leukemia, bone marrow aspirate

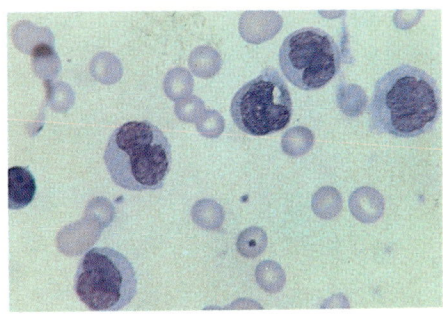

64. Acute monocytic leukemia, peripheral blood

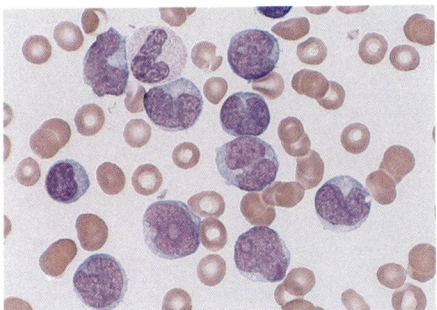

65. Acute myelomonocytic leukemia, peripheral blood. Occasional myeloblasts, with nucleoli, and many immature monocytes (with lobulated nuclei)

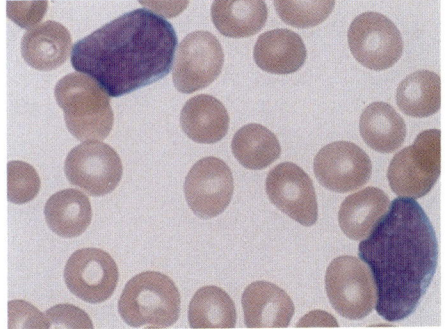

66. Acute lymphocytic leukemia (common early pre−B cell type), peripheral blood

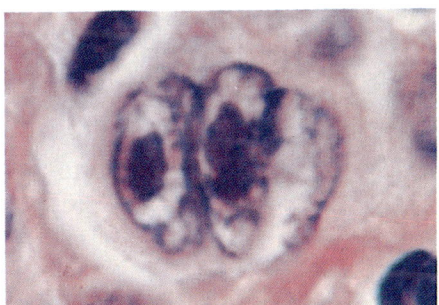

67. Reed-Sternberg cell in Hodgkin's disease, H&E

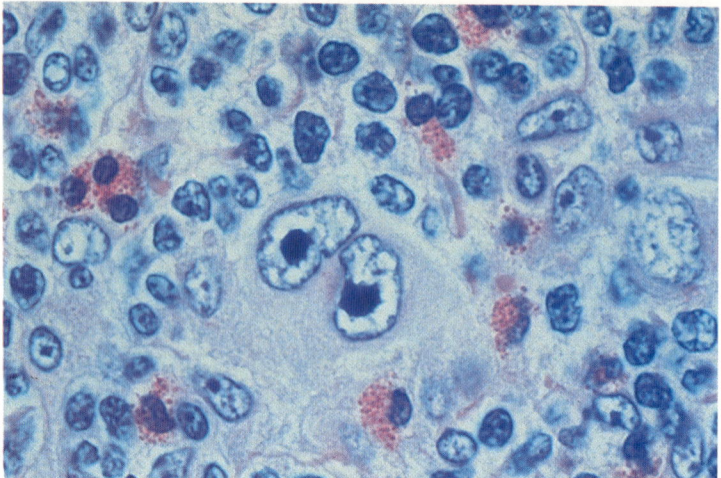

68. Mixed cellularity Hodgkin's disease, lymph node biopsy

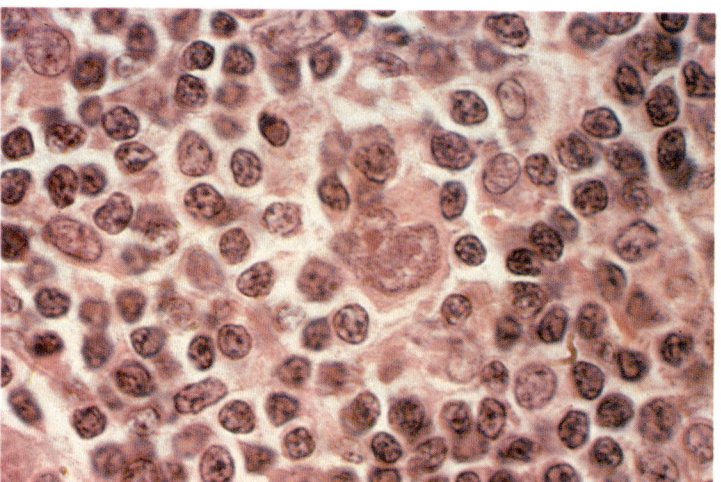

69. Lymphocyte predominance Hodgkin's disease, lymph node biopsy

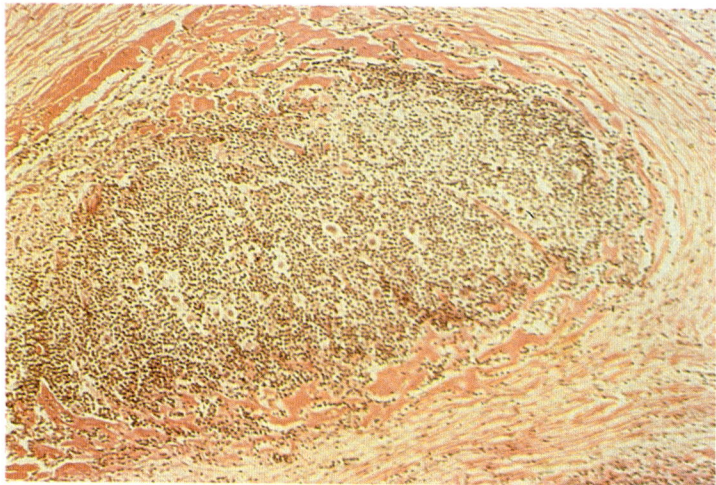

70. Nodular sclerosis Hodgkin's disease, lymph node biopsy

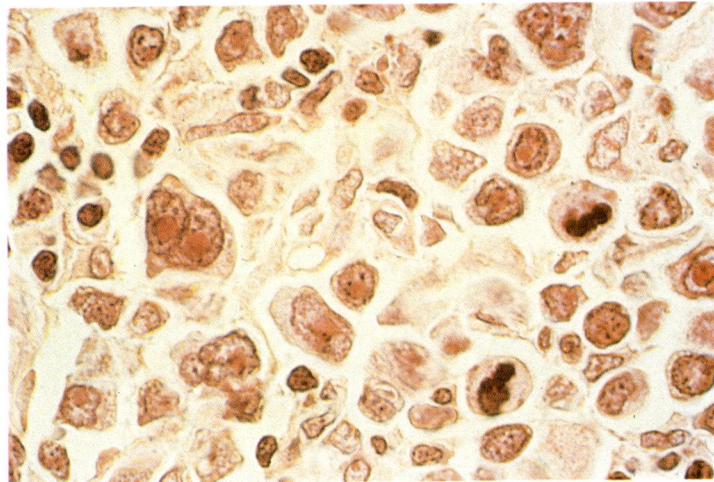

71. Lymphocyte depletion Hodgkin's disease, lymph node biopsy

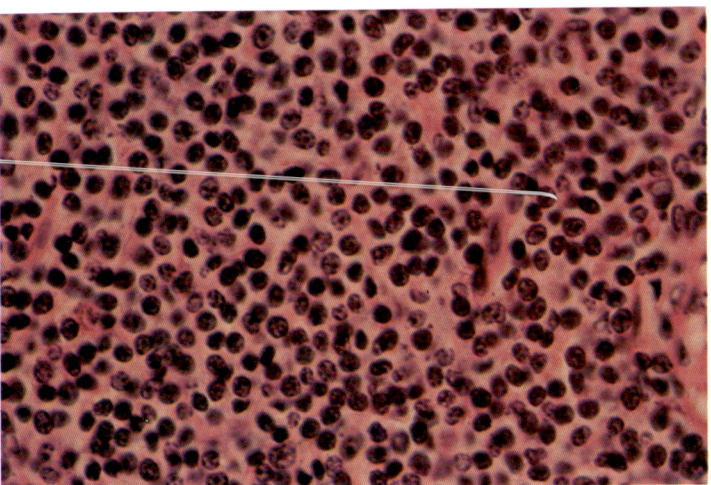

72. Well differentiated lymphocytic lymphoma, lymph node biopsy

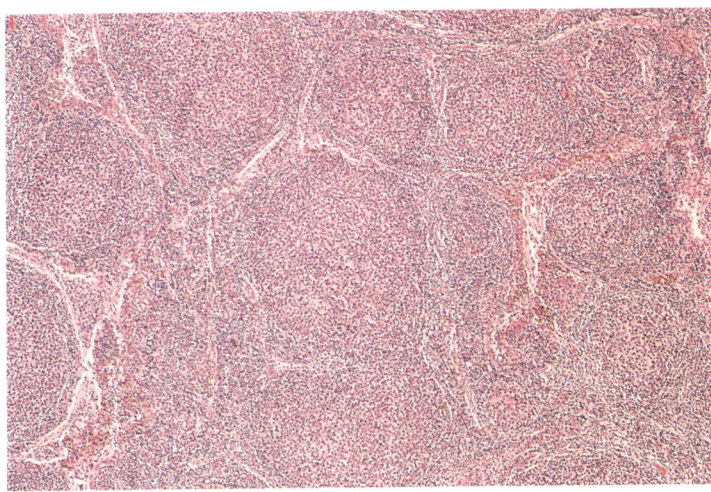

73. Follicular (nodular) lymphoma, lymph node biopsy

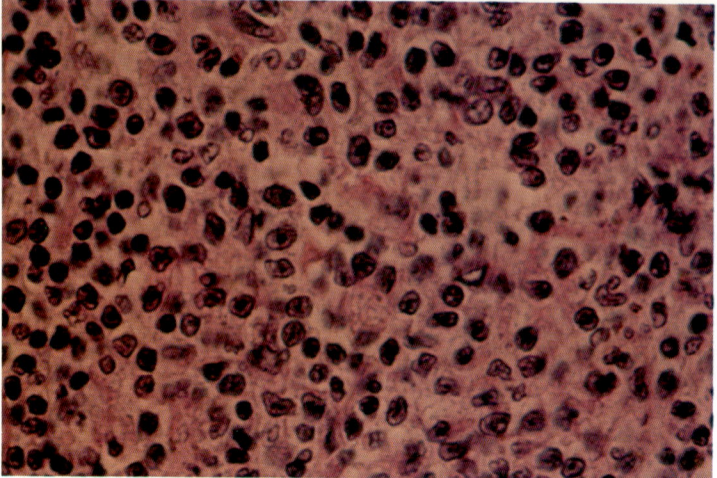

74. Diffuse poorly differentiated lymphocytic lymphoma, lymph node biopsy

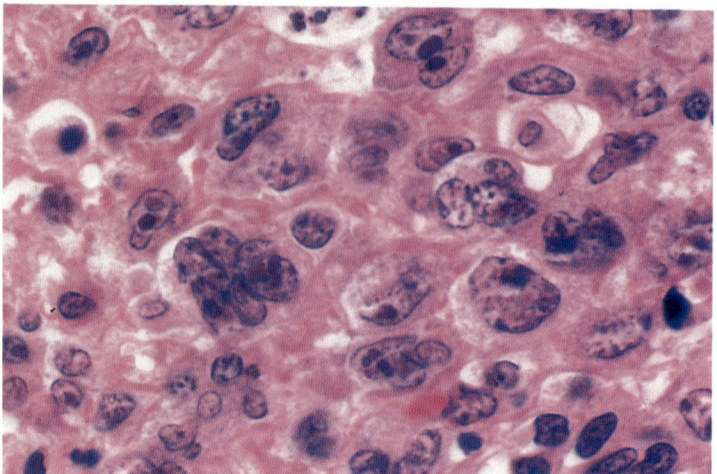

75. Large cleaved cell lymphoma, lymph node biopsy

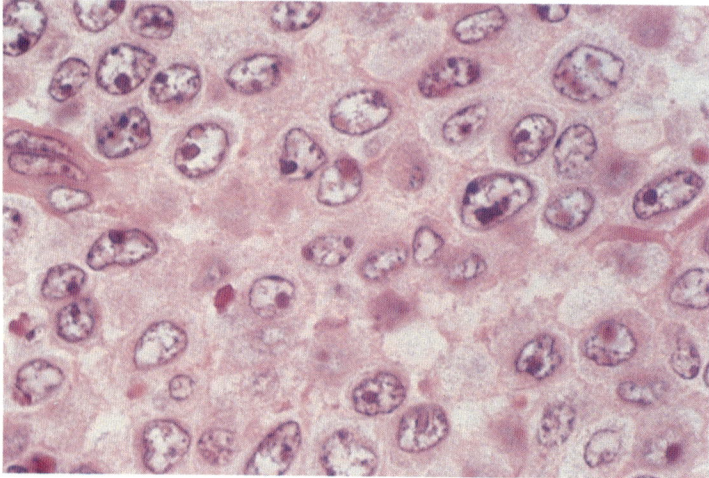

76. Large noncleaved cell lymphoma, lymph node biopsy

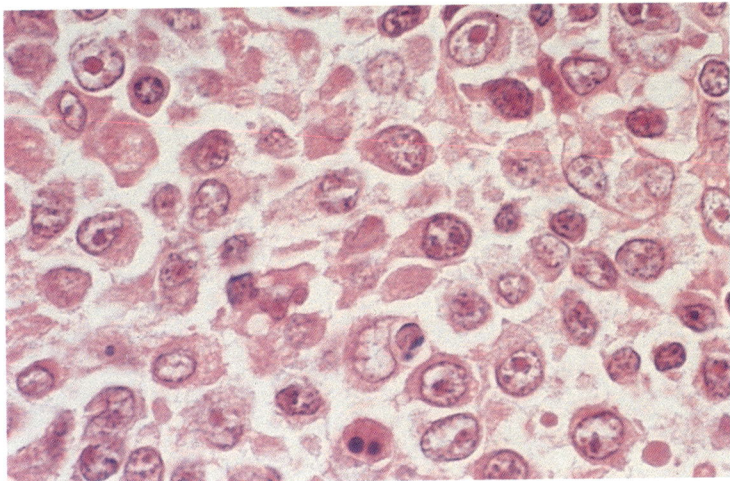

77. Immunoblastic lymphoma or sarcoma, lymph node biopsy

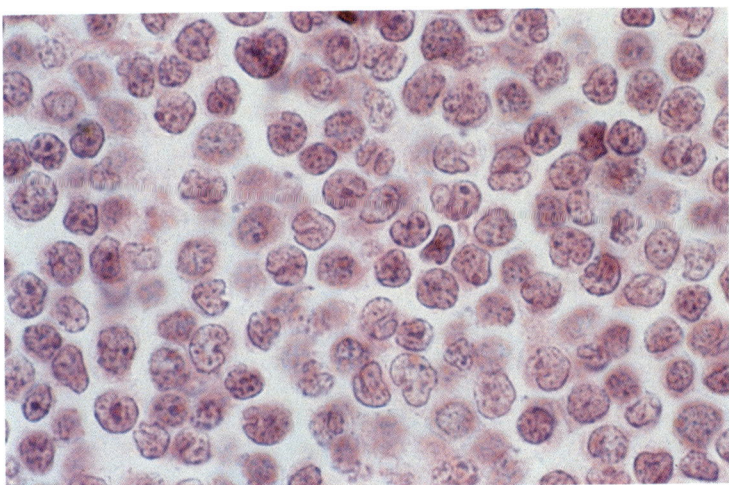

78. Lymphoblastic lymphoma, lymph node biospy

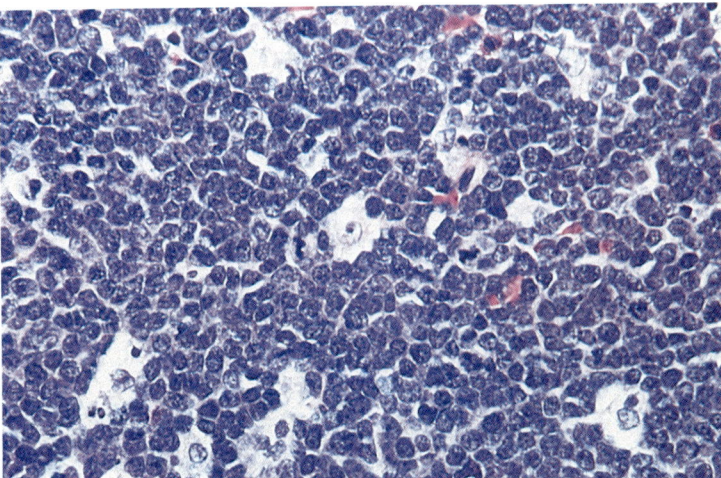

79. Burkitt's lymphoma, lymph node biospy

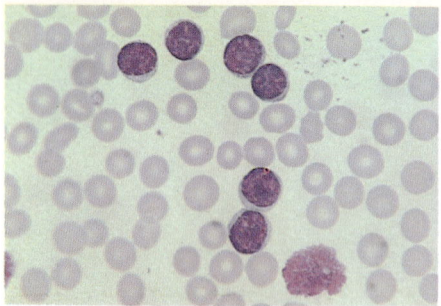

80. Chronic lymphocytic leukemia (CLL), peripheral blood

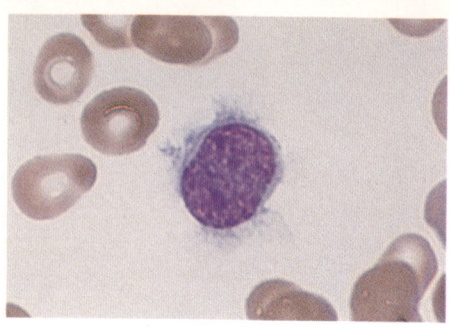

81. Hairy cell leukemia, peripheral blood

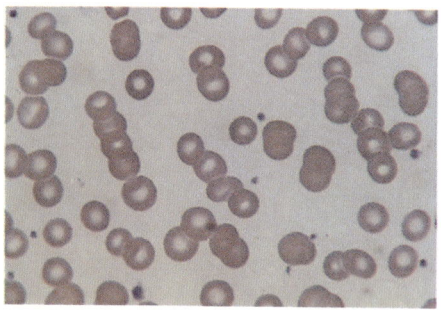

82. Rouleaux in patient with multiple myeloma, peripheral blood

Plates 72 and 74 are adapted from P. R. Reich: *Adria Manual of Lymphomas & Leukemias.* Columbus, Ohio: Adria Laboratories Inc., 1982.

gelsolin, which chops up actin lattices, thereby causing a change from a gel to a sol (disassembled lattice) state; *calmodulin,* a calcium-binding protein; and calcium gradients.

Movement also requires cytoskeletal stability, apparently provided by microtubules that radiate from the centriole region near the nucleus to the periphery of the cell. Colchicine, a microtubule-disrupting agent, causes impaired granulocyte chemotaxis.

The next stage involves a process called *opsonization* (preparation for eating). Opsonization is important for allowing granulocytes to recognize which particles should be ingested and which should not; for example, leukocytes should ingest bacteria, but not normal erythrocytes. Immunoglobulin G antibodies and complement participate in a process by which particles to be ingested are coated and thereby recognized by the leukocyte as particles to be ingested. Fibronectin is another plasma component that binds to bacteria and other particles, facilitating their ingestion. Opsonization also leads the phagocyte to prepare its metabolic machinery for engulfment and digestion. Some bacteria are ingested on direct contact without need for opsonins.

During the next stage of phagocytosis, *ingestion,* the leukocyte pseudopods engulf microorganisms and encase them within phagocytic vesicles, or *phagosomes.* The vesicles move from the cell periphery into the more central part of the leukocyte, where they will fuse with first neutrophilic and then azurophilic granules. Just as leukocyte motility is energy dependent, so too is ingestion, and as a result glycolysis and glycogenolysis are increased in phagocytizing leukocytes.

During *degranulation,* the next stage of phagocytosis, the fusion of phagosomes and granules results in the disappearance from the cytoplasm of the azurophilic, or primary (these are not seen under the light microscope in adult neutrophils), and neutrophilic, or secondary, granules. As a result of this process, digestive enzymes are delivered into the phagosome without affecting the cytoplasm and membrane of the phagocyte itself. The cytoplasmic granules release enzymes, including acid and alkaline phosphatase, nuclear elastase, lactoferrin, and lysozyme. These and other enzymes break down the various constituents of microorganisms and other ingested particles.

In the final stages of phagocytosis, the phagocytes generate hydrogen peroxide and other oxygen metabolites that kill and digest microorganisms. Superoxide (O_2^-) and free hydroxyl radicals (OH·) participate in these killing operations. It appears likely that the enzyme glucose-6-phosphate dehydrogenase (G-6-PD) and the hexose monophosphate shunt are necessary to produce nicotinamide adenine dinucleotide phosphate (NADPH) in order to make hydrogen peroxide, superoxide, singlet oxygen, and free hydroxyl radicals. Lactoferrin participates in the reactions necessary to make free hydroxyl radicals. The microbicidal activity of hydrogen peroxide is potentiated by myeloperoxidase, which reacts with halide (iodide) to produce oxygen metabolites that are even more toxic to microorganisms than hydrogen peroxide itself. Catalase and other enzyme systems are required by the phagocyte to detoxify peroxides and prevent autoperoxidation. The hydrogen peroxide–myeloperoxidase–halide antimicrobial system is very important, since patients who have an abnormal system have difficulty destroying microorganisms such as staphylococci, gram-negative bacteria, and *Candida* pathogens.

Reports of endogenous neutrophil proteins that inhibit chemotaxis or inhibit cellular departure from sites of active inflammation suggest a complex system of inflammation homeostasis, the details of which remain to be discovered.

OTHER LEUKOCYTE FUNCTIONS

Leukotrienes are a class of compounds that mediate some of the inflammatory functions of leukocytes. These compounds are derived from a precursor molecule, arachidonic acid, which in turn is a product of phospholipid metabolism. Substances, such as prostaglandins, which mediate inflammatory reactions, and compounds like thromboxane A_2 and prostacycline, which regulate platelet functions (see Chap. 15), including platelet aggregation and vasoconstriction, are derived from arachidonic acid. Leukocytes transform this precursor to form a number of leukotrienes with various functions, including bronchoconstriction, increasing vascular permeability and mucus secretion, adhesion and chemotactic movement of leukocytes, and stimulation of leukocytes to aggregate, release enzymes, and generate superoxide. Some of these functions were originally ascribed to an impure material called *slow reacting substance of anaphylaxis (SRS-A)*. This material was thought to be released together with histamine and chemotactic factors after an interaction between immunoglobulin E molecules, which are bound to membrane receptors, and antigens such as pollen. Antiinflammatory drugs, for example, aspirin, inhibit the enzyme (cyclooxygenase) responsible for the conversion of arachidonic acid into prostaglandins and thromboxanes. On the other hand, adrenal corticosteroids, as part of their antiinflammatory function, inhibit the release of arachidonic acid from phospholipid stores.

DISORDERS OF NEUTROPHIL FUNCTION

Qualitatively defective neutrophil function occurs in several inherited and acquired diseases. Abnormal serum opsonization due to decreased complement activity or hypogammaglobulinemia and disorders related to defective hydrogen peroxide formation are most commonly found.

Some patients with diabetes mellitus, Chédiak-Higashi anomaly, or myeloproliferative disorders have an impaired cellular response to chemotaxis. Abnormal chemotactic activity is seen in patients deficient in certain complement components, in patients with sepsis, and in patients with *Job's syndrome,* a disease associated with high serum IgE levels, recurrent abscesses, and eczema. An increasing number of drugs have been found to impair chemotaxis as well as other leukocyte functions.

Leukocyte mobility may be impaired in diseases such as rheumatoid arthritis, hepatic cirrhosis, and chronic granulomatous disease. Poor leukocyte mobility has also been found in patients receiving corticosteroids, in patients with defective neutrophil actin function, and in those with the *lazy leukocyte syndrome.* This last is characterized by infections, poor granulocyte locomotion, poor chemotactic responses, and neutropenia that is presumably due to an inability to mobilize marrow granulocytes.

Defective opsonization has been documented in patients with abnormal complement components, immunoglobulin deficiency, systemic lupus erythematosus, hepatic cirrhosis, sickle cell anemia, glomerulonephritis, and the postsplenectomy state.

Patients with diabetic acidosis, acute infections, and chronic granulomatous disease may have impaired ingestion of properly opsonized particles. Usually this dysfunction is seen in conjunction with abnormal migration and chemotaxis.

Abnormal degranulation can result from acquired or inherited deficiency of neutrophilic granules or granule enzymes or from failure of granules to secrete their contents into phagosomes. There appears to be an unusual abnormality in degranulation of neutrophils in the Chédiak-Higashi anomaly: Giant primary granules fail to fuse with phagosomes. Abnormal microtubular assembly may explain this failure.

Chronic granulomatous disease, an often fatal disease seen mainly in young males, is characterized by dermatitis, granulomas, pulmonary infiltrates, hepatosplenomegaly, hypergammaglobulinemia, and death from overwhelming sepsis, usually with staphylococci. The neutrophils have a defect in ability to produce hydrogen peroxide. This defect is paralleled by inability of the phagocytes to reduce a yellow dye, nitroblue tetrazolium, to a blue formazan (NBT test). In most patients with chronic granulomatous disease, there is absense of a component of the cytochrome b system that is necessary for the *oxidative burst* in neutrophils. Because of their inability to form enough hydrogen peroxide to kill staphylococci and other organisms containing catalase (which breaks down hydrogen peroxide), these patients have chronic and often fatal infections. Treatment with interferon-γ has been shown to markedly reduce the rate of infection in patients with this disorder; the mechanism is not entirely clear. Since the hexose monophosphate shunt is required for production of hydrogen peroxide, patients who have a marked decrease in G-6-PD in their white cells may suffer from a syndrome similar to chronic granulomatous disease.

Eosinophils

The *eosinophil* (Plate 44) usually has a two-lobed nucleus and its cytoplasm is filled with large, distinctive granules. These granules stain red with common hematologic stains and it is the affinity of these granules for staining with eosin that accounts for the eosinophil's name. Eosinophils go through the same stages of development as neutrophilic granulocytes, but the contents of the cytoplasmic granules and their staining properties distinguish these two types of granulocytes. The poly has neutrophilic, or indistinct pink, granules, whereas the eosinophil has large, red refractile granules.

Normally, there are 0.05 to 0.45 $\times$ 10^9 eosinophils per liter in the peripheral blood of adults. Eosinophilia ($> 0.60 \times 10^9$ cells per liter) is associated with allergic, parasitic, and other, often idiopathic, diseases (see p. 249). Allergic diseases associated with eosinophilia include those mediated by IgE-dependent mechanisms as well as those with less certain mechanisms, such as adverse reactions to medications. Parasites, specifically the multicellular metazoan "worms," elicit eosinophilia, which is especially prominent during tissue migrations of the parasites. In contrast, unicellular protozoan parasites rarely elicit eosinophilia. Uncommonly, eosinophilia can develop with tuberculosis. Hodgkin's disease and some other lymphomas, occasional carcinomas, and myeloproliferative disorders can be associated with eosinophilia. Because of the absence of endogenous corticosteroids, eosinophilia can develop with Addison's disease. Blood eosinophilia can be seen with prominent eosinophil infiltration of specific organs in some syndromes, such as the range of diseases that can cause pulmonary eosinophilia.

The idiopathic hypereosinophilic syndrome is a disorder characterized by both eosinophilia, persisting in excess of 6 months and not attributable to other etiologies, and signs and symptoms of organ involvement. Cardiac involvement with endomyocardial fibrosis and mitral regurgitation is common in this syndrome. The central nervous system can be involved due either to thromboemboli arising from the heart or local tissue and vessel infiltration with eosinophils. In contrast to the spectrum of disease that can be associated with the hypereosinophilic syndrome, true eosinophilic leukemia is rare.

Eosinophils are recruited to sites of allergic reactions by chemoattractant factors, the most potent of which is the lipid called platelet-

Causes of eosinophilia
Allergic disorders
Drug reactions
IgE-mediated diseases
Other immunologic mechanisms
Neoplastic disorders
Hodgkin's disease
Some non–Hodgkin's lymphomas
Some carcinomas
Chronic myelogenous leukemia and other myeloproliferative disorders
Eosinophilic leukemia (rare)
Infections
Metazoan parasitic infections
Sometimes tuberculosis
Vasculitis
Churg-Strauss variant of polyarteritis nodosa
Idiopathic
Syndromes with specific organ involvement
Idiopathic hypereosinophilic syndrome

activating factor. In addition, lymphokines and interleukin-5 can cause the accumulation of eosinophils in tissues. If eosinophils degranulate in tissues, several eosinophil granule-derived cationic proteins, including major basic protein, are released from the cell. These cationic proteins can be beneficial when they are released as part of the eosinophil's multiple mechanisms of killing larval parasites, but can be toxic to other cell types when they are released in association with other disease processes. Thus, eosinophils may contribute to local tissue damage in diseases such as asthma and the hypereosinophilic syndrome.

Low eosinophil counts develop during most bacterial and viral infections. Stress, endogenous secretion of adrenal corticosteroids, and administration of glucocorticosteroids suppress the number of blood eosinophils.

Basophils

Another type of leukocyte with specific granules is the basophil (Plate 45). Granules within the cytoplasm of basophils are large and coarse, and stain blue or black with common stains. Basophil granules have a high content of histamine and apparently play a role in acute, allergic reactions. Unlike neutrophils and eosinophils, basophils have high-affinity Fc receptors for IgE. Binding of antigen to adjacent cell-bound IgE triggers the release of mediators from basophils.

Normally, 0.02 to 0.05 $\times$ 10^9 basophils per liter are found in adult peripheral blood. Elevation of the basophil count, or basophilia ($> 0.05 \times 10^9$ cells per liter), is most often encountered with chronic myelocytic leukemia and other myeloproliferative disorders.

Mast cells also contain histamine-containing granules and have a function similar to that of basophils. Mast cells, however, are not present in the blood, but are found in the bone marrow and in mucosal and connective tissues. Degranulation of mast cells can be mediated by IgE, which can also elicit the release of newly formed lipid mediators, including prostaglandin D_2 and leukotrienes. The events resulting from the release of the contents of basophil or mast cell granules include: increased vascular permeability, smooth-muscle spasm, mucus secretion, eosinophil and neutrophil chemotaxis, pruritus, and vasodilatation. Urticaria (hives), rhinitis (inflammation and secretion of the nasal mucus membranes), asthma, or dermatographism (wheal formation after mild skin trauma) may result from this process, depending on the location and extent of the basophil or mast cell degranulation and mediator release.

Systemic mast cell disease (mastocytosis) is characterized by pancytopenia, hepatosplenomegaly, dermatographism and urticaria, and syncope from the release of vasodilatory compounds. Skeletal lesions consisting of infiltrates of mast cells may be present. The diagnosis can be made by finding increased urinary excretion of mast cell–derived mediators (histamine, prostaglandin D_2) or by demonstrating increased numbers of mast cells in bone marrow or tissue biopsies.

Monocytes

The monocyte (Plate 46) in the peripheral blood is a large cell with a muddy gray cytoplasm containing scattered well-defined granules and a kidney-shaped or enfolded nucleus with a fine reticular chromatin pattern. The cell is produced from a committed progenitor cell, the CFU-M, which is derived from the CFU-GM, the common progenitor cell for both the granulocytic and monocytic cell series. Mature monocytes are released into the circulation, enter the tissues, and there transform into the macrophages of the reticuloendothelial system. These macrophages, or *histiocytes,* are large cells with filmy cytoplasm containing vacuoles and inclusions and an eccentric nucleus, sometimes with two or more small, robin's egg blue nucleoli. Because RES macrophages are derived from monocytes, the term *mononuclear–phagocyte system* is used as an alternative to *reticuloendothelial system.*

Monocytes and especially macrophages play a large role in removing foreign substances from the tissues. They function in a manner very similar to that of granulocytes, but there are important differences. Monocytes and macrophages are more efficient than neutrophils at phagocytizing mycobacteria, fungi, macromolecules, and sensitized erythrocytes and less effective in ingesting pyogenic bacteria. They are long-lived cells and can synthesize digestive enzymes. Complement components, transferrin, interferon, endogenous pyrogen, lysozyme, colony-stimulating factors, and many other substances can be synthesized and secreted by the monocyte–macrophage system. The cells in this system assist in the removal of aged or damaged cells, such as erythrocytes and tumor cells, and also are interwoven with lymphocytes in cellular immunity and humoral antibody production. Their specific role is described later.

Monocytosis is usually defined as an "absolute" monocyte count greater than 1.0 to 1.5 × 10^9 per liter. On a relative basis monocytes normally account for 1 to 10 percent of blood leukocytes. Monocytosis is often found in patients with chronic infections, such as tuberculosis and subacute bacterial endocarditis, and in inflammatory diseases, including collagen vascular conditions and inflammatory bowel disorders. Preleukemia, myelocytic leukemias, lymphomas, and the myeloproliferative diseases are also causes of monocytosis. Patients with aplasia or hypoplasia of granulocytic marrow elements may have monocytosis, often preceding the return of neutrophils.

Malignancies of cells in the mononuclear–phagocyte system include so-called true histiocytic lymphomas and *histiocytic medullary reticulosis,* a related disease characterized by phagocytosis of hematopoietic cells (see Chap. 13). The diseases lumped under the term *histiocytosis X* are more indolent forms of neoplasia of the mononuclear–phagocyte system. The bone marrow, skin, and lungs are the organs most commonly affected.

Lymphocytes

Origin

The precursor of the lymphocyte is believed to be the primitive multipotential stem cell that also gives rise to the pluripotential myeloid (bone marrow) stem cell for the granulocytic, erythroid, and megakaryocytic cell lines. Lymphoid precursor cells travel to specific sites, where they differentiate into cells capable of either expressing cell-mediated immune responses or secreting immunoglobulins. The influence for the former type of differentiation in humans is the thymus gland; the resulting cells are defined as thymus-dependent lymphocytes, or *T cells.* The site of the formation of lymphocytes with the potential to differentiate into antibody-producing cells has not been identified in humans, although it may be the tonsils or bone marrow. In chickens it is the bursa of Fabricius, and for this reason these bursa-dependent lymphocytes are called *B cells.* B cells ultimately differentiate into morphologically distinct, antibody-producing cells called *plasma cells.*

Cytology

Wright-stained lymphocytes are not distinguishable as B or T cells. They vary from the size of a red cell to two or three times as large. They have a smooth blue or gray cytoplasm and clumped or smudgy nuclear chromatin. If they have a small amount of cytoplasm, they are called small or mature lymphocytes (Plate 47); if they have a large amount, they are called large lymphocytes (Plate 48). In normal persons both small and large lymphocytes are found in the peripheral blood; the former far exceed the latter cell types. The earliest recognizable lymphoid precursors are called lymphoblasts. Atypical lymphocytes, as seen in viral illnesses such as infectious mononucleosis, have vesicular blue or blue-gray cytoplasm (Plate 49), folded-over or monocytoid nuclei (Plate 50), and sometimes nucleoli (Plate 51). They are characterized also by abundant cytoplasm that piles up along adjacent red blood cells.

Besides B and T cells, there is a smaller subset of lymphocytes called *large granular lymphocytes* or natural killer (NK) cells. These cells are large and contain distinct reddish granules. They are committed to destroying foreign cells, such as tumor cells or virus-infected cells. These cells are closely related to T cells. They may be associated with an indolent, presumably neoplastic disease often accompanied by autoimmune cytopenias (LGL syndrome).

Surface Markers

Certain surface markers have been useful in differentiating among the numerous subsets of human T and B lymphocytes (Table 10-4). B cells have membrane-bound immunoglobulins (SIg), particularly IgM and lesser amounts of IgG and other immunoglobulins, detectable with fluorescent antiimmunoglobulin sera. They also have receptors for the Fc portion of immunoglobulins and for the third component of complement (C3 receptor), demonstrable by the B cell's ability to bind red cells coated with complement and to form erythrocyte–antibody–complement, or EAC, rosettes. Not all B cells have all these markers. Most B cells have a short life span, probably days to weeks, but others are long-lived and programmed to react quickly to specific antigens. These cells mediate the so-called anamnestic response. B cells are located in the germinal centers of lymph nodes and spleen, in the medullary cords of lymph nodes, and in the bone marrow.

Human T cells have receptors for normal sheep erythrocytes. When human lymphocytes are mixed in vitro with sheep red cells, many of the lymphocytes become surrounded by erythrocytes arranged in rosette formation (erythrocyte, or E, rosette). T cells are found in thymus; blood; thoracic duct lymph; perifollicular,

Table 10-4. Identification of immune cells by surface markers

Cell type	Surface markers[a]			
	SIg	C3 (EAC)	Fc (EA)	E rosette (E)
T	−	+[b]	+[b]	+
B	+	+	+	−
K (killer)	−	+	+	
Mononuclear phagocyte	+	+ (nonspecific)	+	−

[a]Use of these surface markers has largely been replaced by monoclonal antibodies to surface antigens (see Table 10-6).
[b]C3 and Fc found on some subsets of T cells.
SIg = Surface immunoglobulins. Identified by fluorosceinated antisera raised against antigenic components on Ig molecules.
C3 = Complement receptor. Detected by ability to form EAC rosettes with sheep red cells (E) coated with antibody (A) and complement (C).
Fc = Fc receptor. Binds Fc portion of immunoglobulins and demonstrated by lymphocyte's ability to bind fluorosceinated, aggregated immunoglobulins, or by rosette formation with erythrocytes coated with antierythrocyte antibodies.

medullary, and paracortical areas of the lymph node; periarteriolar areas of the spleen; and virtually all tissues to which lymphocytes have access.

Gene Rearrangements

B and T cells undergo gene rearrangements as part of their maturation. Recently the ability to detect this rearrangement has provided scientists with a powerful tool to determine whether a proliferation of B or T cells is monoclonal or polyclonal; that is, if all cells undergo the same rearrangement then we believe that the proliferation is monoclonal or derived clonally from one cell, rather than polyclonal or arising from multiple different lymphocytes with different gene rearrangements. Monoclonal proliferations are generally characteristic of neoplastic diseases.

Rearrangements of genes that code for the chains that make up immunoglobulins are studied by comparing DNA from lymphoid tissues with DNA from nonlymphoid or *germline* tissues. The *Southern blot* method is employed. DNA is prepared from tissue cells, and digested with enzymes, endonucleases, which cut the DNA base pairs at known sites. The resultant pieces from each sample are electrophoresed to separate them. Using a radioactive probe known to hybridize (or bind) to a specific gene, it is possible to see whether the DNA is in its usual (or germline) configuration or whether a rearrangement has occurred, resulting in the gene appearing in a different DNA piece.

For example, the genes that code for the heavy chain of the immunoglobulin molecule are located on chromosome 14 (κ light-chain genes are on chromosome 2 and λ on 22). On this chromosome there are multiple genes that code for each of the variable, joining, and diversity portions of the heavy chain. B cells as part of the maturation process rearrange these genes so that only one variable, one joining, and one diversity gene recombine to form a DNA strand that codes, in part, for that cell's immunoglobulin. This immunoglobulin is the same as that detected on the cell's membrane. If a lymphoid cell becomes neoplastic and proliferates so that there are many cells, all with the same gene rearrangement, then the Southern blot method will show that the gene in question (variable, joining, or diversity) is in a DNA fragment different from non-lymphoid or germline tissues. A B cell polyclonal proliferation (each cell has the gene in a different DNA piece) will result in multiple gene rearrangements, each too small to be easily detected by the Southern blot. Polyclonal proliferations are generally not malignant, but not all monoclonal proliferations are necessarily malignant.

Analogous to the B cell immunoglobulin genes are the genes coding for a receptor on T cell membranes. This receptor is made up of at least five chains. Genes on two chromosomes, 14 and 7, code for these chains. The genes on chromosome 7 coding for the β-chain of the T cell receptor are usually studied using the Southern blot method. If a rearrangement has occurred, it confirms the presence of a T cell proliferation. As with B cell immunoglobulin genes, this method indicates whether there is a single rearrangement characteristic of monoclonality or whether there are multiple rearrangements suggestive of polyclonality and hence benignity of the lesion.

Immune Response

Successful humoral immune responses require macrophage and T cell interactions as well as B cells. Macrophages not only phagocytize foreign matter, but also contribute to antibody response in several ways: (1) They store antigens intracellularly and retain processed antigens on their membranes for presentation to lymphocytes; (2) they process antigens to make them more immunogenic; and (3) they activate certain T cells (helper T cells), which by their interaction with B cells or by production of soluble factors enhance B cell proliferation, antibody production, and probably the switch from IgM to IgG antibody synthesis.

Suppression and modulation of antibody production depend in part on another subset of T cells (suppressor T cells). These cells interact directly with other T cells—in some cases with B cells—and elaborate soluble suppressor factors that modulate the humoral immune response. Loss of T helper or suppressor function may cause autoimmunity or immunodeficiency. Macrophages may also suppress immune responses by removing antigen.

IDIOTYPIC–ANTIIDIOTYPIC NETWORKS

In one region of the Fab piece (which carries specificity) of an antibody molecule, there is a unique sequence of amino acids that gives that particular antibody its own identity or *idiotype*. The human immune system can raise "antiidiotypic" antibodies against this hypervariable region. The idiotypic determinants of these antiidiotypic antibodies can themselves elicit the production of other anti-antiidiotypic antibodies. This results in an inhibition of clonal proliferation initially stimulated by an antigen. The targets of suppression by antiidiotypic antibodies are idiotype-bearing B and T cells. Enhancement of suppression of T helper, T suppressor, and B cells may occur in this network of responses, leading to modulation of the immune response.

T CELL FUNCTION

The T cell plays the predominant role in cellular immunity. Cellular immune phenomena result from sensitization of lymphocytes following interaction with cell surface antigens. Immunity in this case is mediated by these sensitized T lymphocytes rather than by humoral antibodies. Delayed hypersensitivity, allograft rejection (histocompatibility), graft-versus-host disease, immunity to tumors and intracellular parasites, and contact allergy are all clinical examples of cellular immune reactions.

Induction of cell-mediated immunity involves the production of cytotoxic T cells capable of killing antigen-bearing target cells, such as tumor cells or foreign (e.g., grafted) cells. Complex interactions among macrophages and subsets of T cells lead to proliferation of T cells, production of soluble mediators (lymphokines) of cell-mediated immunity (Table 10-5), and the capacity of cytotoxic lymphocytes to kill antigen-bearing target cells on contact. Often antibody produced by B cells (plasma cells) binds to target cells and facilitates cell lysis by T cells.

We can now see that lymphocytes are mediators of immunity and are responsible for clearing foreign materials (e.g., antigen-bearing cells and microbes) from the body. B lymphocytes are stimulated to make specific antibody that coats foreign cells or agents, making them susceptible to lymphocytotoxicity or neutrophil and macrophage ingestion. T cells not only aid this humoral or antibody response, but also give rise to cell-mediated immunity whereby sensitized T cells are able to destroy foreign cells directly and to stimulate inflammatory reactions by lymphokines, bringing T lymphocytes, neutrophils, and macrophages into an activated state to destroy foreign cells or ingest cell degradation products and microbes. T cells act as modulators of these immune reactions, so

Table 10-5. Some of the humoral mediators produced by T lymphocytes (lymphokines)

Lymphokine	Regulatory functions*
Interleukin-1	Activates resting T cells Hematopoietic growth factor Mediates inflammatory reactions Endogenous pyrogen
Interleukin-2	Growth factor for activated T cells
Interleukin-3	Growth factor for stem cells (see Chap. 1)
Granulocyte–macrophage colony-stimulating factor (GM-CSF)	Promotes growth of hematopoietic cells of different lineages (see Chap. 1) Activates mature granulocytes and monocytes
Granulocyte CSF (G-CSF)	Promotes neutrophil growth and function
Monocyte CSF (M-CSF)	Promotes monocyte growth and function
Interleukin-4 (B cell stimulating factor)	Growth factor for activated B cells and resting T cells
Interleukin-6 (B cell stimulating factor 2 B cell differentiating factor)	Enhances cytotoxic T cells Induces differentiation of B cells to plasma cells Promotes megakaryocyte and other hematopoietic cell growth
Interferon (α, β, and γ)	Antiviral activity Augments natural killer cell activity
Tumor necrosis factor (cachectin)	Suppresses hematopoietic cell growth Direct cytotoxin for some tumor cells Stimulates production of lymphokines Activates macrophages Mediates inflammatory reactions and septic shock

*Only some of the known functions of these lymphokines are listed. Adapted from C. Dinarello and J. Mier, Current Concepts. Lymphokines. *N. Engl. J. Med.* 317 : 940, 1987.

that along with clearance of antigen by macrophages, death of anti-body-producing plasma cells, certain humoral factors, and anti-idiotypic modulation, the immune response ultimately ceases. Abnormalities in this control system lead to immunodeficiency, autoimmunity, and hematologic neoplasms.

Lymphocyte Cell Markers

In addition to the membrane markers previously discussed, the lymphocyte surface carries a number of other antigens. Sera raised in animals or monoclonal antibodies produced by cells in culture are used to detect these antigens. As lymphocytes mature, differentiate, and activate, antigens appear and disappear. Since correlations exist between antigens or other "cell markers" expressed by the lymphocyte and their maturation stage and function, knowledge of cell markers can help classify lymphoproliferative diseases, such as lymphocytic leukemias and lymphomas. In some cases now, and perhaps more in the future, these classification schemes will help in the selection of therapy. In later chapters the use of the markers to subclassify lymphoproliferative diseases is discussed. Here we describe the cell marker changes that occur as lymphocytes mature and activate or transform under the influence of antigenic stimuli.

Lymphoid stem cells descended from the multipotent stem cell express *Ia antigens* coded for by the HLA-DR locus in the major histocompatibility complex. They also contain the lymphocyte marker enzyme, terminal deoxynucleotidyl transferase (Tdt). Tdt is found in both immature T cells and B cells. Ia antigens are present only in B cells. Under the influence of the thymus, T cells differentiate from the lymphoid stem cell and express the antigen(s) listed in Table 10-6. Cells destined to become B cells, early pre-B cells, acquire the *common acute lymphocytic leukemia antigen* (CALLA). Antibody to CALLA is raised against lymphoblasts from patients with the usual form of acute lymphocytic leukemia. This antigen is lost at the more mature, pre-B stage of maturation.

Various B cell antigens such as CD19 and 22 appear at the early pre–B cell stage and are then found in all B cells except the most mature, that is, the plasma cell (Plate 52). The presence of cytoplasmic heavy chains of the IgM molecule ($C\mu$) characterizes the pre–B cell stage. Membrane or surface complete immunoglobulins, SIg M and SIg D, appear in the subsequent mature B cell stage of development. At this point the B lymphocytes are undergoing idiotypic diversity. Each B cell is manufacturing an immunoglobulin

Table 10-6. T lymphocyte markers and associated diseases

T cell	Antigen(s)[a]	Associated disease(s)
Early thymocyte[b]	CD2, CD5, CD7	T-ALL, LL
Common thymocyte	CD1, CD2, CD4, CD8, CD7	T-ALL, LL
Mature thymocyte	CD2, CD3, CD4 or CD8, CD7	LL
Peripheral T lymphocyte		
Helper/inducer	CD2, CD3, CD5, CD4	PTCL, CTCL, ATL
Suppressor/cytotoxic[c]	CD2, CD3, CD5, CD8	LGL

LL = lymphoblastic lymphoma; T-ALL = T cell acute lymphocytic leukemia; PTCL = peripheral T cell lymphoma; CTCL = cutaneous T cell lymphoma; ATL = adult T cell leukemia/lymphoma; LGL = leukemia/lymphocytosis of large granular lymphocytes.
[a]In order to identify cell antigens, monoclonal antibodies are reacted with cell preparations. Cell-bound antibody is detected with an immunofluorescence microscope or a fluorescence-activated cell sorter, a machine that assays single cells for fluorescence after activation with ultraviolet light. The antigen(s) detected on thymocytes and T cells by some of the currently available monoclonal antibodies are shown (using CD nomenclature from the Third International Workshop, September 1986).
[b]Thymocytes are lymphoid cells that originate in the bone marrow, migrate to the thymus where they become functionally competent, and then enter the peripheral lymphoid compartment (blood, spleen, and lymph nodes).
[c]Suppressor/cytotoxic cells can function as antigen-dependent killer cells, and they inactivate inducer cells as well as effector cells, such as macrophages. They also suppress B cell immunoglobulin production. They are different from natural killer (NK) cells, which can function as antigen-independent killer cells. These NK cells can be recognized by their cytoplasmic azurophilic granules and expression of NK-related antigens, e.g., CD16.

against one of several million possible antigens. When the mature B cell encounters its corresponding antigen (determined by the Ig on its surface), it will "turn on" or transform and proliferate, and its progeny in the form of plasma cells will produce large amounts of cytoplasmic IgG, IgA, or IgD with the original B cell's SIg specificity. When stimulated the mature B cell undergoes morphologic transformation into a large immunoblast with prominent nucleoli in the nucleus. Plasmacytoid lymphocytes (Plate 53), with characteristics of both a lymphocyte and a plasma cell, differentiate from these cells and produce large quantities of cytoplasmic Ig, usually IgM, before transition to plasma cells, which produce the mature IgG, IgA, or IgD antibodies.

Lymphocytosis

Lymphocytosis in the peripheral blood is defined as an "absolute" lymphocyte count (lymphocyte fraction × total WBC) greater than 5.0×10^9 cells per liter, including atypical lymphocytes. A finding of many atypical lymphocytes in the white cell differential count suggests the diagnosis of infectious mononucleosis, infectious hepatitis, cytomegalic virus infection, or drug hypersensitivity. A depression of the granulocyte count may cause a relative lymphocytosis.

A low "absolute" lymphocyte count, 1.5×10^9 cells per liter or less, may be caused by cytotoxic anticancer agents, x-irradiation, or adrenal corticosteroids. Malignant diseases, including carcinomas of the lung or breasts and Hodgkin's disease, can also be responsible for lymphocytopenia. Human immunodeficiency virus (HIV) infection produces lymphocytopenia as well.

Case Development Problem: Leukocytes

A 45-year-old woman is admitted with high fever and signs and symptoms of a kidney and bladder infection. She has been treated for psychiatric problems with a phenothiazine, Thorazine, which she has been taking up until the time of admission. Five years ago she had a gastrectomy for severe gastritis. On examination, besides signs of acute urinary tract infection, splenomegaly is the only finding.

Laboratory Data
Hematocrit: 0.29 (29%)
White blood cell count: 1.2×10^9/L
White cell differential count:
polys, 5%
bands, 10%
metamyelocytes, 5%
myelocytes, 2%

promyelocytes, 0
blasts, 0
lymphs, 20%
monocytes, 58%
Platelets: 75×10^9/L
Reticulocyte count: 3%

1. Describe at least four pathogenetic mechanisms to explain this clinical picture.

    a. Phenothiazine-induced neutropenia leading to acute urinary tract infection

    b. Leukopenia due to severe infection and excessive utilization of white cells at the site of inflammation, particularly if the phenothiazine is suppressing neutrophil production by the bone marrow

    c. Leukopenia secondary to gastrectomy, malabsorption of vitamin B_{12}, and megaloblastic anemia

    d. Splenomegaly (of unknown cause) causing hypersplenism and depression of the white count, thereby predisposing to kidney infection

2. How would you distinguish among these pathophysiologic mechanisms?

A bone marrow examination could confirm the diagnosis of phenothiazine-induced myeloid hypoplasia. If megaloblastic anemia secondary to vitamin B_{12} deficiency is causing neutropenia, then red cell and white cell precursors should be megaloblastic. Hypersplenism should be manifested in the bone marrow by increased cellularity, usually of all cell series. Peripheral utilization of white cells at the site of infection should also lead to a hypercellular marrow; the granulocytic series may be severely shifted to the left due to premature release of young white cells. The results of urinalysis would show whether white cells are reaching the urinary tract. Presumably if the patient can produce white cells, they would appear in the urine.

Bone marrow examination shows the erythroid series to be normal in number and morphology. Granulocytic elements are markedly depressed, and only a few blasts and promyelocytes can be found. Megakaryocytes are present. The peripheral blood smear shows only toxic granulations and Döhle bodies in addition to a paucity of neutrophils and some immature forms. Urinalysis shows five to ten white blood cells per high power field.

3. On the basis of these findings, what is the most likely diagnosis?

Phenothiazine-induced granulocytic hypoplasia leading to severe leukopenia and infection.

4. If the granulocyte elements of the bone marrow were hyperplastic, how could you distinguish between hypersplenism and excessive peripheral white cell destruction due to infection?

In many cases it is necessary to treat the patient's infection and observe the white count. When infection is controlled, the white count should rise toward normal. On the other hand, if hypersplenism is present, even after control of infection the white count will remain low; in addition, one would expect anemia and thrombocytopenia to be present. (Since anemia and thrombocytopenia *are* present, an element of hypersplenism is probably present, as well as drug toxicity.)

In this patient the infection is controlled with antibiotics, but the white count remains 1.2×10^9 per liter.

5. How would you treat this patient?

All drugs potentially toxic to bone marrow should be stopped. Infections should be appropriately treated. If this is drug-induced neutropenia, the neutrophil count will rise 1 to 2 weeks after the offending drug is discontinued.

Topics for Discussion: Leukocytes

Composition of leukocyte granules
Control mechanisms of granulocytopoiesis
Leukocyte kinetics
Mechanism of phagocytosis
Leukotrienes
Myeloperoxidase–halide–hydrogen peroxide system
Mechanisms of neutrophilia
Drug-induced neutropenia
Function of eosinophils
Function of basophils
Mononuclear–phagocyte system
Lymphocyte function
Lymphocyte antigens
Immunoglobulin gene mapping and rearrangements

Selected Readings

General Considerations

England, J. M., and Bain, B. J. Total and differential leucocyte count. *Br. J. Haematol.* 33:1, 1976.

Jandl, J. H. Granulocytes, Section 16; Monocytes and Macrophages, Section 17; Lymphocytes and Plasma Cells, Section 18; and Leukocyte Anomalies, Section 19. In J. H. Jandl, *Blood.* Boston: Little, Brown, 1987.

Johnston, R. B., Jr. Current concepts: Monocytes and macrophages *N. Engl. J. Med.* 318 : 747, 1988.

Lichtman, M. A. (ed.) Granulocyte and monocyte abnormalities. *Clin. Haematol.* 4 : 1, 1975.

Wintrobe, M. M. et al. Leukocytes—The Phagocytic and Immunologic Systems, Section 3; Granulocytes—Neutrophils, Eosinophils, and Basophils; Mononuclear Phagocytes (Monocytes and Macrophages); The Reticuloendothelial (Mononuclear Phagocyte) System and the Spleen; The Lymphatic System; Immunoglobulins and Complement; Cell Mediated Immunity; Methods of Examining the Immune System. In M. M. Wintrobe et al. (eds.), *Clinical Hematology* (8th ed.). Philadelphia: Lea & Febiger, 1981.

Granulocytes

Baehner, R. L., and Boxer, L. A. Disorders of Granulopoiesis and Granulocyte Function. In D. G. Nathan and F. A. Oski (eds.), *Hematology of Infancy and Childhood.* Philadelphia: Saunders, 1981.

Bainton, D. F. Neutrophil granules. *Br. J. Haematol.* 29 : 17, 1975.

Dresch, C., Najean, Y., and Banchet, J. Kinetic studies of ^{51}Cr and DF^{32}P labelled granulocytes. *Br. J. Haematol.* 29 : 67, 1975.

Fauci, A. S. et al. The idiopathic hypereosinophilic syndrome: Clinical, pathophysiologic, and therapeutic considerations. *Ann. Intern. Med.* 97 : 78, 1982.

Glasser, L., and Fiederlein, T. L. Functional differentiation of normal human neutrophils. *Blood* 69 : 937, 1987.

Groopman, J. E. et al. Effect of recombinant human granulocyte–macrophage colony-stimulating factor on myelopoiesis in the acquired immunodeficiency syndrome. *N. Engl. J. Med.* 317 : 593, 1987.

Hohn, D. C., and Lehrer, R. I. NADPH oxidase deficiency in X-linked chronic granulomatous disease. *J. Clin. Invest.* 55 : 707, 1975.

Jacob, H. S. et al. Complement-induced granulocytic aggregation: An unsuspected mechanism of disease. *N. Engl. J. Med.* 302 : 789, 1980.

Johnston, R. B. Defects of neutrophil function. *N. Engl. J. Med.* 307 : 434, 1982.

Keller, H. U., Hess, M. W., and Cottier, H. Physiology of chemotaxis and random motility. *Semin. Hematol.* 12 : 47, 1975.

Klebanoff, S. J. Antimicrobial mechanisms in neutrophilic polymorphonuclear leukocytes. *Semin. Hematol.* 12 : 117, 1975.

Klebanoff, S. J. Oxygen metabolism and the toxic properties of phagocytes. *Ann. Intern. Med.* 93 : 480, 1980.

Lehrer et al. Neurophils and host defense. *Ann. Intern. Med.* 109 : 127, 1988.

Logue, G. Felty's syndrome: Granulocyte-bound immunoglobulin G and splenectomy. *Ann. Intern. Med.* 31 : 191, 1976.

Logue, G. L., and Shimm, D. S. Autoimmune granulocytopenia. *Ann. Rev. Med.* 31 : 191, 1980.

Malech, H. L., and Gallin J. I. Neutrophils in human diseases. *N. Engl. J. Med.* 317 : 687, 1987.

Michet, C. J., Doyle, J. A., and Ginsburg, W. W. Eosinophilic fasciitis: Report of 15 cases. *Mayo Clin. Proc.* 56 : 27, 1981.

Miller, M. E. Pathology of chemotaxis and random mobility. *Semin. Hematol.* 12 : 159, 1975.

Nathan, C. F., Murray, H. W., and Chon, Z. A. The macrophage as an effector cell. *N. Engl. J. Med.* 303 : 622, 1980.

Nutterworth, A. E., and David, J. R. Eosinophil function. *N. Engl. J. Med.* 304 : 154, 1981.

Petz, L. D., and Fudenberg, H. H. Immunologic mechanisms in drug-induced cytopenias. *Prog. Hematol.* 9 : 185, 1975.

Pisciotta, A. V. Immune and toxic mechanisms in drug-induced agranulocytosis. *Semin. Hematol.* 10 : 279, 1973.

Quie, P. G. Pathology of bacteriocidal power of neutrophils. *Semin. Hematol.* 12 : 143, 1975.

Robinson, W. A., and Mangalik, A. The kinetics and regulation of granulopoiesis. *Semin. Hematol.* 12 : 7, 1975.

Samuelsson, B. Leukotrienes: Mediators of immediate hypersensitivity reactions and inflammation. *Science* 220 : 568, 1983.

Senn, H. J., and Jungi, W. F. Neutrophil migration in health and disease. *Semin. Hematol.* 12 : 27, 1975.

Stohlman, F., Queensberry, P. J., and Tyler, W. S. The regulation of myelopoiesis as approached with in vivo and in vitro techniques. *Prog. Hematol.* 8 : 259, 1973.

Stossel, T. P. Phagocytosis. *N. Engl. J. Med.* 290 : 717, 774, 833, 1974.

Stossel, T. P. Phagocytosis: Recognition and ingestion. *Semin. Hematol.* 12 : 83, 1975.

Sullivan, T. J. The role of eosinophils in inflammatory reactions. *Prog. Hematol.* 11 : 65, 1979.

Tauber, A. I. Current views of neutrophil dysfunction. *Am. J. Med.* 70 : 1237, 1981.

Vincent, P. C. The measurement of granulocyte kinetics. *Br. J. Haematol.* 36 : 1, 1977.

Ward, P. C. The myeloid leukocytoses. *Postgrad. Med.* 67 : 219, 1980.

Weetman, R. M., and Boxer, L. A. Childhood neutropenia. *Pediatr. Clin. North Am.* 27 : 361, 1980.

Young, G. A., and Vincent, P. C. Drug-induced agranulocytosis. *Clin. Haematol.* 93 : 483, 1980.

Lymphocytes

Cooper, M. D. Current concepts. B lymphocytes: Normal development and function. *N. Engl. J. Med.* 317 : 1452, 1987.

Dinarello, C. A., and Mier, J. W. Current concepts. Lymphokines. *N. Engl. J. Med.* 317 : 940, 1987.

Fauci, A. S. et al. Activation and regulation of human immune responses: Implications in normal and disease states. *Ann. Intern. Med.* 99 : 61, 1963.

Fudenberg, J. H., and Smith, C. L. The lymphocyte in health and disease: II. *Semin. Hematol.* 17 : 1, 1980.

Geha, R. S. Regulation of the immune response by idiotypic-antiidiotypic interactions. *N. Engl. J. Med.* 305 : 25, 1981.

Janossy, G. (ed.). The lymphocytes. *Clin. Haematol.* 11 : 291, 1982.

Reinherz, E. L., and Schlossman, S. F. Regulation of the immune response-inducer and suppressor T-lymphocyte subsets in human beings. *N. Engl. J. Med.* 303 : 370, 1980.

Reinherz, E. L. et al. Discrete states of human intrathymic differentiation: Analysis of normal thymocytes and leukemic lymphoblasts of T-cell lineage. *Proc. Natl. Acad. Sci. USA* 77 : 1588, 1980.

Ross, G. D. Identification of human lymphocyte subpopulations by surface marker analysis. *Blood* 53 : 799, 1979.

Royer, J. D., and Reinherz, E. L. Current concepts. T lymphocytes: Ontogeny, function, and relevance to clinical disorders. *N. Engl. J. Med.* 317 : 1136, 1987.

Zacharski, L. R., and Linman, J. W. Lymphocytopenia: Its causes and significance. *Mayo Clin. Proc.* 46 : 168, 1971.

11 Myeloproliferative Disorders

Stephen H. Robinson

General Aspects

By strict definition the term *myeloproliferative disorder* refers to a disorder of bone marrow cell growth. A variety of diseases could be so classified, including the various forms of acute nonlymphocytic leukemia and the myelodysplastic syndromes (refractory anemias). However, the term is usually reserved for four chronic diseases that have many qualities in common: chronic myelogenous leukemia, polycythemia vera, agnogenic myeloid metaplasia with myelofibrosis, and essential thrombocythemia. Each of these diseases is characterized by "autonomous" or purposeless proliferation of one or more of the three major cell lines that normally develop in the bone marrow: erythrocytes, granulocytes, and megakaryocytes. These disorders may also be associated with an increase in the number of eosinophils and, particularly, basophils in the peripheral blood. We now know that all of these marrow-derived cell lines develop from the pluripotential hematopoietic stem cell (see Chap. 1), and it has become clear that the myeloproliferative disorders are neoplastic (or perhaps preneoplastic) disorders of the pluripotential stem cell that lead to clonal expansion of this cell and the differentiated cells that are derived from it. The acute nonlymphocytic leukemias and myelodysplastic syndromes are also clonal disorders of the pluripotential stem cell or, in some instances of acute myelogenous leukemia, more committed progenitor cells, but in these disorders marrow cell differentiation is more abnormal and the clinical course of the disease more acute and problematic.

Table 11-1 shows that the three major cell lines derived from the pluripotential stem cell may all be affected to a greater or lesser extent in the myeloproliferative disorders. For example, in polycythemia vera, although an increase in red blood cell proliferation is most conspicuous, the production of white blood cells and platelets is usually increased as well. Fibrosis of the bone marrow may occur in any of these disorders, although it is most prominent in agnogenic myeloid metaplasia with myelofibrosis. Initially, it was thought that the increase in fibroblasts also emanated from the pluripotential

Table 11-1. Major distinguishing features of the myeloproliferative disorders

Disorder	RBCs	WBCs	Platelets	Marrow Fibrosis
P. vera	+++	++	++	+ (late)
CML	±	+++	++	± (late)
AMM + MF	±	±	±	+ to +++
Thrombocythemia	±	±	+++	± (late)

P. vera = polycythemia vera; CML = chronic myelogenous leukemia; AMM + MF = agnogenic myeloid metaplasia with myelofibrosis.
The number of +'s refers to the degree of increased proliferation in each cell line, ± indicates that the cell number may be either increased or decreased.

stem cell, but there is now evidence, as reviewed below, that the fibroblastic proliferation is reactive and not directly related to the underlying stem cell defect.

Since the four chronic myeloproliferative disorders may all be associated with increased proliferation of the major marrow cell lines to variable extents, it has been suggested that these disorders may represent points in the spectrum of a single disease process. This argument is strengthened by the fact that patients may present with one disorder that seems to evolve into another. Thus, a patient who has had a high platelet count and carried a diagnosis of essential thrombocythemia may later develop a high hematocrit and all of the features of polycythemia vera. In this example it is then difficult to know whether the elevated platelet count was an early manifestation of the disease process that eventually manifested itself, or whether one disorder was transformed into the other. In other instances a transformation phenomenon is clear. Thus, late in the course of polycythemia vera some patients will gradually become anemic and all of the stigmata of myeloid metaplasia with myelofibrosis will develop.

Three of the myeloproliferative disorders—polycythemia vera, agnogenic myeloid metaplasia with myelofibrosis, and essential thrombocythemia—share many clinical and biologic characteristics and appear to be closely related disorders. In contrast, chronic myelogenous leukemia is clearly a separate nosologic entity; it has a specific chromosomal marker, the Philadelphia (Ph') chromosome, and the clinical course of these patients is quite unfavorable as compared to that of patients with any of the other three myeloproliferative disorders.

Nature of the Stem Cell Defect

The conclusion that the myeloproliferative disorders are due to clonal expansion of a neoplastic pluripotential stem cell is based on studies of chromosomal abnormalities and of patients who are heterozygotes for different forms of the enzyme glucose-6-phosphate dehydrogenase (G-6-PD). In chronic myelogenous leukemia the Ph' chromosome, which initially was thought to be present only in white blood cell precursors, was soon found as well in early marrow cells of the erythroid and megakaryocytic series. Thus, the Philadelphia chromosome must reside in a common precursor cell, the pluripotential stem cell of the bone marrow, that imparts this abnormality to all of its progeny.

The gene for G-6-PD is carried on the X chromosome. There are multiple isozymes of G-6-PD, many of which function quite normally and a few, which are usually unstable, that are associated with G-6-PD deficiency. Blacks often inherit a normally functioning type A isozyme of G-6-PD in addition to the most common normal B form. Thus, some black females will be heterozygotes for type A and type B G-6-PD enzymes, carrying the gene for type A on one X chromosome and the gene for type B on the other. Early during fetal life one of the two X chromosomes in each cell is inactivated, so that approximately 50 percent of the cells in such a person will be type A and 50 percent type B. This distribution applies to all somatic cells, including the stem cells of the bone marrow and the progeny of these stem cells in the marrow and peripheral blood. In black female patients heterozygous for type A and B G-6-PD who also have a myeloproliferative disorder, non–bone marrow cells such as skin fibroblasts demonstrate the usual array of both type A and type B cells (Table 11-2). However, all of the cells in the peripheral blood—red cells, white cells, and platelets—are only of a single G-6-PD type, either A or B. Thus, it must be concluded that a type A or B pluripotential stem cell in the bone marrow became neoplastic and developed a growth advantage over the accompanying normal type A and B stem cells. Because of this proliferative advantage and the capacity of neoplastic stem cells to suppress the growth of normal marrow cells, the bone marrow became repopulated by stem cells derived from the type A or B neoplastic cell and the progeny of these clonally derived cells usurped both the bone marrow and peripheral blood.

The observation that a single isozyme of G-6-PD, either A or B, characterizes the bone marrow and peripheral blood has been made in patients with all four of the myeloproliferative disorders, indicating that in each of these disorders there is clonal expansion of

Table 11-2. Clonal origin of myeloproliferative disorders

G-6-PD A/B patients	RBCs	WBCs	Platelets	Other cells (e.g., skin)
Hematologically normal	50% A 50% B	50% A 50% B	50% A 50% B	50% A 50% B
With chronic myelogenous leukemia*	100% A	100% A	100% A	50% A 50% B

*In other patients with CML, the blood cells might be 100 percent B.

an abnormal pluripotential stem cell. Similar findings have been made in many patients with acute nonlymphocytic leukemia and in patients with the myelodysplastic syndromes as well.

Manifestations Common to the Myeloproliferative Disorders

Table 11-3 shows a variety of manifestations that are common to the four myeloproliferative disorders and, to some extent, to the non-lymphocytic leukemias and myelodysplastic syndromes as well. Since the pluripotential stem cell is the site of disease, there is often involvement of multiple marrow cell lines. Moreover, both basophils and eosinophils are also derived from the pluripotential stem cell, and it is not surprising that these cells are also often increased in a number in these disorders. The myeloproliferative disorders are often associated with splenomegaly, sometimes massive in proportion. Patients may have symptoms of hypermetabolism, for example, sweating, weight loss, and mild fever, due to the increased metabolic burden of the excessive numbers of cellular elements that are produced in these disorders. Similarly, increased nucleic acid turnover accounts for hyperuricemia and a predilection to formation of uric acid stones or manifestations of gout. In all of these disorders, there is the possibility of transformation to acute non-lymphocytic leukemia; fortunately, this complication is relatively uncommon in all but chronic myelogenous leukemia, in which most patients eventually succumb to a so-called blast crisis. In addition, marrow fibrosis may supervene in any of these patients. It has been demonstrated that the fibrous tissue in these instances is not of one G-6-PD type. Thus, the fibroblastic growth appears to be reactive rather than neoplastic in nature. It has been hypothesized that this may occur in response to the production of fibroblast mitogens such as platelet-derived growth factor, a major source of which is megakaryocytes and platelets, cells that are typically increased in the myeloproliferative conditions.

Finally, a variety of qualitative platelet abnormalities have been described in patients with the myeloproliferative disorders, most nota-

Table 11-3. Common features of the myeloproliferative disorders

Excessive or diminished proliferation of red cells, granulocytes, platelets
Basophilia, eosinophilia
Hypermetabolism (fever, sweats, weight loss)
Hyperuricemia
Increased transcobalamin, serum B_{12}
Qualitative platelet abnormalities
Splenomegaly, often massive
Possible termination in acute myelogenous leukemia
Possible development of myelofibrosis

bly in polycythemia vera, myeloid metaplasia, and essential thrombocythemia. Although this is somewhat debatable, abnormal platelet number or function, or both, may contribute to the tendency of some of these patients to have either thrombotic or hemorrhagic complications.

Chronic Myelogenous Leukemia

Chronic myelogenous leukemia (CML) is a fascinating but eventually devastating hematologic disorder in which one can trace the evolution of a benign neoplasm of hematopoietic progenitor cells into an acute malignancy. Studies of molecular genetics are beginning to provide an understanding of the pathogenesis of the disease. Table 11-4 shows the major clinical manifestations. CML may occur in any age group but usually affects adults of young to middle-age. These patients are often asymptomatic at the onset of the chronic, benign phase of this disease, although they may sometimes complain of symptoms of hypermetabolism (weight loss, sweating, and perhaps mild fever) or they may have symptoms referable to an enlarged spleen (a sensation of fullness in the left upper abdomen or easy satiety after eating small amounts of food). The physical examination is usually unrevealing except that splenomegaly is detected in perhaps 60 to 70 percent of patients at the time of diagnosis.

Table 11-4. Chronic myelogenous leukemia: chronic phase

Age	Usually young to middle-aged adults
Symptoms	Often asymptomatic at onset
	Fatigue
	Weight loss
	Fever, sweats
Examination	Splenomegaly
Laboratory findings	Neutrophilic leukocytosis with immature cells
	↑ Basophils, often ↑ eosinophils
	Anemia; rarely polycythemia in early phase
	Platelets usually ↑, occasionally ↓ or normal
	↓↓ Leukocyte alkaline phosphatase
	Ph' chromosome
	Marrow–granulocytic hyperplasia, occasionally mild fibrosis
	↑ Uric acid
	↑ Transcobalamin, occasionally ↑ serum B_{12}
Therapy	Sometimes none required
	Chronic phase easily controlled by alkylating agents or hydroxyurea
	Splenic irradiation ("abscopal" effect)
	α-Interferon
	Allogeneic bone marrow transplantation

Laboratory Manifestations

The hallmarks of this disorder are found in the laboratory examination of the peripheral blood. There is a marked neutrophilic leukocytosis and, in well-established cases, the white count may be as high as 500,000 or even 1 million cells per cubic millimeter of blood. Typically, unless the disease is detected early in its course when the white blood cell count is still not very high, the entire granulocytic maturation series that characterizes granulocytopoiesis in the bone marrow is present in the peripheral blood—but in the absence of significant numbers of erythroid precursor cells or megakaryocytes. Thus, the peripheral blood will contain a rare myeloblast and occasional promyelocytes, but progressively larger numbers of myelocytes, metamyelocytes, band forms, and mature neutrophils (Plate 54). The orderly sequence of white cell maturation in the bone marrow is intact, at least from a morphologic point of view, but it is so excessive that it spills out into the peripheral blood. In addition, there are often increased numbers of eosinophils and, particularly, basophils in the peripheral blood—a finding that helps to differentiate leukocytosis as a manifestation of a myeloproliferative disease from that resulting from an excessive reaction to an underlying infectious or inflammatory process.

The platelet count is often elevated at the time of diagnosis, although it can be normal or occasionally decreased. Anemia is the rule at presentation, although, rarely, there may be transient erythrocytosis at the onset of the disease.

The differential diagnosis of CML includes all of the other chronic myeloproliferative disorders, any of which can be accompanied by leukocytosis, although usually not to the degree present in chronic myelogenous leukemia. Thus, a total white blood cell count in excess of 50,000 cells per cubic millimeter of blood strongly suggests CML. Eosinophilia, basophilia, and an elevated platelet count can also be observed in the other myeloproliferative disorders, as can splenomegaly on physical examination. In addition to the other myeloproliferative disorders, an excessive bone marrow response to infection, inflammation, or possibly neoplasia may sometimes give rise to a peripheral blood picture that mimics CML. This phenomenon is referred to as a leukemoid reaction. In leukemoid reactions as compared to CML, however, the shift-to-the-left in the peripheral blood elements usually does not extend much beyond the late myelocyte level (i.e., myeloblasts, promyelocytes, or early myelocytes are not commonly present in the peripheral blood), there is usually no eosinophilia or basophilia, the platelet count is typically normal although it may be elevated in reaction to the underlying disorder, and splenomegaly is unusual unless it is a manifestation of the underlying disorder that stimulated the leukocytosis.

Two additional tests are very useful in confirming the diagnosis of CML and differentiating it from other myeloproliferative disorders or a leukemoid reaction. These are the leukocyte alkaline phosphatase score and assay of immature cells in the peripheral blood or bone marrow for the Ph' chromosome.

LEUKOCYTE ALKALINE PHOSPHATASE

Leukocyte alkaline phosphatase (LAP) is an enzyme associated with the granules of neutrophilic leukocytes, and it is usually assayed by a cytochemical staining method in which granules containing LAP appear dark blue. In CML the LAP score is characteristically lower than normal, that is, very few bands and mature leukocytes contain any enzyme activity and those that do stain only lightly. In contrast, the LAP score is higher than normal in leukemoid reactions and is generally, but not invariably, elevated as well in the three other chronic myeloproliferative disorders, polycythemia vera, agnogenic myeloid metaplasia with myelofibrosis, and essential thrombocythemia.

PHILADELPHIA CHROMOSOME

The Philadelphia (Ph') chromosome is an abnormal number 22 chromosome that appears to have lost one of its long arms. This chromosomal abnormality is present in 80 to 90 percent of patients with CML and represents virtually conclusive evidence of the presence of this disorder. However, there are some other diseases, particularly some forms of acute lymphocytic leukemia (ALL), in which an analogous chromosomal abnormality exists.

Recent investigation of the translocation that leads to the presence of the Ph' chromosome in patients with CML and in some patients with ALL has provided potential insight into the pathogenesis of the proliferative defect in CML and has helped to clarify why a small minority of patients who present with what appears to be CML do not have the Ph' chromosome.

Although it was first thought that the Ph' chromosome resulted from the loss of material from the long arm of chromosome 22, modern banding techniques of chromosome analysis revealed that it is due to a reciprocal translocation of material from chromosomes 9 and 22. As a result of this translocation, there is a fusion of the c-*abl* oncogene from chromosome 9 with the *bcr* (break point cluster region) oncogene on chromosome 22. This genetic fusion leads to the production of a unique chimeric protein of molecular weight 210 kd. This protein has tyrosine kinase activity, as is true for many proteins that are associated with receptor function in cell membranes. The c-*abl*–*bcr* fusion gene is clearly important in the pathogenesis of CML since transfection of this gene into mice leads to the development of a disorder that closely resembles CML. One might speculate (and, indeed, there is some evidence) that the 210-kd protein product of this fusion gene may render CML cells abnormally responsive to hematopoietic growth factors such as GM-CSF; such a mechanism could explain the proliferative advantage of CML as compared to normal hematopoietic cells.

Approximately 90 percent of patients with CML by clinical criteria are found to have the Ph' chromosome when their cells are karyotyped. The remaining 10 percent of patients who are apparently Ph'-negative were originally found to have a generally more rapid and aggressive course, entering the acute leukemic phase of this disease more rapidly than patients with Ph'-positive CML. It has now been determined that some patients who fail to demonstrate the Ph' chromosome when their cells are karyotyped in fact have the c-*abl–bcr* fusion oncogene on examination of DNA from their blood cells; these patients are thus Ph'-positive on a molecular if not on a karyotypic basis, and they have a clinical course similar to that of patients who are Ph'-positive by classic chromosomal analysis. The remaining Ph'-negative patients who do not demonstrate the c-*abl–bcr* fusion gene perhaps have another disorder, chronic myelomonocytic leukemia, which has a comparatively poor prognosis.

Patients with ALL whose cells demonstrate the Ph'chromosome tend to fare poorly as compared to patients with the more common form of this disease. It has recently been determined that the c-*abl–bcr* fusion in these patients takes place in a genetic region somewhat different from that found in Ph'-positive CML and, indeed, the chimeric protein produced by the ALL cells is of 190 rather than 210 kd. Thus, at a molecular level the Ph' chromosome in CML apparently differs from that found in Ph'-positive ALL.

Clinical Course

The median survival of patients with CML is about 3.5 years. After about 1 year to an outside limit of perhaps 10 to 14 years, chronic-phase CML transforms either gradually or more suddenly into acute leukemia that is highly refractory to therapy. Virtually all patients with CML who do not die of nonrelated causes eventually succumb to this "blast transformation." Most patients go through an intermediate "accelerated phase," which lasts from several weeks to several months before final transformation to acute leukemia takes place. In a minority of patients, there is the rather sudden development of a clone of acute leukemic blast cells that rapidly usurps the bone marrow and peripheral blood. Table 11-5 summarizes the clinical findings associated with this transformation from a benign neoplasm to a malignant disorder of the blood-forming tissues.

Transformation of chronic-phase CML to the accelerated phase is usually associated with weight loss, fever and sweats, often a rapidly

Table 11-5. CML → accelerated phase → blast phase

Symptoms	↑ Fatigue, weight loss, fever
Examination	↑↑ Spleen size
	Often lymphadenopathy
Laboratory findings	↑ Anemia
	↑ or ↓ in platelet count
	Progressive or abrupt shift to immaturity of white cells
	↑ Basophils
	Leukocyte alkaline phosphatase may ↑
	Myelofibrosis in some patients
	New chromosomal abnormalities; Ph' persists or may ↑
Therapy	Accelerated phase: hydroxyurea or 6-MP + prednisone may be partly and temporarily useful
	Blast phase: as for AML or as for ALL (outlook grim in either case)

AML = acute myelogenous leukemia; 6-MP = 6-mercaptopurine; ALL = acute lymphocytic leukemia.

enlarging spleen, and sometimes lymphadenopathy. The patient becomes anemic and the platelet count often rises, although it may fall. There may be bone pain and the marrow may demonstrate the development of myelofibrosis. Often, the number of basophils in the peripheral blood increases and this may be the first evidence of transformation in an otherwise well patient. In the peripheral blood and bone marrow, there is a progressive loss of the orderly granulocytic differentiation that characterized the chronic phase of the disease. There are fewer mature neutrophils and band forms, and progressively increasing numbers of more immature granulocytic elements until finally there is a predominance of myeloblasts and promyelocytes with a paucity of mature neutrophils, signifying the advent of the blast phase of the disease. The development of chloromas, "green tumors" consisting of immature myeloid cells, in different parts of the body may presage or accompany entry into the accelerated or blast phase of CML. Karyotyping continues to demonstrate the Ph' chromosome but now there may be multiple apparent Ph' chromosomes in addition to other abnormalities frequently seen in acute leukemia.

In the majority of instances, the phenotype of the blast cells is that of myeloblasts. However, in perhaps 30 percent of patients the blast phase is lymphoblastic in nature. In these individuals the cells may have the morphologic characteristics of ALL. More importantly, the cells are positive for markers of ALL, including terminal deoxynucleotidyl transferase (Tdt) and the common acute lymphocytic leukemia antigen (CALLA). In addition, the cells may demonstrate immunoglobulin gene rearrangements consistent with a pre–B cell phenotype. Occasionally, the ALL cells may have the characteristics of T lymphocytes. The lymphocytic nature of the blast crisis in some patients with CML strongly suggests that the cell of origin in CML is the very primitive multipotential stem cell, which gives rise to pluripotential stem cells of both the myeloid and lymphoid series (see Fig. 1-1).

Therapy

The chronic phase of CML may be asymptomatic and may require no therapy, at least for some period of time. Most hematologists would treat patients with white counts above 50,000 or 100,000 because of the possibility of leukostatic lesions occluding the small blood vessels in organs such as the brain, heart, and lungs. Other indications for treatment include hypermetabolism, with weight loss and perhaps mild fever, or symptomatic splenomegaly. Treatment consists of hydroxyurea or an alkylating agent such as bulsufan (Myleran). It is usually easy to achieve control of the clinical manifestations of chronic-phase CML with these agents; the white count, differential count, hemoglobin level, and platelet count may all return to normal; the spleen returns to normal size, and the patient usually feels entirely well. However, the Philadelphia chromosome usually remains present in most if not all metaphases in the bone marrow.

Recent studies have indicated that remissions may also occur with the use of α-interferon. If interferon is used early during the course of CML, there may be a reduction or even total disappearance of Ph' chromosome-bearing cells in the bone marrow in some patients. Whether such a "chromosomal remission" will be translated into greater longevity of these patients is yet to be determined. Preliminary uncontrolled observations do suggest that such patients may fare better than their counterparts who retain the Ph' chromosome. Recently, therapy with low doses of cytosine arabinoside is being examined to determine whether this form of therapy may have some specific effectiveness for CML.

Patients in the accelerated phase of CML usually do not respond well to chemotherapy, although they may have partial responses to high doses of hydroxyurea or to combinations of prednisone and 6-mercaptopurine or 6-thioguanine. The blast phase of CML is even more problematic. If this phase is lymphoid in type, patients will often respond to drug therapy that has proved useful for patients with de novo ALL, for example, a combination of vincristine, prednisone, and an anthracycline drug such as daunomycin. These patients may be returned to the chronic phase of CML for a few weeks to several months, but inevitably the blast phase returns and eventually becomes refractory to therapy. Patients with a myeloid blast crisis analogous to acute myelogenous leukemia are very difficult to treat; a minority of these patients achieve remissions of their disease with combinations of drugs such as cytosine arabinoside and daunomycin as used in patients with de novo AML. However, such remissions are usually short-lived. Thus, virtually all patients entering the blast phase of CML will die of this disorder within a few weeks to a few months.

In view of the inevitably fatal outcome of CML, despite its benignity during the chronic phase, the treatment of choice for this condition is allogeneic bone marrow transplantation. Only this form of therapy offers the patient the possibility of cure. Approximately 60 percent of patients with chronic-phase CML who have a histocompatible marrow donor can achieve a complete remission of long duration, presumably a cure, from this disease. If marrow transplantation is undertaken during the accelerated or the blast phase, the prognosis is much more dismal, although perhaps as many as 10 to 20 percent of patients can still be salvaged by marrow transplantation at this advanced stage of their disease.

Polycythemia Vera

Polycythemia vera (PV) is a disorder that usually occurs in middle-aged to elderly subjects and, in its classic form, consists of erythrocytosis accompanied by leukocytosis, thrombocytosis, and splenomegaly.

Differential Diagnosis of Erythrocytosis

Erythrocytosis has multiple causes, of which PV is only one. These are reviewed in the diagram in Figure 11-1. In considering the differential diagnosis of an elevated hematocrit, one must first ask whether this reflects an apparent or real increase in the total body content of erythrocytes. This question is answered either on clinical grounds or with the use of chromium 51–labeled red cells to measure the total body red cell mass. A relative increase in hematocrit due to "dehydration," that is, loss of extracellular fluid and plasma volume, is usually apparent from the history and physical examination. Rehydration will cause the hematocrit to fall into the normal range once again. On the other hand, there is a chronic condition found in well persons in which a moderately elevated hematocrit is associated with a normal red blood cell mass and thus a decreased plasma volume. This condition has been referred to variously as stress polycythemia, spurious polycythemia, or Gaisböck's syndrome. It is usually found in middle-aged men who are plethoric, hypertensive, and generally heavy users of tobacco. Indeed, it is now recognized that excessive smoking may produce either a contraction of plasma volume or an increase in the red cell mass (see below), or both, and it is likely that most patients

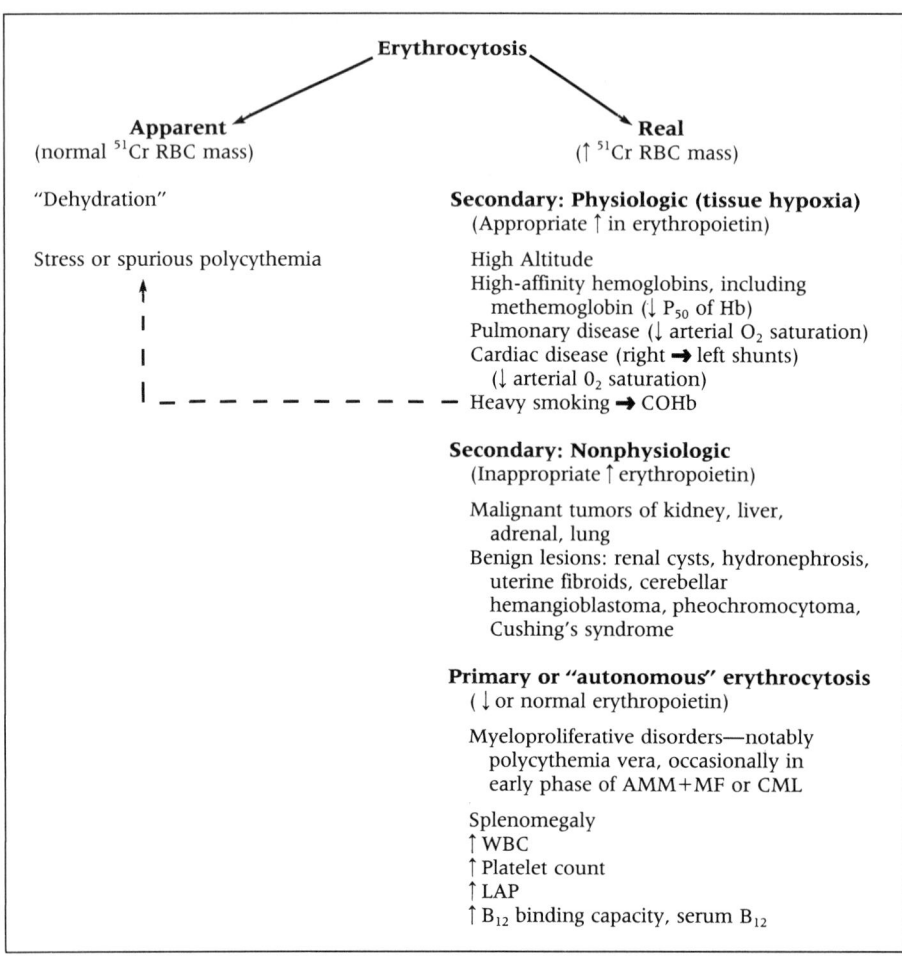

Fig. 11-1. Causes of erythrocytosis. (AMM+MF = agnogenic myeloid metaplasia with myelofibrosis.)

with what was considered stress polycythemia fall within the spectrum of "smoker's polycythemia."

If studies with ^{51}Cr-labeled red blood cells reveal that the total red cell mass is elevated, three general categories of true erythrocytosis should be considered: (1) response of the bone marrow to an appropriate, physiologic increase in the production of erythropoietin, the hormone that is produced by the kidney in response to hypoxia; (2) response of the bone marrow to an inappropriate increase in erythropoietin production by mass lesions, usually tumors, often in the kidney but possibly in other organs; or (3) primary or autonomous erythrocytosis, as in the myeloproliferative disorders, most notably PV. Categories (1) and (2) are considered "secondary" forms of erythrocytosis.

Secondary erythrocytosis resulting from hypoxia and the effect of increased titers of plasma erythropoietin on red cell production by the bone marrow may be observed with severe pulmonary disease, cyanotic congenital heart disease, residence at high altitude, or with hemoglobinopathies in which the hemoglobin molecule has a high affinity for oxygen. In addition, heavy smoking may lead to true erythrocytosis. Carbon monoxide in the inhaled smoke produces carboxyhemoglobin, in which binding sites for oxygen are replaced by carbon monoxide, which has a much higher affinity for hemoglobin than oxygen; moreover, by virtue of the binding of carbon monoxide to some of these sites, conformational changes occur in the hemoglobin molecule that cause the sites not occupied by carbon monoxide to have a high affinity for oxygen. The resulting tissue hypoxia engenders increased production of erythropoietin by the kidney, erythroid hyperplasia of the bone marrow, and subsequently erythrocytosis in the peripheral blood.

As noted above, heavy smoking may also produce contraction of the plasma volume, so that several profiles of smoker's polycythemia are possible: contraction of the plasma volume alone, expansion of the red cell mass alone, or both contraction of the plasma volume and expansion of the red cell mass. The diagnosis of smoker's polycythemia should be suspected when the patient inhales 1 1/2 or more packages of cigarettes or several cigars each day. The diagnosis is supported by elevated levels of carboxyhemoglobin in the blood and a high oxygen affinity of hemoglobin (i.e., a low P_{50}, indicating that little oxygen pressure is necessary to half-saturate hemoglobin with oxygen). Finally, it must be demonstrated that cessation of smoking will cause a return of the hematocrit to normal. This may occur within only a few days since the contraction of plasma volume observed in some smokers is rapidly reversible, whereas expansion of the red cell mass will subside only slowly once smoking is stopped.

Secondary erythrocytosis due to inappropriate production of erythropoietin has been observed with virtually any space-occupying lesion of the kidney, including renal cell carcinoma, renal cysts, hydronephrosis, polycystic disease of the kidney, or medullary sponge kidney. Increased amounts of erythropoietin can often be found in the renal tumor or cyst fluid. Inappropriate production of erythropoietin has also been described with nonrenal neoplasms, including hepatoma, uterine fibroids, adrenal tumors including pheochromocytoma, and cerebellar hemangioblastoma.

Erythrocytosis due to autonomous production of red blood cells in the bone marrow characterizes PV and may also be observed transiently in some of the other myeloproliferative disorders, for example, the early phase of CML or agnogenic myeloid metaplasia with myelofibrosis. In vitro cultures of bone marrow cells from patients with PV or the other myeloproliferative disorders require either no erythropoietin or only very small amounts of this hormone for growth of erythroid colonies as compared to the much larger erythropoietin requirement for growth of erythroid cells from normal bone marrow. Thus, the PV progenitor cells have a proliferative advantage over their normal counterparts. The resulting increase in red cell mass produces a state of hyperoxia that suppresses erythropoietin production by the kidney. The low erythropoietin level in the plasma permits continuing growth of PV, but not normal erythroid progenitor cells, so that the bone marrow becomes repopulated by the abnormal PV clone.

Diagnosis of PV

First, it is usually necessary to distinguish real from apparent erythrocytosis by demonstrating an increase in the red cell mass with ^{51}Cr-labeled red blood cells. One must then distinguish secondary erythrocytosis due to either an appropriate or inappropriate increase in erythropoietin production from autonomous (myeloproliferative) forms of erythrocytosis, as exemplified by PV. The cardinal points of difference between PV and secondary erythrocytosis are shown in Table 11-6. In PV, the classic example of a myeloproliferative disorder, the increase in the red blood cell count is usually accompanied by an increase in the white blood cell and platelet counts as well, and there is commonly but not invariably an increase in basophils and sometimes eosinophils. Moreover, some immature myeloid cells may be present in the peripheral blood. On the other hand, the increase in erythropoietin that underlies secondary erythrocytosis causes an increase only in the red blood cell count. Splenomegaly is characteristic of most patients with PV, but is not present in secondary erythrocytosis unless the latter is associated with a disease that also causes splenomegaly. An elevation in the serum uric acid level, LAP score, and vitamin B_{12} binding capacity, sometimes with an increase in the vitamin B_{12} serum level, are all characteristic of PV as compared to secondary erythrocytosis. A helpful diagnostic clue is the fact that many patients with PV experience severe itching after bathing. The cause of the pruritus is unknown, although it has been attributed to the release of histaminelike materials from basophils during cutaneous vasodilatation. This symptom is not found in patients with comparable degrees of erythrocytosis on a secondary basis.

A bone marrow examination may sometimes be useful in distinguishing PV from secondary erythrocytosis. Typically, in PV the bone marrow shows hyperplasia of all elements, including megakaryocytes, even though the peripheral blood platelet count may not be increased. Also, iron is typically absent. In secondary erythrocytosis, in contrast, the marrow is normal or demonstrates

Table 11-6. Differentiation of polycythemia vera from secondary erythrocytosis

	Polycythemia vera	Secondary erythrocytosis*
WBC	60%	Usually normal
Platelets	60%	Usually normal
Basophils, eosinophils	often	Usually normal
Splenomegaly	75%	Usually none
Uric acid		Occasionally
Leukocyte alkaline phosphatase	80%	Usually normal
B_{12} binding capacity, serum B_{12} level	75%	Usually normal
Pruritus after baths	Sometimes	Absent
Bone marrow	Hyperplasia of all elements or of megakaryocytes; absent Fe	Normal or erythroid hyperplasia only
Serum level of erythropoietin (EP)	or normal	or normal
Erythroid progenitor cells in culture	EP requirement	Normal EP requirement

*Secondary to either hypoxia or inappropriate erythropoietin production.
Percent refers to approximate percentage of patients affected.

erythroid hyperplasia only; iron stores are not depleted, despite increases in the red cell mass comparable to those found in PV. Thus, the iron depletion characteristic of PV is not due only to an expansion of the red cell mass beyond the iron supply, but probably results from the bleeding tendency inherent in PV as well.

The serum erythropoietin level, which can now be measured with great sensitivity by radioimmunoassay techniques, is sometimes helpful; this test is most useful if the level is distinctly high (characteristic of secondary erythrocytosis) or low (characteristic of PV), but often erythropoietin titers fall within the broad range of normal with either type of erythrocytosis.

Finally, in vitro cultures of erythroid progenitor cells may be useful in distinguishing PV from secondary erythrocytosis, since in PV erythroid colonies derived from erythroid colony-forming units (CFU-E) and burst-forming units (BFU-E) will grow in the absence of added erythropoietin, whereas erythropoietin is required for growth of erythroid colonies from the marrow of normal subjects.

Clinical Aspects of PV

One may consider the major clinical features of PV to fall into three categories: (1) those related to the increase in red blood cell mass and blood viscosity; (2) those related to hypermetabolism; and (3) those that are less well explained (Table 11-7). Most important are clinical manifestations of increased blood viscosity. Early descriptions of PV listed headache, blurred vision, nosebleeds, and hypertension as symptoms of this disorder, but most hematologists today find that patients with PV are usually asymptomatic at the time of

Table 11-7. Polycythemia vera

Clinical features
Increased blood volume, blood viscosity
   Headache, blurred vision
   Hypertension
   Congestive heart failure
   Hemorrhage and/or thrombosis—equivocal role of ↑ platelet number,
     abnormal function
Hypermetabolism
   Hyperuricemia—urate stones, gout
   Weight loss, fatigue, sweating, heat intolerance
Unexplained
   Pruritus after bathing
   Peptic ulcer disease
Therapy
Phlebotomy
Myelosuppressive therapy—^{32}P, alkylating agents (leukemogenic risk),
   hydroxyurea, α-interferon
Course
Long survival with therapy
Conversion to AMM + MF ("spent phase")
Conversion to ANNL

AMM + MF = agnogenic myeloid metaplasia with myelofibrosis; ANNL = acute
nonlymphocytic leukemia.

diagnosis. The major risks of increased blood viscosity in this disorder are hemorrhage or thrombosis, or both; patients with essential
thrombocythemia are also at risk from both of these apparently
obverse complications. Indeed, it seems reasonable that the often-
found increased platelet number and abnormal platelet function in
PV may contribute to these complications of this disorder. However,
hemorrhage and thrombosis in patients with PV correlate well with
the height of the hematocrit and only poorly with that of the platelet
count. Hemorrhage is presumably a result of loss of endothelial
integrity as the result of small blood vessel ischemia due to sludging
of blood in the microvasculature. The origin of the thrombotic tendency seems more obvious in view of the hyperviscous condition of
the circulating blood.

    Symptoms referable to hypermetabolism include mild weight
loss, sweating, and heat intolerance; these symptoms are rare in
patients with PV. Complications of hyperuricemia, including renal
stones and actual attacks of gouty arthritis, are somewhat more
common.

    Less well-explained aspects of PV include pruritus after bathing,
which has been described earlier in this chapter, and a probable
increase in the incidence of peptic ulcer disease, which also has been
ascribed to the release of biologically active amines from the
increased numbers of circulating basophils in this disorder, perhaps
in conjunction with hyperviscosity in blood vessels supplying the
gastrointestinal mucosa.

Treatment of PV

Therapy consists of physical removal of the excess red cell mass and/or use of cytotoxic agents to suppress the excessive proliferation of red blood cells, and perhaps platelets as well. Although the ideal form of therapy is yet to be determined, it is clear that treatment of PV allows most patients to survive without morbidity for many years. Studies performed by the Polycythemia Vera Study Group have indicated that therapy with phlebotomy (i.e., periodic removal of a unit of whole blood) can effectively reduce the hematocrit in many patients with PV; however, phlebotomy when used alone is associated with an increased incidence of thrombosis during the first 3 to 5 years of therapy, as compared to the findings with myelosuppressive agents. Myelosuppression can be effected with radioactive phosphorus (^{32}P), alkylating agents such as busulfan or chlorambucil, hydroxyurea, or, more recently, α-interferon. Use of these agents results in a lower incidence of thrombosis during the first few years of therapy, but ^{32}P and alkylating agents lead to a high incidence of acute myelogenous leukemia, approaching 10 percent, after several years. Whether hydroxyurea has a leukemogenic effect is under evaluation as patients treated with this agent are followed for several years; however, if such an effect is associated with the use of hydroxyurea, it is clearly much smaller than that associated with ^{32}P or alkylating drugs. Even patients treated with phlebotomy alone have an increased incidence of leukemic transformation with time. Thus, PV is intrinsically associated with a risk of leukemic transformation, but that risk is magnified greatly by the use of radioactive agents or alkylating drugs.

In view of the findings just described, many hematologists now prefer to treat their patients with PV with hydroxyurea, supplemented by periodic phlebotomy when necessary, the goal being to maintain the hematocrit in the low 40s. Hydroxyurea is particularly useful if frequent phlebotomies are required to maintain the hematocrit at this optimal level or if the platelet count is very high. However, there are no conclusive clinical data to indicate that control of the platelet count in PV has any salutary effect in this disorder.

Course and Prognosis

Most patients with PV survive for long periods, often without complication. The risks of thrombosis, hemorrhage, or transformation to acute nonlymphocytic leukemia have already been described. In addition, usually after many years, PV may evolve into the so-called spent phase, which is virtually identical to agnogenic myeloid metaplasia with myelofibrosis (see section to follow). Thus, the patient with long-standing PV may no longer require phlebotomy and soon needs transfusion as he or she enters an anemic phase of the disease.

At the same time, the spleen grows progressively larger and the marrow becomes fibrotic, with a leukoerythroblastic (myelophthisic) peripheral blood picture. It is sometimes in the context of these changes that acute nonlymphocytic leukemia also appears. Acute leukemia supervening in a patient with PV is generally refractory to chemotherapy.

Agnogenic Myeloid Metaplasia with Myelofibrosis

The cardinal features of agnogenic myeloid metaplasia with myelofibrosis (AMM + MF) are summarized in Table 11-8.

Pathology

As implied by the name of this entity, AMM + MF is characterized by extramedullary hematopoiesis in the spleen, liver, and potentially a variety of other tissues, in addition to fibrosis of the bone marrow. The clinical and laboratory manifestations of this disorder follow from an understanding of this pathology.

Extramedullary hematopoiesis may occur in response to severe anemia, for example thalassemia, or compromise of the bone marrow, for example by metastatic carcinoma. In AMM + MF, in contrast, the myeloid metaplasia is an autonomous rather than a reactive process. Indeed, the marrow cells and peripheral blood elements that are generated in both the bone marrow and the extramedullary sites are clonal, as assayed in black female heterozygotes for G-6-PD.

Table 11-8. Agnogenic myeloid metaplasia with myelofibrosis

Agnogenic = primary, essential, idiopathic
Myeloid metaplasia = extramedullary hematopoiesis
Hepato-, splenomegaly
Ineffective hematopoiesis
Lack of normal BM/PB barrier
^{59}Fe uptake in spleen, liver

Myelofibrosis
Marrow varies from fibrotic to hypercellular
Bone marrow aspiration → "dry tap"
Biopsy required to demonstrate fibrosis
Distortion of BM/PB barrier

Blood picture (all cell lines may vary from high to low)
Anemia the rule, erythrocytosis rarely (early)
Platelets high, normal, low
WBC normal, low, high (rarely > 50,000)
LAP variable, usually high
"Leukoerythroblastic" blood picture + giant platelets or megakaryocyte fragments in PB
Marked poikilocytosis, teardrop RBCs

BM = bone marrow; PB = peripheral blood; LAP = leukocyte alkaline phosphatase.

The bone marrow in patients with AMM + MF varies from densely fibrotic to markedly hypercellular from patient to patient and sometimes within the same patient. Even in patients with hypercellular bone marrows, some fibrotic reaction almost invariably is present. It may be necessary to demonstrate this with special stains for reticulin, an early form of collagen (Plate 55).

Full-blown collagen formation may be seen in patients with more advanced degrees of fibrosis (Plates 56 and 57). The fibrosis is apparently reactive to the underlying myeloproliferative process, since the marrow fibroblasts do not share in the G-6-PD isozyme clonality that can be demonstrated for the hematopoietic cells. It has been suggested that the marrow fibrosis might possibly be due to the fibroblast-stimulating activity of a factor such as platelet-derived growth factor, which is produced by the increased numbers of (qualitatively abnormal) megakaryocytes in this disorder.

A clinical and pathologic picture virtually identical to that of AMM + MF may be seen in the spent phase of polycythemia vera. Occasionally, a similar picture may emerge during the accelerated phase of CML; in this instance the number of poorly differentiated granulocytic cells is conspicuously increased. Metastatic carcinoma in the bone marrow may produce a very similar "myelophthisic" blood picture (see below), but the spleen is characteristically not enlarged.

Clinical Features

Patients with AMM + MF may be initially asymptomatic, may complain of symptoms referable to hypermetabolism, or may experience abdominal discomfort or easy satiety due to an enlarged spleen. The most notable finding on physical examination is splenomegaly, which is almost invariable in this disorder, and which may be massive in proportions, particularly as the disease progresses. The liver may also be enlarged.

Laboratory Manifestations

The hematopoiesis that occurs in extramedullary sites is largely ineffective; that is, the immature cells do not develop normally and presumably die in situ without giving rise to effective peripheral blood cells. Moreover, the barrier that maintains immature cellular elements within the normal bone marrow is defective or absent in these extramedullary sites, and thus nucleated red blood cells, immature granulocytes, and giant platelet forms or megakaryocyte fragments are found in the peripheral blood (Plate 58). To complete this "leukoerythroblastic blood picture," highly characteristic teardrop-shaped red blood cells are present in the peripheral blood (Plate 59); these are derived from both the fibrotic bone marrow and extramedullary hematopoiesis in the spleen, particularly the latter since the number of teardrop forms decreases substantially if the spleen is removed.

Since the bone marrow is at least partially fibrotic in virtually all cases of AMM + MF, attempts at bone marrow aspiration usually give rise to a "dry tap," and a bone marrow biopsy is required for examination of the marrow contents. The marrow biopsy may show quite a variable picture from one patient to another, or often in different areas of bone marrow from the same patient. Some areas may demonstrate marked hypercellularity, with hyperplasia of all of the cellular elements and a notable clustering of megakaryocytes. Other areas may be marked by dense fibrosis, often with deposition of collagen, as may be demonstrated by special stains such as Mallory's trichrome stain (Plate 57). When the fibrosis is more subtle, it may be necessary to do a silver stain to demonstrate increased deposition of reticulin (Plate 55), an early form of collagen that helps to form the stromal latticework of the normal bone marrow. The fibrosis disrupts the normal barrier that maintains immature cells within the marrow compartment. Thus, the myelofibrosis as well as the extramedullary hematopoiesis accounts for the presence of immature elements and red cell poikilocytosis, including teardrop red cell forms, in the peripheral blood (Plates 58 and 59). A very similar leukoerythroblastic (or myelophthisic) blood picture may be seen when the marrow contains metastatic cancer, particularly when there is a desmoplastic (fibrotic) reaction to the cancer cells. These patients often have some reactive extramedullary hematopoiesis, but, in distinction to patients with AMM + MF, the spleen is usually not enlarged. The metastatic cancer cells will be apparent on bone marrow biopsy, or more rarely bone marrow aspiration (Plate 60), differentiating the problem from AMM + MF.

Most patients with AMM + MF are anemic, often severely so, although mild erythrocytosis has been observed in some patients during the early phase of this disease. There is usually a mild reticulocytosis, sometimes as high as 5 to 7 percent, due to the early release of reticulocytes from extramedullary sites and from a bone marrow compromised by fibrous tissue. The platelet count is characteristically high, but may be normal or even low, and there is usually considerable heterogeneity of platelet morphology on the peripheral blood smear, with the presence of some giant platelet forms. Similarly, the white blood cell count is variable and may be low, high, or normal. Characteristically, as noted previously, immature granulocytic elements are seen on the peripheral smear. Thus, when the white count is high, AMM + MF must be distinguished from CML. In CML, however, the peripheral blood smear does not usually contain large numbers of nucleated red blood cells, platelet morphology is usually normal, and there is no teardrop poikilocytosis of the erythrocytes. Moreover, the LAP score in AMM + MF is usually high (although it may be normal or even low), whereas it is typically quite low in CML. Finally, the Ph' chromosome characteristic of CML is not found in patients with AMM + MF.

Demonstration of extramedullary hematopoiesis with the use of isotopic iron (or indium, which like iron is also taken up by the transferrin receptor on early erythroid cells) has been occasionally used as a diagnostic test for AMM + MF. The iron or indium is taken up by developing erythroid cells and the demonstration by scanning techniques of uptake in the spleen or liver provides evidence of extramedullary hematopoiesis in these organs. This test, however, is rarely necessary to make a diagnosis of AMM + MF. Many patients with AMM + MF have osteosclerosis, which is evident on skeletal x-rays.

Prognosis, Course, and Therapy

Although the median survival after diagnosis is about 5 years, many patients with AMM + MF live for a long time. Anemia is often a significant problem, and many patients with this disorder become transfusion-dependent, with all of the problems that occur with multiple transfusions, such as allosensitization, febrile transfusion reactions, and exposure to blood-borne viral diseases. The anemia may sometimes respond to therapy with androgens, for example, norethandrolone given in large doses of 100 to 300 mg per week intramuscularly. Some patients with marked thrombocytosis may have complications resulting from hemorrhage or thrombosis, or both. In these instances, and in efforts to control symptomatic splenomegaly or hypermetabolism, therapy with antimetabolites may be useful. The drug most commonly used today is hydroxyurea, which is usually successful in controlling the thrombocytosis and sometimes in reducing spleen size. Recent studies indicate that α-interferon may have a beneficial effect in some patients with AMM + MF, particularly those with exuberant blood cell production.

Many patients with AMM + MF eventually require surgical splenectomy. Although the spleen is a site of extramedullary hematopoiesis, the latter is generally ineffective and increased destruction of mature red blood cells in the spleen more than offsets the production of new red blood cells in that organ. Thus, removal of the spleen is often associated with improvement in regard to anemia. Some physicians believe that it is necessary to demonstrate residual hematopoiesis in the bone marrow by the use of scanning techniques for uptake of radioactive iron or indium before splenectomy is undertaken, in order to ensure that the spleen has not become the primary site of erythropoiesis; however, these scanning techniques are not currently performed in many hospitals, and it has been reported rarely if at all that splenectomy has led to a permanent failure of erythropoiesis. Particularly if the spleen has become very large, splenectomy may be a formidable surgical undertaking and thus should not be put off too long.

If AMM + MF is observed in a young patient, consideration should be given to allogeneic bone marrow transplantation. However, most patients with this disorder are in an older age group and hence are not eligible for this form of therapy.

In a small number of patients with AMM + MF, 10 percent or fewer, acute nonlymphocytic leukemia eventually develops. This may occur whether or not the patient has received cytotoxic drugs in the past, and it is typically highly refractory to antileukemic chemotherapy.

Essential Thrombocythemia

Essential thrombocythemia (ET) is characterized by a predominant increase in the platelet count, although mild abnormalities may be found in the hematocrit or white blood cell count, or both, as well. This disorder seems to be closely related to polycythemia vera and AMM + MF. Indeed, isolated thrombocytosis sometimes evolves into one of these other disorders. More rarely, it may evolve into CML, although CML has many features that distinguish it from these other three, more closely related myeloproliferative disorders. In most patients, however, thrombocytosis remains the primary clinical problem.

Clinical and Laboratory Features

In addition to evidence of bleeding and/or thrombosis, which affects only a minority of patients with ET, the only notable finding on physical examination is splenomegaly; this is present in about 30 percent of patients with this disorder (Table 11-9). Thus, there are often no symptoms or physical signs of ET and the disorder is commonly detected only with routine blood testing. Characteristically, the platelet count is high, sometimes several million. The peripheral blood smear usually reveals considerable heterogeneity in the morphology of the platelets, some of which are very large and sometimes bizarre in appearance. As with the other myeloproliferative disorders, the platelets are often qualitatively abnormal when examined with tests of platelet aggregometry; demonstration of qualitative platelet abnormalities may help to distinguish thrombocytosis due to a myeloproliferative disorder from secondary (reactive) thrombocytosis, in which platelet morphology and function are both usually normal, but does not help to predict whether a given patient with ET will manifest hemorrhagic or thrombotic complications.

Table 11-9. Features of essential thrombocythemia

Platelet count often over 1.0 million
Abnormal platelet morphology, function
Marrow examination sometimes useful
Splenomegaly ($^1/_3$ of patients)
Course: benign, vs. hemorrhage and/or thrombosis; occasionally
  "conversion" to PV, AMM + MF, CML
Therapy: plateletpheresis (acutely); hydroxyurea, ^{32}P, alkylators; ? role for
  low-dose aspirin; anagrelide

The white blood cell count is sometimes elevated, with an increase in the number of basophils, although usually it is normal. Similarly, the hematocrit is usually normal but may be slightly increased or decreased in patients with ET.

Differential Diagnosis

To a large extent, the diagnosis of ET is one of exclusion of causes of secondary thrombocytosis. These are listed in Table 11-10. In addition, the presence of splenomegaly and the results of certain laboratory tests can be helpful in distinguishing myeloproliferative from reactive causes of thrombocytosis. The platelet count in patients with secondary causes of thrombocytosis is usually not very high and rarely exceeds 1 million platelets per cubic millimeter of blood; a broad range of platelet counts may be seen in ET and in the other myeloproliferative disorders, with values often reaching several million per cubic millimeter of blood. Thus, a very high platelet count favors the diagnosis of ET. Platelet aggregometry to look for evidence of qualititative platelet abnormalities has been mentioned previously. Similarly, marked morphologic abnormalities of the platelets in the peripheral blood smear (Plates 12 and 58) favor a diagnosis of ET. Platelet function and morphology are usually normal in secondary thrombocythemia. The leukocyte alkaline phosphatase score is usually elevated in patients with ET, although it can be normal or depressed; the LAP score may, of course, be elevated with secondary or reactive thrombocytosis if the underlying cause (for example, chronic infection) is associated with an increase in leukocyte turnover. A bone marrow examination is sometimes but not invariably helpful; in ET it may demonstrate a hypercellular bone marrow, clustering of megakaryocytes, and sometimes mild fibrosis, demonstration of which may require use of the reticulin stain. On the other hand, the bone marrow in ET often fails to show any diagnostic abnormalities.

Course and Therapy

Most patients with ET have a good prognosis. Indeed, it is a matter of controversy whether such patients require therapy at all and

Table 11-10. Differential diagnosis of thrombocytosis

Primary ("autonomous")
Myeloproliferative disorders—essential thrombocythemia, CML, PV,
AMM + MF
Secondary (reactive)
With severe infection or inflammatory disease
After surgery
With major hemorrhage
With malignancy
Iron deficiency anemia
Postsplenectomy

---

whether there is a level of the platelet count above which (e.g., 1.5 or 2.0 million platelets per cubic millimeter of blood) therapy should be instituted. Some experts suggest that the patient's history is the best guide, and it is certainly clear that any previous history of hemorrhage or thrombosis, or both, the major complications of ET, make it mandatory that the platelet count be lowered by physical or pharmacologic means. However, this approach suffers from the disadvantage that one may fail to treat the previously asymptomatic patient who is destined to develop a morbid hemorrhagic or thrombotic complication. Thus, although many patients may live with platelet counts in the many millions without problem, some hematologists prefer to treat all patients whose platelet counts exceed 1.0, 1.5, or 2.0 million per cubic millimeter of blood in order to prevent such a complication in a few such patients. There are no firm guidelines and such decisions are to be considered part of the art rather than the science of medicine.

There is a subset of patients with ET who are relatively young women. Initially, these patients were considered to have quite a good prognosis and, because of this and their age, therapy was often omitted. More recently, it has been demonstrated that these patients, too, may have complications related to bleeding or thrombosis, or both, so that they are also potential candidates for therapy aimed at reducing the blood platelet count. Indeed, because of these observations, many hematologists are now more inclined to treat most or all patients with ET in order to normalize their platelet counts.

If the need to reduce the platelet count is urgent, for example, in the setting of ongoing thrombotic disease or when surgery is necessary, modern techniques of blood separation, i.e., plateletpheresis, can be used to rapidly decrease the blood platelet count. Chronic control of thrombocytosis is achieved with the use of agents that suppress increased platelet production by the bone marrow. In the past a variety of agents have been used for this purpose, including ^{32}P or alkylating agents such as busulfan, melphalan, or even nitrogen mustard. Most commonly hydroxyurea is now used for this purpose. Large doses of hydroxyurea, in the range of 2 to 4 gm per day, will reduce the blood platelet count over a few days. Smaller doses, in the range of 0.5 to 1.5 gm per day, usually suffice to maintain the platelet count at a level less than 400,000 to 500,000. Some hematologists believe that low doses of aspirin may be helpful in preventing thrombosis in ET until the time that the platelet count is reduced to an acceptable level, but this is a controversial subject; in larger dosages of three tablets per day, aspirin has been shown to increase the bleeding tendency in polycythemia vera and might be expected to do so as well in ET. Aspirin therapy is clearly effective, however, in a rare manifestation of either ET or polycythemia vera; this is so-called erythromelalgia, a disorder in which the patient experiences painful, red, and swollen fingers or toes as the result of microthrombi in the digital vasculature. These patients respond well to aspirin therapy, followed by reduction of the platelet count or hematocrit, or both, by pharmacologic means.

A new drug, anagrelide, selectively decreases the platelet count in patients with ET or other myeloproliferative disorders without affecting the other cell lines. This agent may become highly useful in treating the thrombocytosis of these conditions since it appears to have relatively little toxicity.

We have already alluded to the observation that patients who present with an isolated elevation of the platelet count and are thought initially to have ET may eventually develop polycythemia vera, AMM + MF, or even CML. It seems likely that the thrombocytosis in these patients was simply the initial manifestation of the final disorder, even though there may have been an interval of several years before the latter became clinically evident. Alternatively, it is possible that this represents a transition of one myeloproliferative disorder to another, particularly within the triad of polycythemia vera, AMM + MF, and ET, which have many characteristics in common.

Case Development Problems: Myeloproliferative Disorders

A 65-year-old man has headache and his face appears flushed. His hematocrit is 0.64 (64%); hemoglobin, 16 gm/dL, and red blood cell count, 8×10^{12} cells per liter.

1. On the basis of these data alone, what tentative diagnoses can you make and what diagnostic procedures would you undertake to confirm them?

The clinical situation is that of erythrocytosis. The red cell mass should be determined by a radiochromium, isotope dilution method to confirm that it is indeed increased. Calculation of red cell indices yields a mean corpuscular volume of 80 femtoliters and mean corpuscular hemoglobin concentration of 25 gm/dL.

These indices indicate the presence of a hypochromic, microcytic anemia. Iron deficiency sometimes complicates polycythemia vera, so the serum iron and total iron-binding capacity (TIBC), and perhaps the serum ferritin level, should be measured, or a bone marrow examination for iron stores done.

The red cell mass is significantly above that predicted. Thus, the patient has true polycythemia. A diagnosis of polycythemia *vera* cannot be made, since patients with secondary polycythemia also have an increased red cell mass. The patient does not have relative polycythemia due to a decreased plasma volume, since the red cell mass is actually abnormally high.

The patient has an enlarged spleen. His white blood cell count is 20×10^9 per liter with no immature white cells or nucleated red cells seen on peripheral smear; his platelet count is 700×10^9 per liter. An LAP score is high, 280.

2. What diagnosis is suggested by these findings, and what further tests should be done?

This compilation of findings is virtually diagnostic of polycythemia vera. Additional tests for causes of secondary erythrocytosis are probably superfluous.

3. What therapy for his polycythemia would you recommend?

Most hematologists would treat with phlebotomy to reduce the hematocrit acutely, and also use hydroxyurea to suppress the excessive production of red cells (and platelets) on a chronic basis, with periodic phlebotomy as needed to maintain a hematocrit in the low to mid 40s.

The patient is treated successfully for 8 years, with his blood counts maintained at normal levels and his spleen normal in size. He has been asymptomatic. Now, 8 years after initial diagnosis, his spleen begins to enlarge again, and he becomes anemic.

4. On the basis of your knowledge of polycythemia vera, what abnormal findings would you look for in his peripheral blood smear?

Two possibilities exist: He is developing (1) acute leukemia or (2) myeloid metaplasia and myelofibrosis. The presence of immature white cells in the peripheral blood would be important, especially if they were mostly blasts, suggesting acute leukemia. Changes in red cell morphology would be of value, since teardrop forms (along with nucleated red cells, immature leukocytes, and giant platelets) favor the diagnosis of myelofibrosis. The platelet count is usually low in acute leukemia, whereas in myeloid metaplasia with myelofibrosis it is often high or normal.

5. How would you distinguish the clinical picture of myeloid meta-plasia with myelofibrosis from that of CML?

Myeloid metaplasia sometimes develops late during the course of polycythemia vera, whereas CML is not often (and is probably never) associated with preceding polycythemia. A very high white count, in excess of 50,000, favors a diagnosis of CML. Patients with myeloid metaplasia have a high LAP score and no Philadel-phia chromosome. Patients with CML have the Philadelphia chromosome and a low or zero LAP score. The most massively enlarged and firmest spleens are seen in myeloid metaplasia, whereas in CML the spleen usually does not become very large until late in the course of the disease. Teardrop red cell forms, a leukoerythroblastic blood picture, and marrow fibrosis are aspects of agnogenic myeloid metaplasia, but may also occur in the accelerated phase of CML.

The patient now has a hematocrit of 0.25 (25%) and a white count of 30×10^9 per liter with 1 percent blasts, 4 percent myelocytes, 6 percent metamyelocytes, and the rest bands and polys. There are numerous nucleated red cells and giant platelets on the blood smear, in addition to teardrop red cell forms. His platelet count is 600×10^9 per liter. His spleen is massively enlarged and fills the whole abdomen.

6. What is the likely diagnosis?

The most likely diagnosis is myelofibrosis with myeloid meta-plasia.

7. List the various therapies that might be used to treat this patient, and describe their advantages and disadvantages.

Androgens, hydroxyurea, and splenectomy. Splenectomy re-lieves cytopenias, but is associated with an operative risk. Andro-gens may improve anemia, but do not often affect the other blood counts or shrink the spleen. Hydroxyurea may shrink the size of the spleen, but can also cause severe cytopenias. Red cell transfu-sions are probably indicated. In sum, therapy for this patient's current condition is problematic at best.

The patient's spleen is removed in an attempt to ameliorate his anemia. This is unsuccessful, however; he not only remains anemic, but develops a white blood cell count of 100×10^9 per liter with 90 percent myeloblasts.

8. What is likely to have occurred, and how can this complication be treated?

The patient has developed acute myelogenous leukemia, another possible late complication of polycythemia vera, which may occur in the context of the development of myelofibrosis with myeloid metaplasia. Chemotherapy is usually not successful in such secondary forms of acute leukemia. A younger patient might have been a candidate for bone marrow transplantation.

Topics for Discussion: Myeloproliferative Disorders

The role of the c-*abl–bcr* gene rearrangement in the pathogenesis of CML

The pros and cons of treating a high platelet count in asymptomatic patients with a myeloproliferative disorder

The pathogenesis of marrow fibrosis in AMM + MF and other myeloproliferative disorders

The mechanisms underlying the bleeding tendency due to a high hematocrit or high platelet count

Selected Readings

Adamson, J. W., and Fialkow, P. J. The pathogenesis of myeloproliferative syndromes. *Br. J. Haematol.* 38 : 229, 1978.

Berk, P. D. et al. Therapeutic recommendations in polycythemia vera based on Polycythemia Vera Study Group protocols. *Semin. Hematol.* 23 : 132, 1986.

Castro-Malaspina, H. et al. Characteristics of bone marrow fibroblast colony-forming cells (DFU-F) and their progeny in patients with myeloproliferative disorders. *Blood* 59 : 1046, 1982.

Golde, D. W. et al. Polycythemia: Mechanisms and management. *Ann. Intern. Med.* 95 : 71, 1981.

Kurzrock, R., Gutterman, J. U., and Talpez, M. Molecular genetics of Philadelphia chromosome-positive leukemias. *N. Engl. J. Med.* 319 : 990, 1988.

Prchal, J. F. et al. Polycythemia vera. The in vitro response of normal and abnormal stem cells to erythropoietin. *J. Clin. Invest.* 61 : 1044, 1978.

Schafer, A. I. Bleeding and thrombosis in the myeloproliferative disorders. *Blood* 64 : 1, 1984.

Smith, J. R., and Landaw, S. A. Smokers' polycythemia. *N. Engl. J. Med.* 2988 : 6, 1978.

Ward, H. P., and Block, M. H. Natural history of agnogenic myeloid metaplasia (AMM) and a critical evaluation of its relationship with the myeloproliferative syndrome. *Medicine* 50 : 357, 1971.

12 Acute Leukemias and Myelodysplastic Syndromes

David M. Mastrianni
Catherine Wheeler

Acute leukemia is the result of the clonal proliferation and impaired differentiation of immature hematopoietic cells originating at the stem cell level. This proliferation results in the appearance of large numbers of immature cells ("blasts") in the marrow and peripheral blood, and in rapid bone marrow failure. These immature blast cells generally retain some features indicative of their origin in the hematopoietic lineage. If the blasts have lymphoid features, the leukemia is acute lymphocytic leukemia (ALL). If myeloid features predominate, the disease is acute myelogenous leukemia (AML, often referred to as acute nonlymphoblastic leukemia, or ANLL).

The myelodysplastic syndromes (MDS) are a heterogeneous group of diseases in which the clonal proliferation and failure of normal maturation are more subtle and insidious.

In this chapter, we review acute myelogenous leukemia, acute lymphocytic leukemia, and the myelodysplastic syndromes. The discussion of AML includes a review of bone marrow transplantation, a topic relevant to all three areas.

Acute Myelogenous Leukemia

Acute myelogenous leukemia (AML) is manifested by the clonal proliferation of immature cells that resemble precursors of normal myeloid cells. "Acute" refers to the short life expectancy of untreated patients. Although the true definition of "myeloid" (pertaining to the bone marrow) is broad, AML commonly refers to a disorder of hematopoietic cells that are *not* of lymphoid origin. Thus, in different forms of AML the blasts resemble precursors of granulocytes, monocytes, red cells, or platelets.

Acute myelogenous leukemia is uncommon; approximately 10,000 cases are diagnosed in the United States each year. The median age of patients is 60 years, and 90 percent of acute leukemias in adults are AML. Although in most patients no cause can be identified, certain risk factors for development of AML have been identified. Ionizing radiation is leukemogenic. Patients treated with radiotherapy for ankylosing spondylitis and survivors of the

293

atomic bombings of Hiroshima and Nagasaki share an increased risk of AML. Chemotherapy, particularly with alkylating agents, procarbazine, or nitrosoureas, predisposes to AML. As is discussed later, these treatment-related leukemias often evolve from a myelodysplastic syndrome and may contain deletions in chromosome 5 or 7. Exposure to chemicals such as benzene may predispose to AML. Several congenital disorders are associated with an increased risk of AML. Many of these disorders, which include Klinefelter's syndrome, Bloom's syndrome, Fanconi's anemia, von Recklinghausen's disease (neurofibromatosis), or the immunodeficiency states of ataxia–telangiectasia and X-linked agammaglobulinemia, share a predisposition toward chromosomal fragility. Children with Down's syndrome (trisomy 21) also have an increased incidence of AML (as well as ALL).

Other hematologic disorders may terminate in AML. The most obvious is chronic myelogenous leukemia (CML). As discussed elsewhere, all patients with CML will eventually develop acute leukemia and in two thirds the leukemic blasts will appear myeloid. Later in this chapter we review the myelodysplastic syndromes, which may also evolve into AML. In a small number of patients with polycythemia vera or agnogenic myeloid metaplasia, AML may develop. In general, patients with secondary AML evolving from these disorders have a dismal prognosis. Our discussion is directed at de novo AML.

Clinical Presentation

Patients with AML often seek medical care for symptoms due to the loss of normal blood elements. Neutropenia may lead to fevers or overwhelming infection. Anemia may result in fatigue and dyspnea. Thrombocytopenia predisposes to bleeding. Occasionally, symptoms may result from accumulation of the leukemic blasts. In 20 percent of patients, peripheral blast counts are over 50,000 per cubic milliliter. These blast cells are rigid and may increase blood viscosity, agglutinate with one another, and adhere to vascular endothelium, thus causing leukostatic complications involving the central nervous system (CNS), heart, lungs, and kidneys. Uncommonly, focal collections of leukemic blasts in tissues (chloromas) may be the presenting finding. Metabolic derangements secondary to the rapid cell turnover include hyperuricemia, hyperkalemia, and hyperphosphatemia.

The diagnosis of acute myelogenous leukemia is usually made by the identification of myeloblasts in the peripheral blood and greater than 30 percent myeloblasts in the bone marrow. The differential diagnosis is limited. Myeloblasts may be seen in the peripheral blood in CML or a leukemoid reaction. In these conditions, myeloblasts form only a small percentage of cells and are accompanied by intermediate forms (myelocytes and metamyelocytes) and by large numbers of mature polymorphonuclear leukocytes or band forms, which are usually absent or decreased in AML. Bone marrow replacement with myeloblasts does not occur in these conditions. The distinction of AML from ALL, however, may be difficult. In 1976, the French-American-British (FAB) cooperative group classified acute leukemias based on morphologic examination of bone marrow and blood with the addition of the cytochemical myeloperoxidase stain. This classification remains in widespread use today. In addition, multiple other cytochemical stains and surface membrane phenotyping are usually available to supplement the initial morphologic analysis. Chromosomal analysis or studies of molecular gene rearrangements may aid in classification, but these studies require extra time and are not usually available when initial therapeutic decisions are made.

For the clinician, the distinction of AML from ALL is critical to therapy. Table 12-1 summarizes differences between AML and ALL. The morphologic identification of myeloblasts may be aided by the presence of cytoplasmic granules (Plate 61), which may coalesce to form Auer rods (elongated, red refractile inclusions) (Plate 62). AML blasts (with the exception of megakaryoblastic leukemia) generally stain with myeloperoxidase and express myeloid surface markers. In contrast, lymphoid leukemic cells often are shown to contain large inclusions when stained with periodic acid–Schiff (PAS) reagent and express T or B lymphocyte antigens and often the

Table 12-1. Distinction of acute myelogenous from acute lymphocytic leukemia

	AML	ALL
Clinical features		
Age	Commonly adults	Commonly children
Lymphadenopathy	Rare	Common
Central nervous system involvement	Unusual	5%
Cytochemical stains		
Myeloperoxidase	Positive	Negative
Periodic acid–Schiff	Negative (except M6)	Positive
Other studies		
Surface markers	Myeloid	Lymphoid
CALLA	No	In early pre–B lineage ALL
Tdt	Absent	Present
Gene rearrangement studies		
T cell receptor	Absent	Present in T cell ALL
Immunoglobulin	Absent	Present in B cell ALL
Common cytogenetic abnormalities		
	t(9,22)	t(9,22)
	t(8,21)	t(4,11) null cell ALL
	t(15,17) in AML-M3	t(8,14) B cell Burkitt's type
	5q-, 7q-	t(11,14) B cell
	inv 16 in AML-M4Eo	t(1,19) B cell

common lymphoblastic leukemia antigen (CALLA) and the nuclear enzyme terminal deoxynucleotidyl transferase (Tdt). Five to 10 percent of leukemias cannot be classified by these methods. These leukemias may either have features of both AML and ALL or lack features of either lineage (acute undifferentiated leukemia).

Once the diagnosis of AML is made, subtyping is accomplished by defining the lineage features of the dominant leukemic blasts (granulocytic, monocytic, erythrocytic, or megakaryocytic), as summarized in Table 12-2. In general, morphologic appearance, cytochemical stains, and surface membrane antigens are assessed to determine cell lineage. Distinct clinical syndromes are associated with several subtypes. In nearly all patients with acute promyelocytic leukemia (AML-M3 or APML) (Plate 63), laboratory evidence of disseminated intravascular coagulation (DIC), sometimes with overt hemorrhage, is seen as the granules of the cells are released. The DIC, which may worsen with chemotherapy-induced cell lysis, may require factor replacement with plasma and cryoprecipitate. Heparin can be utilized when laboratory evidence of DIC is accompanied by severe thrombosis or bleeding, or both, despite factor replacement. Routine anticoagulation in APML does not seem indicated given the good results obtained with blood product support and prompt administration of chemotherapy. The diagnosis of APML now also has implications for treatment with trans-retinoic acid, discussed later. Another AML subtype, the myelomonocytic AML variant designated M4Eo, is characterized by atypical eosinophilia in the bone marrow and myeloblastomas of the central nervous system or leptomeningeal infiltration. The monoblasts of monocytic (AML-M5) (Plate 64) and less commonly myelomonocytic (AML-M4) leukemia (Plate 65) may infiltrate the skin and gums. In addition, elevations of urinary and serum lysozyme levels may be seen. Erythroleukemia (AML-M6) often evolves from a myelodysplastic state and hepatosplenomegaly is not unusual. Megakaryoblastic leukemias (AML-M7) are associated with marrow fibrosis, which may result in a "dry" bone marrow aspirate.

Biology

Normal hematopoietic cells arise from pluripotential stem cells. The pluripotential stem cell undergoes self-renewal, but more mature progenitor cells and their progeny lose this ability. Though they still proliferate, these more mature progenitor cells are committed to the myeloid lineage. With further maturation, bone marrow cells acquire lineage traits ("differentiation") and ultimately lose the ability to proliferate. Leukemia may arise at various points in the hematopoietic hierarchy. Chronic myelogenous leukemia, for example, arises in an early stem cell common to both myeloid and lymphoid

Table 12-2. Subtypes of acute myelogenous leukemia

Subtype	Cytochemical staining	Common surface antigens	Clinical or cytogenetic
M0: Undifferentiated*	None	Granulocytic markers CD13, CD33 (or CD14)	
M1: Myeloid wihout maturation	Myeloperoxidase (MPO) in a few cells	CD13, CD33	
M2: Myeloid with maturation (Plate 61)	MPO in most cells	CD13, CD33	t(8,21) in 10%
M3: Acute promyelocytic (Plate 63)	Marked MPO in nearly all cells	CD13, CD33, +CD15	t(15,17) in almost all; can be treated with trans-retinoic acid; DIC common
M4: Myelomonocytic (Plate 65) M4Eo variant	MPO Monocyte esterase	Granulocytic and monocytic markers	Inversion 16 with marrow eosinophils and reports of CNS disease
M5: Monocytic leukemia (Plate 64)	MPO Monocyte esterase	Monocytic markers CD11b, My8, CD14	Gum/skin infiltrates and increased lysozyme
M6: Erythroleukemia (Plate 31)	MPO Periodic acid–Schiff	Glycophorin	
M7: Megakaryoblastic	None	Factor VIII antigen	Myelofibrosis common

*The M0 subtype was proposed by a National Cancer Institute workshop. It does not appear in the FAB classification.

cells. AML may arise from a pluripotential stem cell or from a more mature progenitor cell committed to the myeloid lineage. These "leukemic stem cells" in turn give rise to more mature marrow cells, which are nonetheless unable to differentiate beyond the myeloblast or promyelocyte stage or the comparable stage of monocytic, erythroid, or megakaryoblastic development. As was discussed previously, the leukemic blast cells usually retain at least some of the morphologic, cytochemical, and surface membrane features of their normal counterparts.

On a genetic level, malignancies probably result from multiple alterations of critical genes. Of particular interest are the highly conserved proto-oncogenes (c-*onc*). When inserted into a susceptible host, altered proto-oncogenes may cause tumors. Alteration of these critical genes may result in gene amplification, gene loss, or creation of an abnormal gene producing abnormal proteins. Point mutations, translocations, or deletions are common mechanisms for such alterations. Mutations of the N-*ras* oncogene on chromosome 1 can be demonstrated in 25 percent of patients with AML. This gene family encodes a signal-transducing protein that may cause signal overexpression if mutated. Translocation of an active gene near a second gene may result in a fusion protein, as appears to occur in APML (AML-M3), discussed below. Deletions may inactivate genes required for normal differentiation, as apparently occurs in the AML associated with the loss of chromosome 5 or 7, also discussed later.

Clues to the various genetic alterations responsible for AML have been suggested by chromosomal analysis. Cytogenetic abnormalities are detected in the blasts of 60 to 90 percent of patients with AML. In brief, the cytogeneticist stains dividing cells in metaphase ("chromosomal banding") to allow visual analysis of the chromosomal structure. In chromosomal banding nomenclature, "q" designates the long arm of a chromosome and "p" the short arm. Large chromosomal deletions (del), inversions (inv), and translocations (t) of chromosomal material may be identified, but individual genes and their alterations will not be detected. Cytogenetic abnormalities in AML have suggested molecular–clinical syndromes, which are now being analyzed on the gene level using techniques familiar to the molecular biologist. The most dramatic of these to date is the translocation t(15,17)(q22,q12)—the cytogenetic hallmark of promyelocytic leukemia (AML-M3). Recently, this translocation has been defined on the molecular level. The translocation splits the retinoic acid receptor (RAR)-α gene on chromosome 17. Normally, retinoic acid plays a significant role in cell differentiation via specific receptors, including RAR-α, and is involved in the regulation of the rate of transcription (of DNA into RNA) of target genes. In the 15,17 translocation, critical elements of the receptor are replaced by DNA sequences from chromosome 15 (termed the *myl* gene). This translocation thus creates a fused *myl*/RAR-α gene, which produces a novel protein. The fusion protein may suppress the normal RAR-α allele and thus block expression of retinoic acid–controlled genes required for differentiation. Treatment of patients with acute promyelocytic leukemia with all trans-retinoic acid has been effective and morphologic complete responses have been obtained. Parallel studies of leukemic cells from patients treated with trans-retinoic acid have demonstrated differentiation in vitro that correlates with the response in vivo.

The most common translocation in AML is the t(8,21)(q22,q22), seen in 10 percent of patients with M2 leukemias. These patients are typically young and are reported to respond well to chemotherapy, although their overall survival is not clearly better than average. Again, a proto-oncogene, Hu-*ets*-2 (the human counterpart of the transforming gene of the avian erythroblastosis virus), is postulated to be involved since it is translocated from chromosome 21 to chromosome 8. However, proof of involvement of this oncogene in the pathogenesis of the leukemia awaits definitive study. Another, less common, cytogenetic abnormality in AML is the inversion of fragments of chromosome 16 (inv16 [p13,q22]) seen in the myelomonocytic subtype with marrow eosinophilia (M4Eo). These patients appear to have a generally good survival and have been reported to have an increased incidence of disease in the central nervous system. The inversion results in two break points on chromosome 16, but at present the genes involved remain unidentified. Also common in AML are the deletions of the long arm of chromosome 5 (5q-) or 7 (7q-), seen in about 8 percent of patients with AML. These abnormalities are often associated with previous chemotherapy or exposure to mutagens or ionizing radiation, and prognosis is often poor. The region of the 5q deletion contains the genes encoding such proteins as M-CSF, GM-CSF, interleukin-3 (and other interleukins), and their receptors including c-*fms* (the receptor for M-CSF). Loss or alteration of these critical genes required for normal bone marrow cell differentiation may result from these deletions. Defining these cytogenetic events on a molecular level will be critical to understanding the pathophysiology of leukemia as has been done for the t(15,17) translocation in AML-M3.

In addition to molecular and genetic studies of AML, cell culture studies have provided important insights into the biology of AML. Although one might assume that all leukemic cells would proliferate rapidly in culture, most leukemic blasts are hypoproliferative. Thus, the majority of leukemic blasts is the hypoproliferative progeny of a small population of rapidly dividing malignant progenitor cells.

In vitro, growth of colony-forming progenitor cells from normal bone marrow requires the addition of exogenous hematopoietic growth factors. The hematopoietic growth factors include the glycoprotein granulocyte colony-stimulating factor (G-CSF), which induces granulocytic growth and differentiation; macrophage colony-stimulating factor (M-CSF), which induces macrophage growth and differentiation; erythropoietin (Epo), which induces growth and differentiation of erythroid cells; granulocyte–macrophage colony-stimulating factor (GM-CSF), which induces growth and differentiation of multiple cell types; and interleukin-3 (Il-3), which influences a broader spectrum of generally less mature cells. A growth factor that acts on early hematopoietic stem cells, termed *stem cell factor* (SCF), has recently been identified. Stem cell factor is the ligand for the tyrosine kinase–type receptor c-*kit*, a receptor known to mediate stem cell proliferation. These growth factors are further discussed in the chapter on hematopoiesis (see Chap. 1).

The role of growth factors in the pathogenesis of leukemia is not yet clear. In general, Il-3 and GM-CSF increase leukemic blast proliferation in vitro, an effect enhanced by G-CSF. Erythropoietin increases proliferation of erythroid cells from many patients with erythroleukemia. These effects suggest roles for these factors in maintaining growth of the leukemic clone in vivo. The number of growth factor receptors on leukemic blasts appears to be normal. Expression of GM-CSF by cultured leukemic blasts has been reported in some cases, suggesting an "autocrine" loop of stimulation of leukemic cell growth. It is also possible that abnormal secretion of colony-stimulating factors by subclones of the leukemic population (particularly monocytic cells) or marrow stromal elements is important. Internal activation of growth factor receptors that bypasses normal membrane signals might be another mechanism by which abnormalities in growth factors contribute to leukemia.

Therapy

Initial medical management of the patient with AML includes prompt administration of broad-spectrum antibiotics in the febrile neutropenic patient, transfusion of red cells and platelets, and correction of electrolyte abnormalities. Typically, an indwelling central venous catheter is inserted for administration of chemotherapy and other medications, and to aid in blood drawing. Several medical issues warrant comment. In approximately 20 percent of patients, peripheral blast counts are over 50,000 per cubic milliliter. Increased blood viscosity, the rigidity of the blast cells, and their tendency to agglutinate and adhere to vascular endothelium place these patients at risk for leukostatic complications. Central nervous system hemorrhage and pulmonary, cardiac, and renal failure may be devastating. The risk markedly increases when the blast count is greater than 100,000. In such cases, leukapheresis and administration of the antimetabolite hydroxyurea are indicated until the blast count is rapidly reduced. Uric acid nephropathy may result from cell lysis, and prophylactic administration of allopurinol and maintenance of ample urine output are mandatory before chemotherapy is administered. The DIC associated with APML (AML-M3) or other forms of AML may require factor replacement, particularly once cytocidal therapy is begun.

CHEMOTHERAPY

AML becomes clinically evident only when approximately 10^{10} tumor cells exist; a lethal tumor burden is 10^{12} to 10^{13} cells. Treatment of AML begins with intensive induction chemotherapy designed to ablate the leukemic clone. It is expected that the normal bone marrow will also be ablated during this stage of therapy. Induction with a continuous infusion of cytosine arabinoside for 7 days and an anthracycline (usually daunorubicin) administered for 3 days by bolus infusion forms the commonly used "7 and 3" regimen. A complete remission (CR) is defined as the inability to detect leukemia using light microscopy after marrow cellularity is restored. This induction therapy achieves a CR in 60 to 80 percent of patients. Yet, despite this vast cell kill, 10^7 leukemic cells, including 10^4 leukemic stem cells, may remain and be undetectable by light microscopy. Thus, further intensive treatment (variously referred to as "consolidation" or "intensification" therapy) attempts to eradicate the remaining leukemic stem cells once a CR has been obtained. Long-term disease-free survival is reported in 15 to 20 percent of patients. The most aggressive consolidation therapies, which involve multiple cycles of high-intensity chemotherapy and often include high doses of cytosine arabinoside, result in 3-year disease-free rates of 40 to 50 percent in patients less than 45 years old who achieve a complete remission with induction treatment. The improved results with these highly aggressive therapies may represent treatment advances or reflect patient selection (exclusion of older patients and patients who do not survive initial therapy).

Most patients will eventually suffer relapse of their leukemia in the bone marrow. Adverse prognostic features include increasing age and history of a preceding myclodysplastic syndrome. Other prognostic factors, such as chromosomal abnormalities, have limited clinical utility at present, but in the future may be critical for selecting proper therapy. The median duration of complete remissions is 1 to 2 years; the response to further chemotherapy after relapse is usually poor. Multiple agents have been tested in relapsed leukemia and the best complete remission rates in selected patients are approximately 40 percent. These remissions rarely last longer than one year.

One obstacle to eradicating leukemic stem cells is drug resistance. This may be increased by a mutation or an increase in expression of the multidrug resistance (MDR) gene, alterations in drug transport, changes in the inactivation or detoxification of the drug, or mutations in drug targets. Currently, dose escalation and the use of multiple agents represent approaches to these problems. Extreme dose escalation is possible with bone marrow transplantation.

ALLOGENEIC BONE MARROW TRANSPLANTATION

The observation that the effectiveness of chemotherapy appears dose-related provided the rationale for using doses of chemotherapy that are lethal to the bone marrow, followed by hematologic rescue through marrow infusion. Allogeneic bone marrow transplantation is the infusion of marrow harvested from another person. In general, the majority of transplant patients are treated while they are in remission with regimens such as high-dose cyclophosphamide and total body irradiation or busulfan and cyclophosphamide, and rescued with marrow provided by an HLA-identical sibling. Although chemotherapy dose escalation provided the rationale for allogeneic transplantation, the efficacy of bone marrow transplantation in fact depends on both the high-dose chemotherapy and a complex graft-versus-leukemia (GVL) interaction. The existence of GVL is confirmed by the higher rate of relapse in patients with syngeneic transplants (marrow harvested from an identical twin) and in patients given T cell–depleted marrow to decrease graft-versus-host disease (GVHD) (see below). This GVL effect is probably mediated by cytotoxic T cells.

Allogeneic bone marrow transplantation is toxic. One third of patients die during the peritransplant period and the procedure is suitable only for patients under 45 or 50 years old. Prolonged bone marrow aplasia requires specialized blood bank and infectious disease expertise. Failure of the donor marrow to engraft is infrequent, but is more likely with T cell depletion (discussed below). Mucositis is severe and may be accompanied by major organ toxicity including hepatic venoocclusive disease or interstitial pneumonitis (often due to cytomegalovirus). Moderate to severe acute GVHD, which may be evident as a rash, hepatic dysfunction, diarrhea, and fever, is reported in nearly one half of patients transplanted with HLA-identical marrow. Chronic GVHD resembles a collagen-vascular illness, with skin, gastrointestinal, hepatic, and joint involvement accompanied by an immunosuppressed state. Mild cases of GVHD appear to be associated with better survival, presumably because the GVL effect is also increased. Severe GVHD, however, may result in fatal multiorgan disease and is more common in older patients. GVHD can be reduced by immunosuppressive drugs such as methotrexate and cyclosporine. Additionally, GVHD can be reduced by depleting the donor marrow of T cells using monoclonal antibodies, which may be linked to a variety of toxins (such as ricin or diphtheria toxin), density separation, or erythrocyte (E) rosette agglutination. Unfortunately, T cell depletion has been associated with increased rates of graft failure and a higher risk of leukemic relapse. This higher risk of relapse is attributed to a diminution of the GVL interaction.

Despite the toxicity, allogeneic bone marrow transplantation is effective therapy. When used in first remission, many patients can be cured of their leukemia. Relapses after bone marrow transplantation are usually due to a failure to eradicate disease from the host, but leukemia arising in the donor marrow cells has been reported. For young patients who undergo transplantation in first remission with sibling donors who are HLA-identical, the net long-term survival consistently ranges from 40 to 60 percent. Patients in their first remission who undergo transplantation with a single antigen-mismatched sibling appear to have the same prognosis as patients with complete HLA matches. Success is now being reported with transplantation using matched or single-antigen mismatched marrow from unrelated donors.

The proper role of allogeneic bone marrow transplantation in the treatment of leukemia is controversial. Should a suitable patient in first remission undergo the procedure or is transplantation best reserved for patients who suffer a relapse of their leukemia? Most data are from retrospective or, at best, nonrandomized prospective studies. In addition, most studies have been undertaken while transplantation technology was changing and conventional chemotherapy was apparently becoming more effective. Several nonrandomized comparative studies do demonstrate a survival advantage for patients in first remission who undergo bone marrow transplantation as compared with conventional chemotherapy, but these studies are biased by patient selection. Other analyses suggest that, given the cure rate with conventional treatment, overall survival in young patients who would be transplant candidates would be similar if transplantation were delayed until the first relapse. Bone marrow transplantation may be less effective after relapse, but patients already cured by chemotherapy would be spared the potential morbidity and mortality of the transplant procedure. Once relapse occurs, however, the issue is clear. Relapse of AML is invariably fatal when treated with conventional chemotherapy, while bone marrow transplantation may still offer cure in some cases. Finally, it should be emphasized that only 10 percent of patients with AML will be candidates for allogeneic bone marrow transplantation either because of advanced age (the median age of patients with AML is 60), lack of a donor, or failure to survive induction therapy. Unrelated HLA-compatible transplantation is now available through donor registries for some patients without compatible siblings, but the logistical and financial obstacles remain formidable.

AUTOLOGOUS BONE MARROW TRANSPLANTATION

Autologous bone marrow transplantation allows high doses of chemotherapy and radiotherapy to be administered to many patients who are not candidates for allogeneic transplantation. Once in remission, the patient's own bone marrow is removed under general anesthesia, stored during the administration of high-dose chemotherapy, and later reinfused. Because the risk of GVHD is eliminated and marrow engraftment occurs readily, autologous transplantation is less toxic than allogeneic transplantation. On the other hand, its effectiveness is decreased by the probable reinfusion of residual leukemic stem cells and particularly by the absence of a graft-versus-leukemia interaction. Most centers harvest marrow from patients in a complete remission and then administer high-dose treatment similar to that used in allogeneic transplants. To reduce the likelihood of reinfusing occult leukemic stem cells, "purging" the stored marrow of occult leukemic cells can be attempted in vitro. Successful purging of rodent marrows of leukemic cells but not normal stem cells using 4-hydroperoxycyclophosphamide (the active form of cyclophosphamide) encouraged human trials using this and related compounds. Leukemia-associated monoclonal antibodies have been used for the same purpose, as has long-term marrow culture in vitro to select out normal cells for reinfusion. The benefit of these procedures is uncertain.

The published results of autologous bone marrow transplantation include a variety of chemotherapy and purging techniques. Many studies can be criticized for the delay from achievement of complete response to the time of transplantation. This delay may select patients who are already cured. The fact that young patients have been treated in most series also restricts comparison with conventional chemotherapy. Reports of these selected patients undergoing autologous transplantation list a 1- to 3-year disease-free survival rate of 30 to 50 percent for patients in first remission and roughly 20 percent for patients in second remission. Longer follow-up study is needed for significant long-term survival to be demonstrated. Because of the potentially wide applicability and relatively low toxicity of autologous bone marrow transplantation, an increase in antileukemic efficacy by improving treatment regimens and purging techniques would have considerable implications for the treatment of AML.

DIFFERENTIATING AGENTS

Since leukemia is a disease characterized by failure of normal hematopoietic differentiation, inducing differentiation of leukemic blasts is an attractive therapeutic strategy. The induced mature leukemic cells would not replicate and might be functional. As was discussed previously, all trans-retinoic acid has been uniquely successful in inducing differentiation in patients with acute promyelocytic leukemia (AML-M3). Complete clinical and morphologic remissions may be obtained. The persistence of the abnormal and presumably unstable leukemic clone suggests that additional therapy to eradicate the leukemia, such as chemotherapy or bone marrow transplantation, will be required for cure.

Multiple other agents will induce human leukemic cell lines to differentiate in culture; these include compounds such as dimethylsulfoxide and hexamethylene bisacetamide, vitamin D_3, and such cytotoxic agents as cytosine arabinoside and 5-azacytidine. However, agents that cause established cell cultures to differentiate are generally ineffective on heterogeneous fresh leukemic cells in vitro and are usually ineffective and often toxic in vivo.

FUTURE APPROACHES FOR THERAPY

Chemotherapy and bone marrow transplantation (BMT) have clearly advanced the treatment of AML and result in cure of the disease in some patients. Future research in the use of other drug combinations, attempts to synchronize the leukemic cell cycle, and methods of overcoming drug resistance may improve the efficacy of chemotherapy. It is hoped that attempts to separate the graft-versus-leukemia effect from graft-versus-host disease will improve the efficacy and reduce the toxicity of allogeneic BMT. Improved techniques of "purging" bone marrow of leukemic cells before reinfusion in autologous marrow transplantation may improve the efficacy of this procedure. Identification of more precise prognostic factors, particularly chromosomal abnormalities, may help select different treatment strategies for different patients. Further in the future, continued advances in understanding the biology of AML may lead to treatment alternatives that are less toxic and more effective than those available today. The demonstration that promyelocytic leukemia (AML-M3), defined by the t(15,17) translocation, is characterized by a disruption in the retinoic acid receptor-α and that the leukemic cells of these patients (in vivo and in vitro) will differentiate in response to all trans-retinoic acid links the hematologist, cytogeneticist, and molecular biologist. Eventually, treatments tailored to the molecular defect may be designed for other forms of AML as well.

Acute Lymphocytic Leukemia

Acute lymphocytic leukemia (ALL) is a disease characterized by the accumulation of immature lymphoid cells in the blood and bone marrow. Several important features distinguish this disease from AML: the lymphoid origin of ALL, the preponderance of ALL in children, and the success of treatment that allows cure in a substantial percentage of children with this disease.

Clinical Features and Diagnosis

Acute lymphocytic leukemia is the most common cause of death from cancer in children. The disease accounts for 80 percent of childhood and 20 percent of adult acute leukemias. The classic presenting symptoms of ALL (which are similar to those of AML) result from anemia (fatigue), neutropenia (fever and infection), and thrombocytopenia (bleeding). In addition, there are several other common clinical features of ALL. Many patients complain of skeletal or joint pain caused by a "packed" bone marrow or synovial infiltration with leukemic cells. On examination, lymphadenopathy is commonly seen. Rarely, the adenopathy may be combined with significant hepatosplenomegaly to a degree that mimics lymphoma. Blast counts greater than 50,000 are seen in 20 percent of patients. CNS and pulmonary leukostasis is a serious risk in patients with blast counts over 50,000 and prompt leukapheresis is indicated. Mediastinal masses visible on chest radiograph may be seen, particularly in patients with T cell ALL. At diagnosis, CNS involvement is documented in approximately 5 percent of patients. Testicular involvement is detected in 1 percent of males.

The diagnosis of ALL in a patient with immature-appearing cells in the peripheral blood may occasionally be difficult. In young adults and children, the morphologic appearance of the atypical lymphocytes of viral infections such as infectious mononucleosis may be confused with that of the lymphoblasts of ALL by the inexperienced observer. The morphologic distinction between ALL and AML may be unclear and require cell surface marker analysis or special stains (see Table 12-1). Tdt, for example, is expressed in 95 percent of cases of ALL and is rarely seen in AML. The blast cells of ALL will often stain in a chunky or blocklike pattern with PAS stain, a finding that is unusual in AML except in the erythroleukemia subtype (AML-M6). Given the treatment implications, the accurate diagnosis of ALL versus AML is critical and may require the combined efforts of the hematologist and the immunophenotyping laboratory.

Classification

Leukemias are classified by the resemblance of the leukemic cells to normal hematopoietic cells. As we have discussed, the normal bone marrow contains pluripotential stem cells capable of producing myeloid or lymphoid stem cells. Lymphoid stem cells produce B cells and T cells. ALL is manifested by the proliferation of immature lymphoid cells and may have features of B cells or T cells. Since their differentiation is disordered, however, overlapping features may exist. For example, it has been demonstrated that some T cell ALLs undergo immunoglobulin gene rearrangement, which is normally a sign of B cell lineage. As noted in our discussion of AML, a small percentage of leukemias will have features of both ALL and AML (biphenotypic or mixed-lineage leukemia) or neither lineage (undifferentiated leukemia). This may reflect either origin from a multipotential stem cell (the cell that yields both lymphoid and myeloid stem cells) or a defect so severe that features of normal lineage differentiation are lost.

Classification of ALL may be made using the morphologic appearance or immunologic features of the malignant cells. The morphologic classification defined by the FAB group divides ALL into three subtypes: L1 contains small uniform-appearing blast cells (Plate 66), L2 larger pleomorphic blasts, and L3 mature "Burkitt"-appearing cells (basophilic lymphoblasts with cytoplasmic vacuoles). The L1 subtype is common in children. The L2 subtype is more unusual and seen primarily in adults. The Burkitt's L3 subtype is seen mainly in young adults. Many hematologists describe ALL using an immunologic classification to define B cell or T cell ALL. Approximately 80 percent of cases of ALL will have B cell features. Typically, these cells will express B cell antigens and the common ALL antigen (CALLA), and have undergone immunoglobulin gene rearrangement (discussed with the biology of ALL). The stage of production of immunoglobulin allows subdivision of B cell ALL. Most of these leukemias will not produce cytoplasmic immunoglobulin and be considered "early pre–B cell ALL." These leukemias are the common variety characterized by CALLA-positive cells. A minority will produce immunoglobulin in the cytoplasm and be considered pre–B cell ALL. A rare ALL (usually with L3 morphology) will exhibit surface immunoglobulin and be considered "mature B cell ALL." Approximately 20 percent of cases of ALL will have features of T cells, such as the ability to form rosettes with sheep red blood cells via the E rosette receptor (a finding of value to several generations of hematologists but with no known physiologic function), T cell surface markers, and evidence of T cell receptor gene rearrangements. Some reports of ALL (particularly older series) include cases that apparently lacked features of either T or B cells and were termed "null cell" ALL. With the availability of advanced methods of immunologic typing of the leukemic blasts, the null cell category of ALL is obsolete.

Biology

To understand recent advances in the biology of ALL, it is helpful to review several aspects of lymphoid development. Normal lymphocytes include B cells, T cells, and large granular lymphocytes, many of which are natural killer (NK) cells. B cells are immunoglobulin (antibody)-producing cells. The complete immunoglobulin consists of two identical heavy chains (α, ϵ, μ, γ, δ) and two light chains (κ or λ). Immunoglobulin is first expressed in the cell cytoplasm (pre-B stage) and later on the cell surface (mature B cell stage). Each clone of B cells produces a unique immunoglobulin. This is accomplished by rearrangement of immunoglobulin genes. This immunoglobulin gene rearrangement unites separate genes (those for the variable, diversity, and joining [VDJ] antibody regions to those for the constant region) to form a single gene capable of directing production of either the heavy or light chain portion of the antibody. The mechanisms by which gene recombination occur is under intense study and has profound implications for many aspects of molecular immunobiology. For the subsequent discussion of ALL, it is important to note that the heavy chain region is on chromosome 14, the κ light chain region on chromosome 2, and the λ light chain on chromosome 22.

T cell differentiation involves expression of unique T cell antigens and a rearrangement of the T cell receptor genes. The T cell receptor serves a critical role in the identification of antigens and their presentation to the immune system. This receptor is antigen-specific and its production is directed by genes that undergo rearrangements similar to those of the immunoglobulin genes.

In ALL, as in AML, chromosomal derangements visible to the cytogeneticist may offer clues to underlying disease mechanisms. The most common translocation in ALL is the t(9,22), which results in a shortened chromosome 22—the "Philadelphia chromosome," considered the hallmark of CML. This translocation occurs in 5 percent of childhood and 25 percent of adult ALL and imparts a poor prognosis. The transfer of the c-*abl* oncogene from chromosome 9 to the break point cluster region (*bcr*) of chromosome 22 results in the production of a unique fusion protein. Although the chromosomal picture of the t(9,22) in ALL is identical to that of the t(9,22) in CML, differences between the two translocations may be evident when they are analyzed on a molecular level. In ALL, the fusion gene usually produces a 190-kd protein, in contrast to the 210-kd protein observed in CML. This difference is the result of slightly different regions of chromosomal breakage. The role of the 190-kd protein in the pathogenesis of ALL is uncertain, but the 210-kd fusion protein appears to be important in the pathogenesis of CML through its activity as a tyrosine kinase.

Translocations of chromosomal fragments in ALL also frequently occur in the highly active regions of gene rearrangement discussed earlier. B cell lineage ALL may commonly have the translocations t(4,11), t(1,19), or t(11,14). Mature B cell ALL (with the L3 morphology discussed above) may contain translocations found in Burkitt's lymphoma such as t(8,14) or less commonly t(2,8) and t(8,22). In Burkitt's lymphoma and most ALLs with t(8,14), an enhancer for the immunoglobulin gene from chromosome 14 is juxtaposed to the *c-myc* oncogene of chromosome 8. An interesting example of a similar mechanism unique to ALL is the report of a (rare) translocation t(5,14) in a patient with B lineage ALL associated with blood eosinophilia. This translocation juxtaposes the immunoglobulin heavy chain-joining region on chromosome 14 to the region of the promoter of the gene for interleukin-3 on chromosome 5. T cell lineage ALL often involves translocation of the α-chain of the T cell receptor on chromosome 14 or the β-receptor on chromosome 7.

In addition to these translocations, mutations in oncogenes are reported in ALL, for example, altered amounts of RNA transcripts of *c-myc*, *c-myb*, and other oncogenes. The complete relationship between alterations in the structure of genes and their products with the biologic behavior of the malignant cells is not understood. In addition, normal differentiation is influenced by a complex combination of regulatory factors, including the interleukins, interferons, and other growth factors and cytokines. These factors and the bone marrow environment in which they act are almost certainly involved in the leukemic process in ways not yet understood.

Prognosis and Treatment

Patients with ALL are heterogeneous and the recognition of prognostic factors was an important step in the development of therapeutic strategies. Multivariate analyses have demonstrated multiple factors associated with a poor prognosis. The most important are age less than 12 months or greater than 10 years and a markedly elevated leukocyte count (in excess of 20,000). Male sex, CNS disease, and extensive nodal or organ involvement are also adverse clinical features. Children with an L2 or L3 (Burkitt's) morphology have a poorer prognosis than those with the more common phenotype. Cytogenetics are also useful prognostically. The reciprocal translocations described above—t(9,22), t(8,14), t(4,11)—are adverse features, whereas hyperdiploid states (particularly >50 chromosomes) without translocation appear favorable. Immunologic phenotypes have clear prognostic implications, as mature B cell and T cell ALLs have a much poorer outlook than the common CALLA-positive, early pre–B cell ALL in children.

Treatment principles in ALL differ from those in AML in several important respects. (1) ALL is sensitive to vincristine and prednisone, nonmyelotoxic drugs that are minimally active in AML. (2) Many children with ALL can be cured. Thus, patients with a favorable prognosis can be treated in a manner that minimizes toxicity. (3) Maintenance therapy has a clear role in the treatment of ALL. (4) The "sanctuary sites" of the central nervous system and testicles (areas of poor penetration of most systemically administered chemotherapeutic agents) are important sites of relapse in ALL.

Treatment of ALL, as with AML, begins with induction chemotherapy to attempt to eradicate all detectable leukemic cells and obtain a CR. Induction may be followed by high-dose treatment (variously called consolidation, intensification, or postremission therapy) and then low-dose maintenance chemotherapy over 2 to 3 years designed to eliminate remaining undetectable leukemic cells.

CHILDREN WITH ALL

Children with ALL are stratified into standard- or high-risk categories based on the prognostic features described above. For standard-risk patients, induction treatment with vincristine, prednisone, and usually a third agent such as L-asparaginase induces a CR in 90 percent of patients. Unlike induction therapy in AML, this treatment is not myelosuppressive. Following induction, maintenance therapy continues for 3 years in boys and 2 years in girls; boys treated for only 2 years have a higher risk of testicular relapse. This low-dose oral therapy usually consists of weekly methotrexate and daily 6-mercaptopurine augmented by further treatments with vincristine and prednisone. High-dose consolidation or intensification (as in AML) is not widely used in standard-risk children. Cure is possible in 60 to 80 percent of patients.

For high-risk children, initial therapy involves multiple cycles of chemotherapy utilizing vincristine, prednisone, anthracyclines, L-asparaginase, cytarabine, methotrexate, etoposide or tenoposide, and other agents in highly complex protocols. These regimens, in contrast to treatment used in standard-risk children, are highly myelotoxic and organ toxic. However, use of these intensive combinations has allowed remission and survival rates similar to those achieved in standard-risk ALL.

The central nervous system is an important site of relapse despite the low incidence of involvement at presentation. The CNS may act as a sanctuary for leukemic cells since many chemotherapeutic agents do not cross the blood-brain barrier. Thus, CNS "prophylaxis" is used routinely after remission has been induced in order to eliminate initially undetectable leukemic cells. Cranial radiation, intrathecal chemotherapy, and/or high-dose systemic agents that cross the blood-brain barrier can be used. Most centers rely on a combination of cranial radiation (18–24 Gy) and intrathecal methotrexate administered after CR is achieved. Unfortunately, long-term toxicity in the form of learning deficits is an adverse effect of this therapy. For standard-risk children, lower doses of radiation (18 Gy) or intrathecal methotrexate alone are typically employed to decrease these adverse effects. High-dose systemic methotrexate (which crosses the blood-brain barrier) may allow CNS treatment with less toxicity.

Testicular relapse is a significant concern in boys with ALL. Testicular biopsy in boys will demonstrate occult leukemia in approximately 10 percent after systemic therapy, but the management of these patients and the role of prophylactic treatment remain undefined.

In systemic relapse of ALL, the response to retreatment is better in patients who have had a longer remission. A child who has a remission of greater than 18 months has a 50 percent chance of long-term survival when retreated with intensive therapy. Children who suffer relapse within 18 months have a grim prognosis. Children in this group, or those with subsequent relapses, should be considered for allogeneic or autologous bone marrow transplantation. Relapses occurring in the CNS or testis require initial local treatment followed by systemic therapy. Long-term survival rates of 20 percent are reported for children with isolated CNS relapse.

ADULTS WITH ALL

Adults with ALL have a worse prognosis than children. Adult ALL therapy is similar to therapy for high-risk children and usually includes both induction and intensive postremission therapy. The multiple agents outlined previously are administered for periods of 6 months to 2 years. Complete remissions are obtained in 70 to 80 percent of patients and long-term survival (3–5 years) is reported in about 30 percent. The optimal duration of maintenance chemotherapy in adults is unknown, but most patients receive oral maintenance therapy similar to that given to children, with methotrexate and 6-mercaptopurine. Most adults also receive CNS treatment, although its efficacy is uncertain.

ALLOGENEIC BONE MARROW TRANSPLANTATION

A basic description of allogeneic bone marrow transplantation is provided in the review of therapy of AML and the principles of the procedure are similar for ALL. Typically, hematologically lethal doses of chemotherapy with agents such as cyclophosphamide or cytarabine are combined with total body irradiation in an effort to eradicate the leukemic cells. The patient is then hematologically rescued by infusion of normal marrow obtained from a histocompatible donor. The best results of the procedure in ALL are achieved when BMT is done in first remission. However, standard-risk children who have a relatively good prognosis are not candidates for transplantation in first remission because of their good outlook and the toxicity of the procedure. Given the improved prognosis for high-risk patients with intensive protocols, most of these patients will also not undergo BMT in first remission. Selected children with multiple adverse features are considered for this treatment in first remission. Once a relapse has occurred, the length of the initial remission will determine the suitability of BMT. Those patients who had a short CR will be candidates. Survival rates of 30 to 40 percent are reported in these patients. Children with a second relapse are clearly BMT candidates, but it must be remembered that only one third will have an HLA-matched sibling. Transplantation with partially HLA-matched related donors or unrelated matched donors is riskier, but should also be considered for these patients.

For adults with ALL, the role of BMT is incompletely defined. The age restriction of 45 to 50 years deserves reemphasis and results of BMT in adults are not as good as in children. For patients in first remission, the results with BMT or the intensive chemotherapy described previously appear roughly equivalent. Some subgroups with bad prognostic features (such as the Philadelphia chromosome) who are highly likely to relapse may benefit from BMT in first remission. All relapsing patients should be considered for BMT given their poor prognosis.

AUTOLOGOUS BONE MARROW TRANSPLANTATION

Autologous bone marrow transplantation involves removal of the patient's bone marrow followed by administration of high doses of chemotherapy and often total body irradiation. The patients are then hematologically rescued by reinfusion of the stored marrow. Autologous BMT avoids the problems of graft-versus-host disease associated with allogeneic BMT, but lacks the graft-versus-leukemia effect. Another obstacle is the potential for reinfusion of leukemic cells, although it is possible that leukemic recurrence is more commonly due to failure to eliminate the leukemia from the host with the current "conditioning" regimens of chemotherapy and radiotherapy. Elimination of leukemic cells from the preserved marrow by chemotherapeutic or immunologic methods (discussed in the similar section in AML) has been attempted, but with uncertain results. In advanced uncontrolled ALL, relapse after autologous BMT is almost certain. For patients treated in second remission, long-term disease-free survival has been reported in 20 percent of highly selected patients. Autologous BMT may be useful in selected high-risk patients in first remission.

Myelodysplastic Syndromes

The myelodysplastic syndromes (MDS) are a heterogeneous group of disease states that usually present as peripheral blood cytopenias with a hypercellular bone marrow. As in the acute leukemias, the fundamental disorder is the clonal proliferation of stem cells that produce progeny that fail to mature normally. In the acute leukemias the maturation defect leads to the accumulation of blast cells. In MDS, in contrast, the maturation defect is more subtle; mature forms develop but they are often morphologically atypical ("dysplastic") and frequently dysfunctional as well. Although MDS may terminate in acute leukemia, terms such as "preleukemia" or "smoldering leukemia" lack clinical or biologic validity and are no longer used.

Presentation and Diagnosis

Myelodysplastic syndromes are usually diseases of the elderly. In some series, men are slightly more vulnerable than women. MDS in younger patients is typically seen in the setting of prior chemotherapy or radiotherapy, or both, and is a more aggressive disease. Peripheral blood cytopenias are the typical presenting features and result in progressive symptoms related to anemia, thrombocytopenia, and/or neutropenia. MDS may be suggested by findings on the peripheral blood smear that reflect dyspoiesis in the bone marrow. In the red cell line, such findings may include anisocytosis and poikilocytosis, basophilic stippling, and nucleated red cells. The red cells are commonly macrocytic but normocytic, microcytic, and dimorphic populations may be evident. Neutrophil morphology is commonly abnormal, with hypogranulation of the cytoplasm and Pelger-Huët nuclei (bilobed nuclei with a "dumbbell shape" or nonsegmented round or peanut-shaped nuclei, see Plates 41 and 42). Blast forms may be seen at diagnosis in small numbers, or in larger numbers if transformation to acute leukemia occurs. Micro- or macrothrombocytes with low or occasionally high platelet counts may be found. Sometimes, however, the morphology of the peripheral blood is relatively normal.

The differential diagnosis in the typical elderly patient with cytopenias and a blood smear suggestive of MDS includes vitamin B_{12} or folic acid deficiency, an infiltrative process of the marrow (usually by solid tumor or, less commonly, a hematopoietic malignancy such as lymphoma), and toxic or viral injury (e.g., due to alcohol). AIDS may lead to a rather similar picture. The history should specifically address past drug exposure, particularly any chemotherapeutic agents or solvents such as benzene. The physical examination should include a search for splenomegaly. Laboratory studies to exclude vitamin deficiency or the other conditions mentioned above are appropriate.

The diagnosis of MDS is typically made by the bone marrow findings of often striking marrow hypercellularity and dysplastic changes in the marrow cell lines. Dyserythropoiesis with megaloblastic features, sometimes accompanied by multiple fragmented or budding nuclei and ringed sideroblasts (cells containing deposits of iron within the mitochondria), are often but not invariably seen. Dysgranulopoiesis may be manifested by abnormal granulation of neutrophil precursors, which also may have bizarre nuclear shapes, and by a "shift-to-the-left," that is, toward immaturity. A small population of blast cells is present in some patients. Micromegakaryocytes containing single or bilobed nuclei (unlike the normal polypoid nuclei) are common. "Pawnball" megakaryocytes with multiple separate nuclei may be present. In some cases, the marrow may be hypocellular or normocellular, and the marrow pathology may be relatively normal, making the diagnosis difficult.

In addition to a morphologic evaluation of the bone marrow, cytogenetic analysis should be performed. As discussed below, several chromosomal abnormalities are often associated with MDS and may provide diagnostic confirmation and be useful prognostically. This is particularly important in the patients in whom the peripheral blood and bone marrow fail to reveal diagnostic morphologic changes.

Classification and Clinical Course

Classification of MDS is usually according to the French-American-British system summarized in Table 12-3. Although many patients display overlapping features and the criteria are somewhat arbitrary, this classification is useful prognostically. In examining Table 12-3, several features are of note. When the percentage of myeloblasts in the bone marrow exceeds 30 percent, the FAB system considers the diagnosis to be overt AML. In refractory anemia (RA), myeloblasts comprise less than 5 percent of the bone marrow and the various cell lines may or may not show features of dysplasia. Refractory anemia with ringed sideroblasts (RAS) is similar to RA clinically and morphologically except that it is characterized by a marked dysfunction in iron processing with the presence of ringed sideroblasts; these are normoblasts (developing erythroid cells) with iron-laden mitochondria, organelles that have a perinuclear distribution in young erythroid cells (Plate 17). The other states are more aggressive clinically. These disorders are characterized by excess myeloblasts. Refractory

Table 12-3. FAB classification of the myelodysplastic syndromes

Feature	Refractory anemia (RA)	Refractory anemia with ringed sideroblasts (RARS)	Refractory anemia with excess blasts (RAEB)	Refractory anemia with excess blasts in transformation (RAEBt)	Chronic myelomonocytic leukemia (CMML)
Myeloblasts (%)					
blood	0	0	<5	>5 (variable)	<5
marrow	<5	<5	5–20	20–30	<30
Ringed sideroblasts (%)	<3	>15	+/−	+/−	+/−
Blood monocytes	nl	nl	nl	nl	>1 × 10^9/L
Patients developing AML (%)	<10	<10	30–50	>50	30–50
Typical survival	Usually long	Usually long	Few mo to 1 to 3 yrs	Few wk to mo	Variable

anemia with excess blasts (RAEB) and refractory anemia with excess blasts in transformation (RAEBt) differ in the percentage of blasts counted in the bone marrow. Chronic myelomonocytic leukemia (CMML) is in some respects a separate entity involving expansion and dysplasia of the monocytic cell line, often accompanied by erythroid, granulocytic, and megakaryocytic dysplasia, and sometimes an increase in myeloblasts as well.

The myelodysplastic syndromes are usually progressive disorders with considerable variability in natural history. Overall, approximately 5 to 50 percent of patients die as the result of transformation to acute leukemia. The leukemia usually has myeloid characteristics (AML), although rare patients display features of lymphoid (ALL) or mixed phenotypic leukemias. Many patients never develop leukemia, but die as a result of progressive bone marrow failure with pancytopenia resulting in infection and bleeding. Bacterial infections are common. In addition to neutropenia, qualitative abnormalities of neutrophil function have been demonstrated. Opportunistic infections are not characteristic of these patients, although some defects in cell-mediated immunity are evident. Bleeding results from both low numbers of platelets and platelet dysfunction. The remaining patients die of conditions unrelated to MDS, as is expected in an elderly population. In general (see Table 12-3) RA and RAS have a better prognosis, and RAEB, CMML, and RAEBt a worse prognosis. A high percentage of marrow blasts, advanced age, and profound cytopenias predict poor survival. Cytogenetics have prognostic significance: Monosomy 7 (loss of a whole chromosome 7) or complex karyotypes are adverse features, while the isolated 5q- (loss of the long arm of chromosome 5) syndrome, discussed below, confers a better prognosis. It is notable that chromosomal abnormalities in MDS typically involve loss of part of or a whole chromosome, and the translocations seen in AML are unusual.

Treatment-related MDS is seen in the setting of prior chemotherapy (often combined with radiotherapy), particularly with alkylating agents (especially melphalan or chlorambucil) or nitrosoureas (such as methyl-CCNU) and typically occurs after a several-year latency period. These treatment-related MDS have a high incidence of damage of chromosomes 5 and 7. The dismal prognosis of treatment-related MDS should be emphasized; the median survival is only 8 months. Acute leukemia develops in many of these patients.

Biology and Pathophysiology

MDS are clonal disorders arising from a diseased (presumably neoplastic) pluripotent hematopoietic stem cell or cells. This stem cell origin is suggested by the involvement of multiple cell lines. Cytogenetic analysis provides demonstration of clonal defects in some patients. Studies with glucose-6-phosphate dehydrogenase (G-6-PD) heterozygote females, restriction fragment length polymorphisms (RFLP), and methylation-sensitive restriction enzyme analysis have confirmed multilineage clonality in a larger number of patients. The reader is referred to the selected readings for the details of these reports. The result of this stem cell disorder is a clone (or clones) of stem cells with a growth advantage over normal cells in the bone marrow, producing progeny that proliferate and do not differentiate properly. This is similar to the pathophysiology of acute leukemia, except that the defect in differentiation is more complete in the latter condition, with blast cells predominating in the bone marrow and peripheral blood.

Much of our current understanding of the biology of MDS comes from analysis of growth patterns of these cells in culture and attempts to define genetic abnormalities. In most cases of MDS, the number of early progenitor cells in the bone marrow is decreased when assayed using cell culture techniques. Samples from patients with excess blasts (RAEB and RAEBt) placed in culture typically have reduced colony-forming ability. The findings are similar to those in acute myelogenous leukemia. In vitro, these cells are usually dependent on the addition of exogenous colony-stimulating factors for continued growth—as is the case with normal marrow and marrow from most patients with AML. The addition of certain growth factors to cultures may encourage differentiation. In CMML, in contrast, colony-forming ability is enhanced even without stimulation. These findings suggest that abnormalities in growth factor secretion or sensitivity may be involved in the pathogenesis of MDS, but differ among various patients and syndromes. Additionally, production of factors that suppress normal hematopoiesis is possible; this has not been clearly documented for MDS, although there is in vitro evidence that AML blast cells can subvert normal cell growth. Evidence is also developing that abnormalities in the stromal (microenvironmental) cells of the marrow contribute to the development of MDS.

On the genetic level, nonrandom chromosomal abnormalities are commonly found in MDS. In particular, the deletion of a portion of the long arm of chromosome 5 (5q-) occurs in 5 to 10 percent of patients. As an isolated chromosomal defect, this defines the "5q-syndrome," with thrombocytosis, mononuclear megakaryocytes, macrocytic red cells, and, usually, a good prognosis. When additional chromosomal abnormalities are present, however, the prognosis is worsened. The long arm of the fifth chromosome contains multiple genes involved in growth factors, growth factor receptors, and hematopoietic regulatory genes (as discussed in the review of the biology of AML). Less commonly occurring abnormalities include monosomy 7 and trisomy 8. In addition to these gross chromosomal defects, mutations in proto-oncogenes such as the *ras* family and c-*fms* (the receptor for M-CSF) have been reported in a significant percentage of patients. The precise role of these abnormalities is uncertain, but it is tempting to postulate that one or more genetic defects result in a neoplastic or preneoplastic clone of stem cells with a growth advantage over normal stem cells. Further insults yield clones with increasingly deranged maturation. This is illustrated by the worsening of the prognosis of patients with the 5q-syndrome when additional chromosomal abnormalities are found. The poor prognosis of patients previously treated with chemotherapy or radiotherapy, or both, may be explained on a similar basis; the repeated exposure of the marrow to mutagenic influences presumably results in multiple genetic or chromosomal defects.

Treatment

SUPPORTIVE CARE

For the most part there is little effective treatment for MDS, and emphasis is placed on supportive care. Patients with MDS typically manifest anemia, thrombocytopenia, and/or neutropenia. Red cell transfusions are indicated for symptomatic anemia. In patients with a good prognosis, repeated transfusions may eventually result in iron overload, and chelation therapy may be appropriate. Platelet transfusions are indicated for thrombocytopenic bleeding and for surgery, but should be minimized to avoid alloimmunization. Early treatment of infections with appropriate antibiotics is indicated; the use of prophylactic antibiotics is reserved for those with repeated infections. As was noted, most infections are bacterial and opportunistic organisms are infrequently encountered.

STANDARD PHARMACOLOGIC AGENTS

All patients with ringed sideroblasts should receive treatment with high-dose pyridoxine (100–300 mg/day) for at least 3 months. This therapy is nontoxic and some responses have been reported, although they are more common in hereditary or drug-induced sideroblastic anemias (see Chap. 3). Corticosteroids usually have no effect on MDS (though there are rare exceptions) and pose the well-known risks associated with their use—particularly immunosuppression in this population already plagued by infection. Androgen therapy is effective in ameliorating anemia in a minority of patients. The "attenuated" androgen danazol has been helpful in some patients with MDS who have accelerated red cell or platelet turnover.

CHEMOTHERAPY AND BONE MARROW TRANSPLANTATION

Standard aggressive chemotherapeutic regimens used in the treatment of AML are largely ineffective in MDS. Complete remissions are seen in only one third of patients, while nearly half will die during the treatment. The remissions are usually of short duration and patients have an average survival of only several months. The best success has been reported in younger patients.

Given the dismal results with conventional chemotherapy in the treatment of MDS, allogeneic BMT represents the only hope for cure. As discussed in the review of treatment of AML, BMT is restricted to patients under 45 to 50 years of age with an appropriate HLA-matched sibling. Most such young patients will have MDS related to prior chemotherapy or radiotherapy, or both. Overall survival rates of 40 percent in highly selected patients have been reported. It is not necessary to first induce a remission in MDS patients before allogeneic transplantation. Autologous bone marrow transplantation is inappropriate in MDS since it is difficult to achieve a bone marrow remission and the stem cell pool in these patients has presumably been virtually entirely replaced by abnormal progenitor cells.

DIFFERENTIATING AGENTS AND GROWTH FACTORS

Attempts to eradicate the malignant clone(s) in MDS are either unsuccessful (as with conventional chemotherapy) or highly toxic and limited to selected patients (bone marrow transplantation). Much interest has developed in the use of differentiating agents in the treatment of MDS, which, after all, is a disorder of marrow cell differentiation. The malignant clone would remain, but the cells would mature and lose their proliferative potential. The agent most widely used in an attempt to induce differentiation in MDS is low-dose cytosine arabinoside. Improvements in some patients have been reported, but the overall success rate is small. Many hematologists believe that this form of therapy actually works by myelosuppression rather than induction of differentiation in the neoplastic cells. Other agents, such as retinoic acid, vitamin D, or α-interferon, have not demonstrated consistent therapeutic effects. Occasionally, patients treated with retinoic acid will demonstrate a mild to moderate increase in the neutrophil count.

The use of growth factors is a conceptually attractive alternative method of either promoting differentiation of abnormal cells or increasing proliferation of persisting normal clones. In general, those factors that act on more mature committed cells (such as G-CSF or M-CSF) tend to increase differentiation. Growth factors that primarily act on stem cells (such as II-3 or GM-CSF) may increase proliferation of both normal and malignant clones. Thus, the administration of these early-acting growth factors has the potential effect of accelerating the transformation to acute leukemia. The heterogeneity of growth factor responsiveness in MDS both in vitro and in vivo has been emphasized, and it is likely that combinations of factors will be required to achieve maximal therapeutic effect. At present, G-CSF and GM-CSF have been shown to effectively increase granulopoiesis in patients with MDS. Sequential use of Il-3 followed by GM-CSF also seems promising, although there are reports of GM-CSF promoting the development of AML in some patients. Erythropoietin decreases transfusion requirements in a minority of patients. Widespread use of these factors appears inevitable and further studies comparing in vivo results with in vitro growth characteristics may prove useful in developing strategies for tailoring therapy to individual patients.

Case Development Problems: Acute Leukemias and Myelodysplastic Syndromes

Patient History No. 1

A previously healthy 23-year-old woman presents to a walk-in clinic complaining of 5 days of sore throat and low-grade fevers. For 2 days she had noticed gum bleeding when she brushed her teeth. Her examination reveals purpura of the oral mucosa and petechial lesions on her legs. An automated CBC yields a white blood count of 5×10^9 per liter, a hematocrit of 28 percent, and a platelet count of 12,000 per cubic millimeter.

1. What initial tests should be done at this time?

   The initial step in the evaluation of most hematologic disorders is examination of the peripheral blood smear. In this case, the differential diagnosis included viral infection with immune thrombocytopenia (and an unexplained anemia, perhaps due to blood loss) and more serious disorders including acute leukemia and aplastic anemia (although the white blood count is normal).

   Examination of the smear revealed that this patient's peripheral white blood cells are almost exclusively the promyelocytes (large cells with ample cytoplasm containing numerous granules) diagnostic of APML. Some fragmented red blood cells are present. Few platelets are evident. It is worth emphasizing that acute leukemia can present with an elevated, normal, or low total white count and that examination of the peripheral blood smear is essential for diagnosis. The patient is admitted to the hospital and her temperature is found to be 102°F. Initial coagulation tests include a prothrombin time measuring 16 seconds (control 12.0 seconds), a partial thromboplastin time measuring 45 seconds (control 24 seconds), a fibrinogen of 33 mg/dL (normal 150–400 mg/dL), and fibrin split products present in a dilution of 1 : 512. Routine blood chemistries, including uric acid, are normal except for a mild elevation in lactic dehydrogenase (LDH).

2. What initial steps in management are indicated at this time?

Cultures of the patient's blood, urine, and throat are obtained and broad-spectrum antibiotics begun immediately on recognition of the fever. The scenario of fever in a neutropenic patient is considered a true medical emergency. The patient has laboratory evidence of DIC and clinical mucosal bleeding. Fresh frozen plasma and cryoprecipitate are infused to replace her clotting factors. Platelets are administered to raise the platelet count over 20,000. An indwelling central catheter is placed. Intravenous fluids are administered, an ample urine output is established, and allopurinol is given to protect renal function in anticipation of chemotherapy-induced cell lysis causing increased production of uric acid.

3. What further testing is indicated in the patient with acute leukemia?

A bone marrow aspirate and biopsy are routinely obtained when acute leukemia is suspected. The aspirate allows morphologic and cytochemical examination of individual cells and provides dividing cells for metaphase preparations used in chromosomal analysis. The biopsy allows assessment of the degree of marrow replacement by the leukemic clone. Peripheral blood or bone marrow samples are routinely sent for analysis of surface markers. In this patient, however, the findings in the peripheral blood are diagnostic and chromosomal analysis could have been done on the circulating leukemic cells.

This patient's bone marrow is entirely replaced by large promyelocyte-like cells. These cells stain intensely for myeloperoxidase and express CD13, CD33, and CD15. Chromosomal analysis available 2 weeks later reveals the presence of the classic 15,17 translocation seen in APML.

4. What are the initial treatment options for this patient?

This patient would currently be treated with induction therapy consisting of a 7-day continuous infusion of cytosine arabinoside and 3 days of daily bolus infusions of an anthracycline such as daunorubicin. This "7 and 3" regimen will produce a CR in 70 to 80 percent of patients. The patient will typically require hospitalization during the administration of chemotherapy and supportive care during the several-week period of bone marrow suppression. Recently, patients with APML have been treated with trans-retinoic acid. This therapy induces differentiation of the leukemic promyelocytes and often results in morphologic normalization of the patient's bone marrow and peripheral blood. Since most responses are of short duration, the role of this treatment requires further study.

This patient achieves a complete remission after induction chemotherapy. She has two siblings, one of whom is an identical HLA match willing to donate bone marrow.

5. What are the treatment options for this patient following achievement of a CR?

A young person (under 45) who has obtained a CR from AML and who has an HLA-identical sibling willing to donate bone marrow has several treatment options. The patient may continue with conventional chemotherapy ("consolidation"), which involves multiple cycles of various agents, including high doses of cytosine arabinoside. The long-term survival with these therapies is reported to range from 20 to 40 percent. If the patient suffers a relapse of her leukemia, she could then undergo allogeneic bone marrow transplantation. Transplantation is less effective after relapse has occurred, but an additional 10 to 20 percent of patients can be cured. Alternatively, a young patient may undergo allogeneic bone marrow transplantation while in first CR. One third of patients will die from the transplantation procedure and the long-term leukemia-free survival ranges from 40 to 60 percent. Thus, the timing of transplantation remains a controversial issue in this setting.

After considerable discussion, the patient elects not to undergo allogeneic bone marrow transplantation. She completes her consolidation chemotherapy and remains free of leukemia for one year. At that time, the patient suffers a relapse manifested by the appearance of promyelocytes in her peripheral blood.

6. What are the patient's treatment options at this time?

Relapsed AML is invariably fatal when treated with conventional chemotherapy. Young patients with an HLA-matched (or single-antigen mismatched) sibling should undergo immediate allogeneic bone marrow transplantation. It is not necessary to obtain a second remission before the procedure, but often logistical delays require that the patient be treated with conventional chemotherapy before transplantation. Young patients without appropriate siblings should be considered for unrelated donor transplantation or enrollment in studies of autologous transplantation or investigational chemotherapy.

Patient History No. 2

A 70-year-old man is referred for evaluation of anemia that has been present for 6 months. The patient is asymptomatic and has a normal physical examination. A routine CBC reveals a hematocrit (hct) of 32 percent with a mean corpuscular volume (MCV) of 103. The white blood count is 3.2×10^9 per liter and the platelet count is 122,000 per cubic millimeter. Routine chemistries, iron studies, and measurement of vitamin B_{12} and folate levels are normal.

1. What additional studies are indicated at this time?

   Examination of the peripheral blood smear is the first step in the evaluation of this patient.

This patient's peripheral smear demonstrates that the majority of red cells are macrocytic. Mild anisocytosis (variation in size) in the absence of striking poikilocytosis (variation in shape) is noted. The patient's differential count is normal, but abnormal neutrophil morphology with hypogranulation of the cytoplasm is present. Platelets are decreased in number and some large platelet forms are evident. A bone marrow aspirate and biopsy are obtained. The marrow is hypercellular with severe erythroid hyperplasia and mild dyserythropoiesis. Blast cells represent less than 5 percent of cells. Iron stains reveal ample iron stores; no ringed sideroblasts are identified. Chromosomal studies are normal.

2. What diagnosis and prognosis would you give to this patient and his family?

   The patient has evidence of a myelodysplastic syndrome with abnormalities in the erythroid, granulocyte, and platelet lineages. His disorder is classified as RA given the absence of an increase in blasts or ringed sideroblasts. The patient and his family should be told that RA often has a prolonged course and, at present, no treatment is indicated. The risk of transformation to acute leukemia is small.

Over the next 2 years, the patient develops a slowly progressive anemia with preservation of his white count and platelet count. Gastrointestinal or other sources of blood loss are not evident. When his hct falls to 28 percent, angina develops.

3. What treatment options are available for this patient?

   The patient's anemia should be corrected immediately with transfusion of red cells. Further transfusions should be administered as needed. If multiple transfusions are required, iron chelation therapy to prevent iron overload may be appropriate. Androgen therapy may benefit some patients. The growth factor erythropoietin has been used with success in some patients. Aggressive chemotherapy is not appropriate.

Patient History No. 3

A 38-year-old man is referred for evaluation of an abnormal CBC. The patient was treated for Hodgkin's disease 8 years ago with combined MOPP (Mustargen, Oncovin, procarbazine, prednisone) chemotherapy and radiation. He has felt well since the completion of his therapy. A routine CBC reveals a white cell count of 3.0×10^9 per liter with a differential of 57 percent neutrophils, 33 percent lymphocytes, 4 percent eosinophils, 3 percent basophils, and 3 percent blast cells. The hct is 33 percent with an MCV of 105 and platelet count of 124,000 per cubic millimeter. Examination of the peripheral smear confirms the presence of small numbers of myeloblasts. A small percentage of the neutrophils contain Pelger-Huët nuclei. The red cells appear macrocytic and a rare nucleated red cell is seen. The platelet morphology appears normal.

1. What is the likely diagnosis and what further testing is indicated?

   The findings of myeloblasts on the peripheral smear suggest that the patient has either acute leukemia or a myelodysplastic syndrome. The distinction is made by an assessment of the number of myeloblasts present in the bone marrow. The history of prior combined MOPP chemotherapy and radiation treatment place this patient at risk for a myelodysplastic syndrome and for transformation to AML. Such chemotherapy and radiation-induced MDS are often associated with loss of fragments of the long arm of chromosome 5 or 7, and carry a poor prognosis. Thus, chromosomal analysis of metaphase cells obtained from the marrow should be performed.

The patient's bone marrow is hypercellular. Myeloblasts account for 13 percent of cells. Both the maturing white cell and erythroid lineages show evidence of dyspoiesis. Chromosomal analysis discloses a loss of the long arm of chromosome 5.

2. What is the diagnosis? What treatment is indicated at this time?

   This patient's disorder is classified as RAEB. The risk of transformation to acute leukemia in this patient is high. The prior history of chemotherapy and radiation therapy associated with the loss of the long arm of chromosome 5 confers a grim prognosis. Thus, while no immediate treatment is required since the patient is asymptomatic, future allogeneic bone marrow transplantation should be considered when the condition progresses. The patient and his siblings should be HLA typed. If no sibling donor is available, consideration should be given to a search for an unrelated HLA-matched transplant donor. If these patients develop overt leukemia and allogeneic bone marrow transplantation is not available, conventional chemotherapy is often used, but is rarely, if ever, curative.

Topics for Discussion: Acute Leukemias and Myelodysplastic Syndromes

General

Differences between AML and ALL

Mechanisms of leukostasis

Acute Myelogenous Leukemia

Etiologic agents linked to AML

Subtypes in AML: specific syndromes

Chromosomal abnormalities in AML

Acute promyelocytic leukemia (AML-M3 or APML): clinical features, the 15,17 translocation, treatment with trans-retinoic acid

Treatment principles in AML: induction and consolidation treatment

Allogeneic bone marrow transplantation: efficacy, risks, and applicability

Graft-versus-host disease and the graft-versus-leukemia effect

Autologous bone marrow transplantation

Acute Lymphocytic Leukemia

Subtypes of ALL

Chromosomal abnormalities in ALL

The 9,22 translocation in ALL compared with the 9,22 translocation in CML

Treatment of ALL: average- and high-risk patients

CNS prophylaxis: the role of "sanctuary" sites of disease

Allogeneic bone marrow transplantation in ALL

Autologous bone marrow transplantation in ALL

Myelodysplastic Syndromes

Etiology of MDS: risk of prior chemotherapy and radiation therapy

Factors associated with development of acute leukemia

Treatment of MDS: the role of growth factors

Selected Readings

Acute Myelogenous Leukemia

Bennett, J. M. et al. Proposals for the classification of the acute leukemias. French-American-British (FAB) Co-operative Group. *Br. J. Haematol.* 33 : 451, 1976.

Champlin, R., and Gale, R. P. Acute myelogenous leukemia: Recent advances in therapy. *Blood* 69 : 1551, 1987.

Koeffler, H. P. Syndromes of acute nonlymphocytic leukemia. *Ann. Intern. Med.* 107 : 748, 1987.

Santos, G. W. Marrow transplantation in acute nonlymphocytic leukemia. *Blood* 74 : 901, 1989.

Acute Lymphoblastic Leukemia

Bleyer, W. A. Acute lymphoblastic leukemia in children. *Cancer* 65 : 689, 1990.

Champlin, R. and Gale, R. P Acute lymphoblastic leukemia: Recent advances in biology and therapy. *Blood* 73 : 2051, 1989.

Foon, K. A. and Todd, R. F. Immunologic classification of leukemia and lymphoma. *Blood* 68 : 1, 1986.

Jacobs, A. D., and Gale, R. P. Recent advances in the biology and treatment of acute lymphoblastic leukemia in adults. *N. Engl. J. Med.* 311 : 1219, 1984.

Rivera, G. K., and Mauer, A. M. Controversies in the management of childhood acute lymphoblastic leukemia: Treatment intensification, CNS leukemia, and prognostic factors. *Semin. Hematol.* 24 : 12, 1987.

Myelodysplastic Syndromes

Appelbaum, F. R. et al. Bone marrow transplantation for patients with myelodysplasia. *Ann. Intern. Med.* 112 : 590, 1990.

Bennett, J. M. et al. The French-American-British (FAB) Co-operative Group. Proposals for the Classification of the Myelodysplastic Syndromes. *Br. J. Haematol* 51 : 189, 1982.

Beris, P. Primary clonal myelodysplastic syndromes. *Semin. Hematol.* 26 : 216, 1989.

Cheson, B. The myelodysplastic syndromes: Current approaches to therapy. *Ann. Intern. Med.* 112 : 932, 1990.

Kantarjian, H. et al. Therapy-related leukemia and myelodysplastic syndromes: Clinical, cytogenetic, and prognostic features. *J. Clin. Oncol.* 4 : 1748, 1986.

List, A. L., Garewal, H. S., and Sandberg, A. A. The myelodysplastic syndromes: Biology and implications for management. *J. Clin. Oncol.* 8 : 1424, 1990.

13 Lymphoma

Stacey M. Gore
Steven E. Come

The lymphomas are a heterogeneous group of neoplasms that originate from lymphoid cells. A lymphoma may arise within the lymph node itself, in which case it is characterized by infiltration and destruction of the normal lymph node architecture by abnormal, malignant lymphocytes. Additionally, lymphomas may arise within extranodal sites, involving the lymphoid tissue of such diverse organs as the gastrointestinal tract, central nervous system (CNS), and bones. There are two major types of lymphoma, Hodgkin's disease (HD) and so-called non–Hodgkin's lymphoma (NHL), which together account for more than 30,000 new cases annually. Hodgkin's disease accounts for roughly 25 percent of these cases. Non–Hodgkin's lymphoma is three times as common and represents a spectrum of diseases marked by different pathologic features, natural history, and prognosis.

Within the economically developed countries there is a bimodal incidence of Hodgkin's disease, with the first peak occurring in patients in their twenties and the second peak in patients greater than 50 years old. In underdeveloped countries, the late peak is less apparent and there is higher incidence of childhood HD. In all age groups there is a slight male predominance, although within the nodular sclerosis subtype of HD, females are more frequently afflicted. NHL presents at a median age of 42 years, although the incidence begins in childhood and steadily increases with age. Like HD, NHL is more common in males.

Etiology of the Lymphomas

The cause of lymphoma remains unknown in the vast majority of cases, although several etiologic agents are being actively investigated. There is epidemiologic evidence to suggest that HD may be related to exposure to a low infectivity virus or other environmental factors, although direct proof is still lacking. Nevertheless, HD is more common among those with higher socioeconomic status, decreased number of siblings, early birth order, and fewer playmates, suggesting a delayed exposure to a pathologic agent. Additionally, there appears to be a slight but significant increase in HD following an episode of infectious mononucleosis. Although there have been early reports of clusters of HD occurring in areas within the United States, more recent data suggest that this occurrence was merely coincidental.

There is now convincing evidence from animal studies, as well as from humans, that viruses are etiologically important in at least some forms of lymphoma. Epstein-Barr virus (EBV) has been strongly linked with the development of African Burkitt's lymphoma, as EBV DNA has been found incorporated into the genome of these tumors. Further, based on similar molecular data, EBV has been implicated in the etiology of primary CNS lymphoma, as well as in the lymphoid malignancy seen in association with various immuno-suppressed states. Recently the EBV genome has been found in the Reed-Sternberg cells of some patients with Hodgkin's disease. Retro-viruses have also been implicated in the development of lymphoma, with human T lymphotropic (or leukemia) viruses (HTLV) being most important. HTLV-I is related to the adult T cell leukemia/lymphoma (ATL/L) syndrome, and HTLV-II has been isolated from rare cases of hairy cell leukemia. HTLV-III, also known as the human immunodeficiency virus (HIV), causes the acquired immunodefi-ciency syndrome (AIDS). Patients with AIDS have a critical defect in cell-mediated immunity and are at risk for the development of opportunistic infections, as well as numerous neoplasms, including Kaposi's sarcoma, non–Hodgkin's lymphoma, and a particularly aggressive form of Hodgkin's disease. The NHL encountered in AIDS includes B cell immunoblastic sarcoma and small noncleaved cell lymphoma. Frequent extranodal involvement, especially of the cen-tral nervous system, is common in patients with AIDS.

Additional hematologic problems are frequently encountered in patients with AIDS. HIV preferentially infects CD4 lymphocytes, re-sulting in significant lymphopenia, and a characteristic decrease in the CD4 lymphocyte count. More than two thirds of patients will have anemia or granulocytopenia, or both. Thrombocytopenia may be seen in approximately 40 percent of patients. The etiology of these hematologic complications is multifactorial. Bone marrow abnormalities, including hypercellularity, myelodysplastic changes, plasmacytosis, lymphoid aggregates, and granulomas, are quite common, and may result in ineffective hematopoiesis. Bone mar-row culture experiments have demonstrated suppression of growth of granulocyte–macrophage colony-forming units and erythroid burst-forming units by serum containing antibodies to HIV. It has recently been found that the HIV virus may directly infect and suppress both hematopoietic progenitor cells and the stromal cells that support hematopoietic cell growth. These observations help to explain the pancytopenia often observed in patients with AIDS. In addition, immune-mediated destruction of platelets may be especially important in the pathogenesis of thrombocytopenia. Many patients with severe thrombocytopenia have been found to have increased platelet-bound immunoglobulin G (IgG) and circulating immune complexes. Positive Coombs tests and antineutrophil antibodies have also been found. Patients with AIDS are particularly sensitive to hematologic toxicity related to a variety of medications. Neutropenia occurring in patients for whom sulfa-containing antibiotics are prescribed is especially common. Lastly, the lupus anticoagulant has been identified in several patients with HIV-related illness, although thrombotic complications are unusual in this setting.

Congenital or acquired dysfunction of the immune system, such as that found in agammaglobulinemia, ataxia-telangiectasia, Chédiak-Higashi syndrome, and autoimmune diseases such as Sjögren's syndrome, Hashimoto's thyroiditis, and celiac disease, have all been associated with an increased incidence of malignant lymphoma. Therapeutic immunosuppression in renal and cardiac transplant patients is associated with an excess risk of non–Hodgkin's lymphoma. Non–Hodgkin's lymphoma may also occur following the successful treatment of Hodgkin's disease, and appears to be related to the use of certain chemotherapeutic agents. The drug diphenylhydantoin (Dilantin) may be associated with lymph node hyperplasia and rarely with the ultimate development of frank lymphoma.

Cytogenetics and Immunology of the Lymphomas

Cytogenetic studies have demonstrated unique abnormalities in NHL that may be important in the pathogenesis of these disorders. Burkitt's lymphoma is associated with specific translocations involving chromosome 8. In most cases, a portion of chromosome 8, carrying the c-*myc* oncogene, is translocated to chromosome 14, near the region of the immunoglobulin heavy chain gene. Less commonly, the cytogenetic abnormality involves the translocation of c-*myc* from chromosome 8 to either chromosome 2 or 22, near the region of the κ or λ light chain genes, respectively. Active investigation is under way to determine how this specific genetic event relates to the pathogenesis of this disorder. Other nonrandom cytogenetic changes may be observed in other types of NHL, including the 14,18 and 11,14 translocations in follicular lymphomas and trisomy 12 in small lymphocytic lymphoma and chronic lymphocytic leukemia.

The chromosomal translocation t14,18 characterizes the majority of cases of follicular lymphoma, the most common form of indolent non–Hodgkin's lymphoma. This rearrangement juxtaposes the Ig heavy chain gene on chromosome 14 and the *bcl* 2 oncogene on chromosome 18. The *bcl* 2 oncogene is activated and produces the *bcl* 2 protein product in an unregulated manner. Overexpression of *bcl* 2 is thought to lead to interference with a natural process called apoptosis, by which normal cells undergo programmed cell death. Thus, lymphomas characterized by overexpression of the *bcl* 2 oncogene may be due in part to accumulation of immortalized Ig-producing lymphoid cells.

With the advent of molecular biology and monoclonal antibody technology, the cell of origin in most cases of NHL can be identified. For example, the vast majority of nodular or follicular NHL is derived from B cell lymphocytes, as demonstrated by the presence of monoclonal surface immunoglobulin or unique immunoglobulin gene rearrangements. Additional monoclonal antibodies against other specific B cell surface markers, such as B1 or common lymphoblastic leukemia antigen (CALLA), may help characterize the malignant phenotype and identify the normal B cell counterpart. T cell NHL accounts for approximately 30 to 40 percent of cases and may likewise be identified by distinct surface markers or rearrangements of the T cell receptor gene. True histiocytic disorders derived from tissue macrophages and histiocytes are rare and account for fewer than 5 percent of all lymphomas.

Information regarding the cellular origin of Hodgkin's disease is less definite. Although the malignant cell in HD is believed to be the Reed-Sternberg cell and its variants, the origin of this characteristic cell remains controversial. Data from tissue culture experiments have demonstrated that Reed-Sternberg cells may stain with the monoclonal antibodies Leu-M1 and Ki-1, supporting the theory that HD may be derived from either interdigitating dendritic cells or activated lymphocytes. The EB virus genome has been identified in the Reed-Sternberg cells of some patients with HD.

Differential Diagnosis of Lymphadenopathy

The management of patients with undiagnosed lymphadenopathy must be individualized (Table 13-1, Fig. 13-1). Several factors usually determine when enlarged nodes should be biopsied. The history may provide a ready, benign explanation for the lymphadenopathy, such as the presence of an inflammatory condition. In this case, biopsy can be deferred for a 4- to 6-week period of observation. Conversely, if historical or physical findings suggestive of lymphoma or other malignancy are present, biopsy should not be delayed. The physical findings are of primary importance. Lymphomatous nodes are usually rubbery in consistency, matted together, large, and nontender. On the other hand, lymph nodes involved by an inflammatory process, such as viral or bacterial infections, or in allergic reactions, are often tender, discrete, and soft.

Fig. 13-1.
Anatomic location of clinically important lymph node groups.

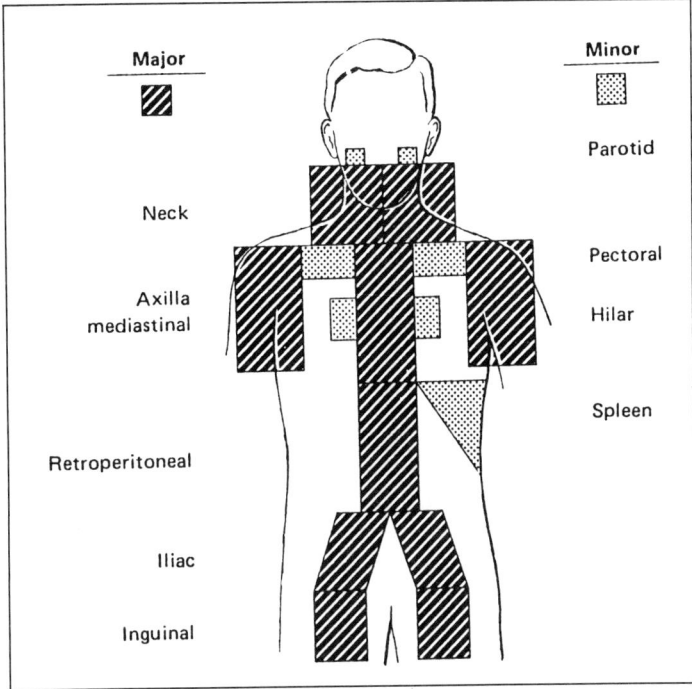

Table 13-1. Diseases that cause lymphadenopathy

I. Infections
   A. Acute infections with localized lymphadenitis
   B. Infectious mononucleosis
   C. Toxoplasmosis
   D. Cat-scratch fever
   E. Tuberculosis
   F. Brucellosis
   G. HIV infection
II. Malignancies
   A. Lymphoma: Hodgkin's disease, non–Hodgkin's lymphoma
   B. Metastatic neoplasms
   C. Leukemia
III. Collagen-vascular diseases
IV. Drug reactions
V. Miscellaneous
   A. Sarcoidosis
   B. Serum sickness
   C. Angioimmunoblastic lymphadenopathy
   D. Lymphomatoid granulomatosis
   E. Dermatopathic lymphadenitis

    Lymphadenopathy may be a sign of other disease states, as well as infections, inflammatory processes, or lymphoma. Unilateral hard nontender submandibular, submental, or cervical nodes in an adult may be related to occult head and neck cancer, and warrant a careful examination of the oral cavity and nasopharynx before node biopsy is carried out. Supraclavicular and scalene node enlargement is always consequential and may be seen in the setting of metastatic carcinoma, frequently of lung or gastrointestinal origin. Unilateral axillary adenopathy may represent spread of breast cancer or melanoma, in addition to benign causes. Inguinal lymphadeno-pathy is frequently reactive, but if unilateral, hard, or progressive, biopsy must be performed. A mediastinal mass is commonly found in lymphomas, but may also be seen in metastatic germ cell tumors, thymomas, substernal thyroids, and primary diseases of the lung. Hilar adenopathy, if bilateral and not associated with other lymph node abnormalities, is commonly found in sarcoidosis. Asymmetric hilar adenopathy raises the possibility of primary bronchogenic carcinoma and other pulmonary disorders.

Pathology of the Lymphomas and Clinicopathologic Correlations

The diagnosis of lymphoma should be made only by biopsy, with careful review of the specimen by an experienced hematopath-ologist. Although needle aspiration may yield cytology suggestive or diagnostic of a lymphoid malignancy, accurate classification gen-erally requires analysis of nodal architecture, necessitating relatively large samples of intact tissue. Proper handling of the biopsy mate-rial to allow for the determination of immunologic surface markers, as well as gene rearrangements, requires close communication among the hematologist/oncologist, surgeon, and pathologist.

Hodgkin's Disease

The diagnosis of Hodgkin's disease requires the presence of the characteristic Reed-Sternberg cell or one of its variants, either the mononuclear "Hodgkin's cell" or the "lacunar cell" seen primarily in the nodular sclerosis subtype of HD. Reed-Sternberg cells are large, with two or more nuclei, each with a prominent eosinophilic nucleolus, giving an "owl's eye" appearance (Plates 67, 68). If Reed-Sternberg cells are lacking, then the diagnosis of HD should rarely be made. However, these cells in and of themselves are not sufficient for the diagnosis of HD. Indeed, cells indistinguishable from Reed-Sternberg cells may be found in patients with some types of NHL, adenocarcinomas, rubeola, and infectious mononu-cleosis. Lymph nodes involved with HD also contain a background of normal inflammatory cells, with frequent eosinophils, neu-trophils, lymphocytes, and plasma cells. Associated fibrosis and necrosis are quite common.

Historically, two major classification schemes have been used for Hodgkin's disease (Table 13-2). The system described by Jackson and Parker divided HD into three groups: paragranuloma, account-

Table 13-2. Two classification schemes for subtypes of Hodgkin's disease

Jackson and Parker	Rye
Paragranuloma	Lymphocyte predominance
Granuloma	Mixed cellularity
	Nodular sclerosis
Sarcoma	Lymphocyte depletion

ing for roughly 10 percent of cases; granuloma, comprising approximately 80 percent of patients; and sarcoma, accounting for the remainder. In the 1960s, Lukes and Butler modified this scheme, which has since been adapted to form the currently used Rye classification. The Rye classification subtypes HD into four histologic groups, which, in addition to providing pathologic data, also provide information related to the natural history and prognosis of this malignancy.

Lymphocyte-predominant HD accounts for 2 to 10 percent of cases and is characterized by a small number of Reed-Sternberg cells amidst a preponderance of normal-appearing lymphocytes (Plate 69). This subtype is associated with a particularly favorable prognosis and generally occurs in young asymptomatic patients with localized disease in peripheral nodes.

Nodular sclerosis HD is the most common type, seen in 40 to 80 percent of patients, and is characterized by several distinct features. Pathologically, nodular sclerosis HD is found to have broad bands of thick collagen fibers that divide the lymph node into nodules. Additionally, one can identify lacunar cells, a Reed-Sternberg variant, formed by cytoplasmic retraction occurring during processing of the lymph node (Plate 70). Clinically, nodular sclerosis HD frequently involves the mediastinal lymph nodes and is the only subtype in which females are affected more commonly than males.

Mixed-cellularity HD accounts for roughly 20 to 40 percent of cases and is characterized by a pleomorphic infiltrate with frequent Reed-Sternberg cells (Plate 68). Lymphocyte-depleted HD comprises 5 to 15 percent of cases and is associated with a paucity of lymphocytes, a large number of Reed-Sternberg cells, and diffuse fibrosis (Plate 71). Although this subtype has traditionally been associated with a worse prognosis, recent data suggest that this conclusion may have been confounded by the previous misclassification of aggressive high-grade NHL within this subtype of HD. Patients with mixed-cellularity and lymphocyte-depleted HD are more likely to be symptomatic and to present with more advanced disease. There is evidence to suggest that within an individual patient, pathologic progression to more aggressive subtypes of HD may occur.

Non–Hodgkin's Lymphoma

Non–Hodgkin's lymphomas are characterized by a greater spectrum of pathologic disorders when compared with the number of subtypes found in HD. To date, at least six classification schemes have been proposed to differentiate among the diverse types of NHL. All have the aim of providing both prognostic and therapeutic information. In discussing the histopathology of NHL, it should be noted that individual patients undergoing multiple biopsy procedures may have evidence of divergent histologies up to 20 percent of the time.

The Rappaport classification is still commonly used and clinicians should therefore be familiar with it (Table 13-3). This system divides the non–Hodgkin's lymphomas into nodular or diffuse subtypes, and further classifies them by whether the infiltrate involves lymphocytes (small cells) or "histiocytes" (large cells), and on how well or poorly differentiated the lymphocytes appear. The nodular and the mature lymphocytic types carry the best prognosis, whereas, in general, the diffuse and "histiocytic" lymphomas carry the worst.

There are several problems, however, in the Rappaport system. For example, well-differentiated lymphocytic lymphoma is always diffuse and yet is marked by an indolent course and a long natural history. Additionally, cells formerly referred to as "histiocytes" are now known to represent transformed or activated lymphocytes, and are not related to tissue macrophages. Lastly, this scheme does not incorporate recently acquired immunologic data regarding NHL.

In 1982, the National Cancer Institute published its report outlining a "Working Formulation" for the classification of non–Hodgkin's

Table 13-3. Classification of non–Hodgkin's lymphoma according to the Non–Hodgkin's Lymphoma Pathologic Classification Project

Working formulation	Rappaport classification (related terms)
Favorable or low grade	
Small lymphocytic	Diffuse, well differentiated, lymphocytic
Follicular small-cleaved cell	Nodular, poorly differentiated, lymphocytic
Follicular, mixed, small-cleaved and large cell	Nodular, mixed, histiocytic–lymphocytic
Intermediate or intermediate grade	
Follicular large cell	Nodular histiocytic
Diffuse small-cleaved cell	Diffuse, poorly differentiated, lymphocytic
Diffuse, mixed, small and large cell	Diffuse, mixed, histiocytic–lymphocytic
Diffuse large cell (cleaved/noncleaved)	Diffuse histiocytic
Unfavorable or high grade	
Diffuse large cell, immunoblastic	Diffuse histiocytic
Lymphoblastic	Lymphoblastic
Small noncleaved cell (Burkitt's and Burkitt's-like)	Diffuse, undifferentiated (Burkitt's and Burkitt's-like)

lymphoma, incorporating features of each of the other six systems (see Table 13-3). The use of this Working Formulation should be encouraged, to allow for the standard and consistent reporting of clinical data. The Working Formulation classifies lymphomas based on their clinical behavior into three groups: low-grade, intermediate-grade, and high-grade. Additional classification is dependent on whether the lymphoma seems to arise from the germinal centers of the node (so-called follicular) or appears to involve the node diffusely. Lastly, cells are described by their size (small vs. large) and by whether or not the nucleus is cleaved. In this chapter the subtypes of NHL are described by their Working Formulation names, although the corresponding Rappaport titles are given in parentheses.

Low-grade NHL include small lymphocytic lymphoma; follicular, predominantly small-cleaved cell lymphoma; and follicular, mixed, small-cleaved and large cell lymphoma. Small lymphocytic (well-differentiated lymphocytic) lymphoma occurs only in the diffuse form and accounts for approximately 5 percent of all NHL. Monotypic, small lymphocytes with dark nuclei and inconspicuous nucleoli replace the normal lymph node architecture (Plate 72). This histologic picture resembles that seen in patients with chronic lymphocytic leukemia. Patients with small lymphocytic lymphoma generally have disseminated disease at the time of diagnosis, with 75 to 95 percent having positive bone marrow examinations. A plasmacytoid lymphocytic variant associated with Waldenström's macroglobulinemia is also seen.

Follicular small-cleaved cell (nodular poorly differentiated lymphocytic) lymphoma (Plate 73) is the most frequent type of NHL seen, accounting for 20 to 30 percent of all cases. Follicular, mixed, small-cleaved and large cell (nodular mixed lymphocytic–histiocytic) lymphoma is less common, comprising less than 10 percent of all NHL. The criteria for mixed lymphoma vary, but generally assume a roughly 50 : 50 distribution of small and large cells. The majority of patients with these low-grade lymphomas has disseminated disease at diagnosis, with greater than 90 percent being Stage III or IV (staging systems are discussed in detail later in this chapter). Generalized lymphadenopathy and splenic, bone marrow, and hepatic involvement are all quite common. These lymphomas are almost exclusively B cell in origin, which can be confirmed by cell surface markers. Circulating mononclonal neoplastic B lymphocytes are commonly identified using sensitive cell-sorting techniques, even when the peripheral blood otherwise appears normal. Typically, patients with these forms of low-grade NHL are middle-aged, with a median age at diagnosis of 45 to 50 years. These lymphomas are associated with an indolent course and a median survival of greater than 5 to 7 years. Transient spontaneous regression may occur in 20 to 30 percent of patients in the early part of their course, while histologic conversion to higher-grade lymphomas may occur in up to 30 percent of patients by 10 years. Despite the high complete remission rates attained with treatment, a continuous tendency to relapse is quite characteristic of follicular small-cleaved lymphoma, and this malignancy is not yet curable with present therapeutic options. However, follicular mixed, small-cleaved, and large cell lymphoma, treated with combination chemotherapy, may on occasion be cured.

Intermediate-grade NHL include follicular, predominantly large cell lymphoma; diffuse small-cleaved cell lymphoma; diffuse, mixed small and large cell lymphoma; and diffuse large cell, cleaved or noncleaved lymphoma. Follicular, predominantly large cell (nodular histiocytic) lymphoma is uncommon, accounting for less than 5 percent of all NHL. This group of NHL has a poor prognosis, characterized by its frequent conversion from the initial follicular to the more aggressive, diffuse large cell lymphoma. Like other follicular lymphomas, this subtype is derived from B lymphocytes. Follicular large cell lymphoma is not a low-grade lesion and durable complete remissions may sometimes be achieved with early aggressive chemotherapy.

Diffuse small-cleaved cell (diffuse poorly differentiated lymphocytic) lymphoma (Plate 74) accounts for 5 to 10 percent of all NHL. This type of lymphoma frequently arises from preexisting follicular small-cleaved cell tumors, although on occasion, it may arise de novo. Most often, diffuse small-cleaved cell lymphoma is derived from a malignant B cell. Like patients with follicular small-cleaved lymphoma, these individuals generally have disseminated disease at diagnosis.

Diffuse, mixed, small and large cell (diffuse, mixed, lymphocytic–histiocytic) lymphoma accounts for 5 to 10 percent of NHL. The immunologic origin of these tumors is heterogeneous, with roughly 70 percent derived from B cells, and the remainder from T lymphocytes. Diffuse, mixed, small and large cell lymphoma presents at a median age of 63 years and is associated with a female predominance. Seventy percent of patients may have extranodal involvement, with cutaneous and gastrointestinal disease being especially common. Response to treatment is generally good, with the majority of patients achieving a complete remission, although late relapses may occur.

Diffuse large cell, cleaved or noncleaved cell (diffuse histiocytic) lymphoma is the most common of the diffuse histologies, comprising more than 20 percent of all cases of NHL. Approximately 70 percent are B cell, 25 percent are T cell, and the remainder arise from true histiocytes. The large-cleaved cell variety (Plate 75) is characterized by round to oval cells, with angulated nuclei and prominent nucleoli. The noncleaved type contains large cells with fine chromatin and distinct nucleoli (Plate 76). Diffuse large cell lymphomas may arise de novo or may occur from the conversion of preexisting, more favorable, nodular or diffuse histologies. Additionally, patients with chronic lymphocytic leukemia may develop large cell lymphoma late in their course, a complication referred to as Richter's syndrome.

Patients with diffuse large cell lymphomas present at a median age of 55 years, although cases in the young and elderly are not unusual. Approximately 30 percent of patients may have localized disease at the time of diagnosis, and presentations involving the gastrointestinal tract, Waldeyer's ring (lymphoid tissue of the pharynx), bone, skin, testis, and central nervous system are relatively common. Untreated, this lymphoma is associated with rapid disease progression and death. Paradoxically, with aggressive combination chemotherapy, cure may be achieved in a significant percentage of patients.

High-grade NHL consists of diffuse, large cell immunoblastic lymphoma; lymphoblastic lymphoma; and small noncleaved cell lymphoma, of either the Burkitt's or non-Burkitt's type. Diffuse, large cell immunoblastic lymphoma or "sarcoma" (Plate 77) accounts for roughly 10 percent of NHL. Seventy percent are of B cell origin and the remainder are derived from T lymphocytes. B cell immunoblastic sarcomas often develop in patients with underlying immune dysfunction, such as Hashimoto's thyroiditis, Sjögren's syndrome, celiac disease, organ transplantation, or AIDS. Almost half of these cases present with extranodal disease. In contrast, T cell immunoblastic sarcoma frequently presents with generalized lymphadenopathy and mediastinal involvement, and, commonly, polyclonal hypergammaglobulinemia may be demonstrated. T immunoblastic sarcoma may also complicate the course of angioimmunoblastic lymphadenopathy.

Lymphoblastic lymphoma (Plate 78) is a disease predominantly of thymic-derived T lymphocytes. Rarely, these lymphomas have immunologic features suggestive of pre–B cells. The typical cell is a lymphoblast characterized by nuclear lobulations that impart a convoluted appearance to the cell. These cells contain terminal deoxynucleotidyl transferase (Tdt), which is occasionally useful as a diagnostic marker. This type of NHL is associated with a striking male predominance and most often presents in adolescence or early adulthood. Anterior mediastinal involvement is especially prominent, and evolution to a leukemia phase indistinguishable from T cell acute lymphoblastic leukemia commonly occurs. Central nervous system involvement is also typical and necessitates prophylactic therapy. However, this histology may also be encountered in older patients with extranodal presentations. Aggressive treatment with combination chemotherapy, radiation therapy, and central nervous system prophylaxis has greatly improved the prognosis of lymphoblastic lymphoma.

Small noncleaved cell lymphoma includes both Burkitt's and non-Burkitt's (diffuse undifferentiated) types. They account for approximately 5 percent of all NHL and are universally derived from B lymphocytes. The cells of Burkitt's lymphoma (Plate 79) are uniform in size and shape, and contain small amounts of cytoplasm and round to oval nuclei with prominent nucleoli. Large macrophages in lacunae create the appearance of clear spaces scattered among the lymphocytes, producing a "starry sky" pattern. As described earlier, distinct chromosomal translocations characterize Burkitt's lymphoma. Endemic Burkitt's lymphoma refers to that found in certain regions of Africa. It generally afflicts children and typically involves the jaw or orbit. Epstein-Barr virus has been found in the genome of these tumors. Sporadic Burkitt's lymphoma, as found in the United States, affects slightly older patients and is characterized by tumors of the gastrointestinal tract and ovaries. Bone marrow and central nervous system involvement occurs in more widespread disease. Staging of Burkitt's lymphoma is different from that used in other NHL. Stage A is disease involving a single solitary extra-abdominal site, Stage B is disease in multiple extra-abdominal sites, Stage C refers to disease that is solely intra-abdominal, Stage D is intra-abdominal disease with one or more extra-abdominal sites, and Stage AR refers to intra-abdominal disease in which greater than 90 percent of the tumor has been resected. With aggressive combination chemotherapy and central nervous system prophylaxis, cure is attainable in many patients.

Small noncleaved lymphoma of the non-Burkitt's variety is characterized by cells that have a greater degree of nuclear variability than in Burkitt's lymphoma. This histologic type is seen more often in adults than is Burkitt's lymphoma, and is the most common form of NHL found in patients with AIDS, patients with organ transplants, and those previously treated for HD.

There are several other types of non–Hodgkin's lymphoma not included in the Working Formulation. These include the adult T cell leukemia/lymphoma syndrome, cutaneous T cell lymphomas, and other related diseases.

Adult T Cell Leukemia/Lymphoma

Adult T cell leukemia/lymphoma is a syndrome etiologically linked to the HTLV-I retrovirus. This disorder was described first in Japan, where it is now known to be endemic. More recently it has been recognized within the Caribbean and southeastern United States. This lymphoma is derived from cells that immunologically mark with the T helper phenotype and are negative for Tdt. Morphologically, the nuclei of the neoplastic cells are quite lobulated, giving them a unique appearance. Clinically, patients are noted to have prominent lymphadenopathy, peripheral blood involvement, skin lesions, hepatosplenomegaly, lytic bone disease, and frequent hypercalcemia. Mediastinal masses are particularly uncommon. Current treatment programs are not effective.

Cutaneous T Cell Lymphoma

Cutaneous T cell lymphomas include mycosis fungoides (MF) and Sézary syndrome (SS), which are two closely allied, if not the same, disorders. The neoplastic cells are immunologically related, and both are derived from postthymic T helper cells. Morphologically, these cells have characteristic irregular cerebriform nuclei. Pathologically, the cells are found infiltrating the skin, with preferential involvement of the epidermis and subepidermal spaces, resulting in the development of classic Pautrier's microabscesses.

Mycosis fungoides may evolve through several different phases. In the initial stage, nonspecific skin lesions, typically erythrodermic or eczematoid, may be present. Over a period of months or years, irregular thickening of the skin or plaques may develop. Finally, the patient may progress to the tumor stage, associated with nodular infiltrations that may ulcerate. Sézary syndrome is a condition characterized by diffuse exfoliative erythroderma in conjunction with circulating abnormal cerebriform T cells in the peripheral blood. Lymphadenopathy in these disorders is not uncommon, although "dermatopathic lymphadenitis," rather than frank lymphoma, may be found on histologic examination of these lymph nodes. Hepatosplenomegaly and other visceral involvement can occur as the disease progresses.

A separate staging system is employed for the cutaneous T cell lymphomas:

Stage I: Cutaneous plaques
Stage II: Plaques with adenopathy *or* cutaneous nodular tumors
Stage III: Generalized erythroderma
Stage IV: Histologic involvement of either the lymph nodes or visceral organs

Mycosis fungoides is an indolent disease with average survival exceeding 5 to 8 years. However, with more advanced disease and visceral involvement, the prognosis is significantly worse. Treatment options are varied and include topical application of nitrogen mustard, ultraviolet light with psoralen administration, electron beam irradiation, and systemic chemotherapy for patients with visceral involvement. Therapy with investigational agents such as α-interferon and monoclonal antibodies is being actively studied.

Diseases Related to the Lymphomas

Several unusual syndromes are related to the lymphomas. These include malignant histiocytosis, lymphomatoid granulomatosis, and angioimmunoblastic lymphadenopathy with dysproteinemia.

MALIGNANT HISTIOCYTOSIS

Malignant histiocytosis, also referred to as histiocytic medullary reticulosis, is a rare neoplasm of true reticuloendothelial histiocytes. The disease is marked by the accumulation of monoclonal histiocytes within the sinuses of lymph nodes, spleen, and liver. Histiocytes with conspicuous erythrophagocytosis are characteristic in this disorder, but are not pathognomonic, as this feature may also be seen in severe viral or bacterial infections. Clinically, patients present with fever, pancytopenia, splenomegaly, and cutaneous lesions. Treatment for malignant histiocytosis has traditionally been disappointing, although recent reports of therapy utilizing anthracyclines, in combination with alkylating agents, have been more encouraging.

LYMPHOMATOID GRANULOMATOSIS

Lymphomatoid granulomatosis is a disorder of uncertain etiology characterized by the accumulation of atypical lymphoreticular cells with plasmacytoid features. In addition, there is pronounced granulomatous inflammation of the small- and medium-sized blood vessels, often resulting in significant necrosis and fibrosis. Most patients with this disorder are adults, in their third to sixth decade, with a definite male predominance. Fever and cough are the most common presenting symptoms, occurring in more than half of the patients. Approximately one third will also report weight loss and dyspnea. Pulmonary involvement is invariably found, although radiographic abnormalities may fluctuate. Other organs affected include the central nervous system, skin, liver, and kidneys. The prognosis of lymphomatoid granulomatosis is poor, with mortality greater than 60 percent. Malignant lymphomas of either the diffuse mixed or immunoblastic type may develop in as many as 50 percent of patients who ultimately die. Treatment of lymphomatoid granulomatosis with alkylating agents such as cyclophosphamide, in combination with corticosteroids, may result in clinical remission.

ANGIOIMMUNOBLASTIC LYMPHADENOPATHY WITH DYSPROTEINEMIA

Angioimmunoblastic lymphadenopathy with dysproteinemia (AILD) is a rare lymphoproliferative disorder characterized by distinct clinical and pathologic features. Lymph node biopsies typically reveal effacement of the normal architecture by a pleomorphic infiltrate consisting of lymphocytes, immunoblasts, and plasma cells.

Abnormal proliferation of arborizing small blood vessels is another distinguishing feature. Rarely, Reed-Sternberg–like cells are present. Similar infiltrates may also involve the spleen, skin, lungs, liver, and bone marrow. Most patients present in the sixth and seventh decades, with the abrupt onset of fever, weight loss, pruritus, and skin lesions that are usually maculopapular. Lymphadenopathy, organomegaly, and pulmonary infiltrates are common. Frequent laboratory abnormalities include polyclonal hypergammaglobuline-mia in 75 percent of patients and Coombs-positive hemolytic ane-mia in 50 percent. The immunologic dysfunction observed appears to relate to polyclonal B cell hyperactivity, resulting from alterations in normal regulatory T cell function. Additionally, defects in cell-mediated immunity are present and may lead to opportunistic infec-tions with unusual organisms.

The natural history of AILD is variable, although in general, pa-tients do poorly, with median survivals of 15 to 30 months. Devel-opment of either B or T cell non–Hodgkin's lymphoma may occur in up to 20 percent of patients. Infrequently, Hodgkin's disease may complicate the course of AILD. Treatment of angioimmunoblastic lymphadenopathy has included the use of corticosteroids alone, or in conjunction with, alkylating agents.

Some investigators now classify lymphomatoid granulomatosis and AILD as belonging to a group of heterogeneous "peripheral T cell lymphomas," referring to the origin of these diseases from mature postthymic T lymphocytes.

Staging of the Lymphomas

Once a diagnosis of malignant lymphoma is made, the next step is to accurately stage the patient, so that the exact extent of the malignant process can be determined. This is especially critical in Hodgkin's disease, where stage has been found to most significantly affect prognosis. Staging is also important in the selection of appro-priate therapy, and in identification of parameters that may be fol-lowed to assess the efficacy of treatment. Although staging is also necessary in patients with non–Hodgkin's lymphoma, the histo-pathologic diagnosis is more important than the stage in predicting prognosis and determining therapy.

Clinical Staging

Clinical staging begins with a detailed history and a complete phys-ical examination. It is important to assess whether the patient has experienced any constitutional symptoms, such as fever, night sweats, or weight loss (more than 10% of body weight). These three systemic complaints are referred to as "B" symptoms and adversely affect prognosis in patients with both Hodgkin's disease and non–Hodgkin's lymphoma. Pel-Epstein fever, a rare manifestation of HD, is a fever that is cyclical, recurring every few days or weeks. In patients with lymphoma, it is crucial to exclude infectious causes before fever is ascribed to the malignancy. Pruritus, which can be severe, may be the presenting symptom in HD or NHL, but in and of itself, does not alter prognosis. Another characteristic symptom in some patients with HD is alcohol-induced pain in areas of lymphomatous involvement; this also has no prognostic significance.

Painless lymphadenopathy is the most common presenting symptom in patients with both HD and NHL. However, there are several differences in the pattern of lymph node involvement. HD typically involves the lymph nodes of the cervical, supraclavicular, axillary, mediastinal, and retroperitoneal areas, whereas NHL, while also involving these sites, frequently affects extra-axial nodes such as those of the epitrochlear, mesenteric, and femoral regions. The lymphoid tissue of Waldeyer's ring is also commonly involved in NHL, but not in HD. The pattern of lymph node spread in HD is relatively predictable, with contiguous involvement from one lymph node–bearing region to the next. Diffuse hematogenous dissemination occurs generally late in its course. This has critical implications for the staging and treatment of HD. NHL, in contrast, is characterized by noncontiguous node involvement, early hematogenous dissemination, and frequent extranodal presentations.

The physical examination should document any abnormalities in the size, consistency, and texture of all lymph nodes. Special attention should be paid to the oropharynx and an assessment of hepatic and splenic size should be made. A detailed neurologic examination must also be performed. Lastly, determination of the patient's general health is important in influencing treatment approaches.

After completing the history and physical examination, clinical staging proceeds with specific laboratory tests. A complete blood count and inspection of the peripheral blood smear should be done. Anemia is common and may relate to chronic disease, bone marrow involvement, blood loss, or autoimmune hemolysis. Leukocytosis with extremely high neutrophil counts may be observed occasionally in HD, along with eosinophilia. Circulating lymphoma cells may be identified on the smear, particularly in NHL. Thrombocytosis or thrombocytopenia may be seen. Low platelet counts may reflect marrow infiltration, hypersplenism, or immune-mediated destruction. Renal and liver function tests, lactic dehydrogenase, uric acid, serum calcium, and serum protein immunoelectrophoresis should all be determined.

Radiographic evaluation is critical in patients with lymphoma. Chest x-rays may reveal adenopathy, pulmonary parenchymal disease, pleural effusions, or abnormalities of the heart or bones. Chest

> **Approach to the patient with Hodgkin's disease and non–Hodgkin's lymphoma***
>
> **I.** History
>   A. Systemic symptoms: weight loss, night sweats, fever
>   B. Symptoms suggesting involvement by extralymphatic lymphoma (nasopharynx, bone, gastrointestinal tract)
>   C. Symptoms of compression or obstruction by large lymph nodes
>   D. Symptoms of spinal cord involvement
> **II.** Examination
>   A. Lymph node enlargement
>   B. Splenomegaly and hepatomegaly
>   C. Abdominal masses
>   D. Signs of extralymphatic involvement
>   E. Signs of obstruction or pressure by lymph nodes (mediastinal, abdominal, pelvic, or femoral)
>   F. Skin infiltration
>   G. Bleeding manifestations
>   H. Signs of neurologic involvement
> **III.** Laboratory data
>   A. Complete blood counts and review of peripheral smear
>   B. Renal function tests
>   C. Liver function tests
>   D. Serum protein electrophoresis
>   E. Uric acid
>   F. Coombs test
>   G. Lactic dehydrogenase level
>   H. Serum calcium
> **IV.** Radiographic studies
>   A. Chest x-ray
>   B. Computed tomography of the chest, abdomen, and pelvis
>   C. Lymphangiogram (rarely used)
>   D. Gallium scan
>   E. Upper gastrointestinal with small bowel follow-through
>   F. Bone scan
> **V.** Invasive procedures
>   A. Lymph node biopsy
>   B. Bone marrow biopsies
>   C. Staging laparotomy with splenectomy, biopsy of abdominal lymph nodes, liver biopsy, and iliac crest biopsy
>   D. Percutaneous liver biopsy
>   E. Skin biopsy

*All of these items do not necessarily apply to all patients.

computerized tomography (CT) has assumed new importance in the evaluation and can more carefully delineate lymphadenopathy and define pericardial abnormalities. The chest CT is also helpful in treatment planning, especially if radiation therapy is to be used.

Subdiaphragmatic staging remains a problem area, especially in the evaluation of HD. Adenopathy in HD is often present in the retroperitoneum and pelvis, and is generally less bulky than that seen in NHL. Lymphangiography (LAG) is a technique designed to evaluate the retroperitoneal lymph nodes. Dye is injected subcutaneously into the leg and finds its way into a lymphatic vessel. This lymph channel can then be cannulated and radiopaque oil injected.

The oil is allowed to distribute itself for about 24 hours through the leg lymphatics and into the abdominal lymph nodes. X-rays of the abdomen are then performed. Replacement of normal lymph nodes by lymphoma gives a characteristic foamy appearance to the node. The LAG is sensitive to abnormalities in the internal architecture as well as in the size of the lymph nodes. The retained dye can guide the surgeon intraoperatively in the choice of biopsy sites, may be helpful in radiation planning, and allows for periodic follow-up study with simple x-rays for 6 months or more. However, several problems are associated with the LAG that limit its usefulness. The LAG does not routinely opacify lymph nodes above the level of the second lumbar vertebra and therefore cannot detect abnormalities in the upper abdomen. Side effects include discomfort, fever, allergic reactions to the oil, and occasional pulmonary insufficiency and wound infections. Finally, the accuracy of the LAG depends on the skill of the radiologist; false positive interpretations may reach 30 percent and false negatives 10 percent.

Abdominal and pelvic CT scans have replaced the LAG in the staging of NHL and are assuming more importance in the evaluation of HD. Indeed, LAGs are rarely used in the staging of HD at present. CT scanning will visualize enlarged nodes above the level of the lumbar vertebrae, and also provides information regarding the size and structure of the liver and spleen. In addition, CT scanning is less morbid than LAG and is more easily repeated during follow-up. However, CT scans are associated with a higher false negative rate than LAG.

Gallium-67 imaging has become very important in the initial evaluation and subsequent follow-up study of patients with certain subtypes of HD and NHL. Gallium scanning is very sensitive in nodular sclerosis HD and in diffuse large cell NHL, but is less often taken up by lymphomatous tissue in other subtypes. Gallium imaging may be helpful in differentiating persistent or recurrent disease from residual fibrosis in treated patients whose lesions were initially gallium-avid. However, gallium scanning is less sensitive in the abdomen because of excretion of gallium into the gastrointestinal tract.

In HD, the spleen is the most difficult organ to assess noninvasively. Indeed, clinical determination of possible splenic involvement based on physical examination and CT scanning is notoriously inaccurate. Roughly one third of patients believed to have splenic HD based on the presence of splenomegaly will be found to have pathologically normal spleens at the time of surgery. Conversely, one third will have occult splenic disease even though the spleen appears normal by noninvasive testing.

Radiographic evaluations of the upper gastrointestinal tract and small bowel are particularly helpful in the staging of patients with NHL involving Waldeyer's ring, symptoms referable to the gastrointestinal region, a palpable abdominal mass, or occult bleeding. However, these studies are rarely required in the evaluation of patients with HD because of the low incidence of intestinal involvement.

Bone scanning may be indicated in patients with lymphoma who have bone pain, elevated alkaline phosphatase, or hypercalcemia.

Pathologic Staging

Bone marrow biopsies may be useful in the staging of patients with lymphomas and are more sensitive in detecting the presence of tumor than are bone marrow aspirations. Bone marrow biopsies are positive in the majority of patients with low-grade NHL and may be abnormal in 5 to 15 percent of patients with large cell NHL. Marrow involvement in HD is also dependent somewhat on the histology of the HD and previous staging results. For example, bone marrows are positive in fewer than 8 percent of patients with lymphocyte-predominant and nodular sclerosis HD, but may exceed 50 percent among patients with lymphocyte-depleted pathology. Marrow involvement may be the sole extralymphatic site of disease in one half to one third of patients with disseminated HD. Bone marrow biopsies should be bilateral, as only one side will be positive in approximately 25 percent of patients with marrow involvement.

The incidence of hepatic involvement varies with the type of lymphoma. Liver disease is present in only 5 percent of asymptomatic patients with Hodgkin's disease and is rarely found in the absence of splenic involvement. The pattern of hepatic involvement is focal in HD, but is more often a diffuse triaditis in NHL. Percutaneous liver biopsy is usually not necessary in the evaluation of low-grade NHL, as bone marrow involvement correlates with hepatic disease. Liver function tests are not specific in the detection of lymphomatous involvement. They may be elevated as a result of a paraneoplastic process, such as that seen in the nonneoplastic granulomas found in the livers of some patients with HD. In NHL, the incidence of hepatic disease varies as a function of the histologic subtype. In low-grade NHL, hepatic involvement may be found in as many as 50 to 85 percent of patients at the time of initial diagnosis, but is seen in fewer than 10 percent of patients with diffuse large cell lymphoma.

Staging laparotomy has provided important information regarding the natural history and pattern of spread in patients with HD. Laparotomy is being performed with decreasing frequency, but should still be done when the findings might modify treatment plans. Despite aggressive noninvasive testing, the results of laparotomy may alter the stage (either up or down) in as many as 35 percent of patients. An adequate staging laparotomy requires splenectomy, wedge and needle biopsies of both lobes of the liver, biopsy of any abnormal nodes demonstrated by either the LAG or CT scans, and random biopsies of the celiac, paraaortic, portal, splenic, mesenteric, iliac, and pelvic nodes, as well as a careful complete abdominal exploration. Open iliac crest bone marrow biopsies can also be performed if the bone marrow was not examined preoperatively. Finally, during laparotomy, the ovaries can be placed behind the uterus or laterally outside the usual radiation field (oophoropexy), if pelvic irradiation is planned. Staging laparotomy should be associated with a mortality of under 1 percent, although substantial morbidity, including pneumonia, pulmonary embolism, pancreatitis, and subdiaphragmatic abscess, may occur in up to 10 percent of patients. Late infectious complications, including pneumococcal sepsis, may occur in splenectomized patients, and preoperative pneumococcal vaccine should be administered. Staging laparotomy is infrequently performed in the evaluation of patients with NHL, as this procedure rarely alters the therapeutic plan. One exception is in the case of gastric lymphoma that is apparently localized to the stomach following noninvasive studies; in this instance, surgery is important in staging and may also be therapeutic.

A clinical stage (CS) is assigned based on the findings of the history, physical examination, laboratory data, and noninvasive radiographic studies. Pathologic staging (PS) refers to the extent of disease as determined by biopsy or laparotomy. The Ann Arbor staging classification is used to express the staging of both HD and NHL. The stages are as follows:

Stage I: Involvement in a single lymph node region on one side of the diaphragm

Stage II: Involvement of two or more lymph node regions on the same side of the diaphragm

Stage III: Involvement confined to nodes, but on both sides of the diaphragm. For patients with HD, Stage III can be subdivided into:

III1 Disease involving the spleen or splenic, celiac, or portal nodes, or any combination of these

III2 Disease involving the paraaortic, iliac, or mesenteric nodes with or without upper abdominal involvement

Stage IV: Disseminated involvement including one or more extralymphatic organs, such as the lung, liver, or bone marrow

The presence of splenic disease is designated by a subscript S. If the patient has one extralymphatic site, usually adjacent to involved lymph nodes, that could be incorporated into a radiation therapy port, this should be noted by a subscript E, and the disease should not be classified as Stage IV on the basis of this extranodal involvement. For example, if the patient has lung involvement adjacent to mediastinal lymph nodes, this may be cured by radical local radio-therapy. Therefore, this condition might be classified as stage II_E. The absence or presence of fever, weight loss, or night sweats is indicated by an A or B appearing after the Roman numeral of this stage, respectively. Patients with advanced stages or B symptoms have a poorer prognosis than those with localized disease or without constitutional symptoms.

It should be emphasized that the Ann Arbor staging classification was first developed for HD and continues to provide important information on prognosis and selection of therapy for patients with this disorder. This classification is less useful prognostically and therapeutically in NHL, in which Stage III or IV disease is the rule, and therapy is guided more by the histologic subtype. The Ann Arbor classification has provided a common language for reporting and comparing data, thus facilitating three decades of fruitful research in lymphoma.

Clinical Findings Associated with Lymphoma

Various combinations of symptoms, physical findings, and disabilities may be produced by the malignant lymphomas, through pressure on or infiltration of organs, by vascular or ductal obstruction, or by overexpression or suppression of a component of the immune system.

Immunologic Abnormalities

Immunologic abnormalities are frequently encountered in patients with lymphomas and contribute to the morbidity and mortality associated with these malignancies. Hodgkin's disease is characterized by defects in cell-mediated immunity. Patients are at increased risk for opportunistic infections with mycobacterial, viral, and fungal pathogens. Indeed, approximately 25 percent of patients with HD develop herpes zoster with a high incidence of dissemination. T cell defects may persist for years in patients cured of HD. Patients who have been splenectomized are at increased risk of bacterial infections, particularly with encapsulated organisms, such as pneumococcus and *Haemophilus,* and have an incidence of herpes zoster that exceeds 60 percent.

Patients with NHL often have abnormalities of the humoral branch of immunity. Monoclonal gammopathies are common and occur in approximately 10 percent of patients with small lymphocytic lymphoma, while hypogammaglobulinemia may occur in as many as 50 percent of patients with this subtype of low-grade NHL. Autoimmune hemolytic anemias and autoimmune thrombocytopenia may also occur.

The Thorax

The mediastinum, lung parenchyma, or pleura may be involved with malignant lymphoma. Anterior mediastinal disease may compress neighboring structures and result in the development of superior vena cava syndrome. Pleural effusions are common and may be due to direct invasion of the pleura or to venous and lymphatic obstruction in the mediastinum. Pleural effusions may be transudative, exudative, or chylous. Cytologic confirmation of lymphomatous involvement should be obtained before the pleural effusion is ascribed to direct invasion by tumor. Pericardial effusions with frank cardiac tamponade may also occur.

Nervous System

Neurologic complications may be seen in both HD and NHL. An epidural mass, usually as a result of extension from the mediastinal or retroperitoneal lymph nodes, may be the initial manifestation of lymphoma or may complicate its course. Back pain, a sensory level, and/or bowel and bladder dysfunction are common findings in this setting. Central nervous system (CNS) involvement is more prevalent in NHL than in HD. Risk factors for this complication include Burkitt's or lymphoblastic lymphoma histology and bone marrow involvement by diffuse large cell lymphoma. Prophylactic therapy is a consideration in these conditions. Primary CNS lymphoma may also occur, especially in patients with immunosuppressive diseases such as AIDS or in organ transplant recipients. Other neurologic problems include lymphomatous meningitis and cranial nerve abnormalities.

Lymphomas are also associated with two types of encephalopathy. Dementia, paralyses, and other neurologic findings characterize progressive multifocal leukoencephalopathy (PML), a disorder that is due to a virus from the papovirus group, known as the JC virus. In subacute cerebellar degeneration, demyelination of nerve fibers results in prominent cerebellar symptoms. No specific therapy is available for these disorders. Rarely, HD may be associated with Guillain-Barré syndrome.

Gastrointestinal System

The gastrointestinal tract may be affected by lymphoma in a variety of ways. Primary gastric NHL accounts for 25 percent of extranodal presentations and may frequently be localized at the time of diagnosis. Gastric lymphoma may occur as a complication of α-heavy chain disease (see Chap. 14), especially in patients from the Mediterranean regions. Patients generally have abdominal pain, weight loss, or bleeding. Involvement of the small intestine may also occur, commonly manifested by malabsorption or intestinal obstruction. Additionally, gastrointestinal involvement may occur in the setting of disseminated NHL, especially among patients with Waldeyer's ring involvement.

Metabolic Abnormalities

Metabolic abnormalities are not uncommon in patients with lymphoma and include renal insufficiency, hypercalcemia, and hyperuricemia. Indeed, renal disorders may result from ureteral obstruction, direct infiltration of the kidneys by tumor cells, nephrotic syndrome, or urate nephropathy. Tumor lysis syndrome, characterized by hyperkalemia, hyperuricemia, hyperphosphatemia, and hypocalcemia, may complicate the treatment of bulky, rapidly growing lymphomas such as Burkitt's disease. Prophylactic therapy with intravenous fluids and allopurinol should be administered before systemic therapy of any lymphoma is undertaken.

Treatment of the Malignant Lymphomas

Treatment of the malignant lymphomas generally involves the use of radiation therapy, chemotherapy, or combinations of both modalities, depending on the histology, stage, and general medical condition of the patient.

Hodgkin's Disease

The majority of patients with Hodgkin's disease is curable with current treatment approaches. Radiotherapy may cure over 80 percent of patients with localized HD and chemotherapy over 50 percent with disseminated disease. Treatment of HD requires an integrated multidisciplinary effort by experienced physicians if the maximum benefit is to be realized.

RADIOTHERAPY

Based on the premise that HD spreads in an orderly fashion to contiguous or adjacent lymph node groups, radiation therapy directed at the involved lymph node region as well as the next contiguous, but uninvolved, site (so-called extended-field therapy) is highly effective in the treatment of Stages I and II HD. While lower doses of radiation will result in tumor regression, a total of approximately 4,000 centigray delivered to the involved nodes over 4 to 4½ weeks is required to ensure eradication of HD. This treatment requires the use of megavoltage machines, such as the linear accelerator capable of generating 4 to 8 megavolts. Radiation therapy of HD can be divided into three ports. The mantle field includes the cervical, supraclavicular, axillary, mediastinal, and hilar lymph node regions. Portions of the lung or heart can be treated if pulmonary or pericardial involvement is present, but careful planning and simulation of the radiation field are required to minimize toxicity to normal tissues. The abdominal or paraaortic field treats the periaortic lymph nodes and splenic pedicle if a staging laparotomy has been performed. If the spleen is still present, the splenic region may need to be included in the field. The pelvic field encompasses the iliac, inguinal, and femoral lymph node regions.

Results of radiation therapy are excellent in early-stage HD. Supradiaphragmatic surgically staged IA HD patients treated with extended-field (mantle and paraaortic) radiation have a 95 percent relapse-free survival and an approximately 100 percent overall survival because of the ability of chemotherapy to salvage the few patients who may relapse. Similarly, supradiaphragmatic surgically staged IIA HD patients treated with similar radiation fields have a relapse-free survival of 75 percent and an overall survival of 95 percent. Surgically staged IIB HD patients have almost equivalent results as patients who are of similar stage but are asymptomatic. However, patients with bulky Stages I and II HD, defined by a mediastinal mass of greater than one third of the transthoracic diameter, have an unacceptably high relapse rate when treated with radiation therapy alone and require combined therapy with chemotherapy and involved-field radiation. Since chemotherapy will be used, staging laparotomy is not indicated in such patients. Patients with more advanced disease generally require chemotherapy.

Complications of radiation therapy are primarily related to the mantle port. Pulmonary reactions are particularly worrisome, but with careful radiation planning, symptomatic radiation pneumonitis should rarely develop. Radiation-induced pericarditis may occur in as many as 4 to 10 percent of patients treated with mantle radiation and presents insidiously with dyspnea 4 to 6 years after therapy. Accelerated atherosclerosis with symptomatic coronary artery disease has also been noted. Transverse myelopathy due to overlapping spinal cord irradiation from the mantle and paraaortic fields should occur rarely. Subclinical hypothyroidism with elevations of the thyroid-stimulating hormone (TSH) may be seen in 50 percent of patients, but frank hypothyroidism requiring hormone repletion is found in only 10 to 20 percent of patients. Sterility associated with pelvic irradiation may occur in women who have not had an oophoropexy. Lastly, a small but significant increase in the incidence of solid malignancies, such as skin neoplasms, bronchogenic carcinoma, and sarcomas, may occur within the radiation field.

CHEMOTHERAPY

Chemotherapy for HD is indicated in patients who relapse after radiation therapy, who have bulky mediastinal masses, or who have advanced Stage III or Stage IV disease. By the early 1960s, at least five different chemotherapeutic agents were found to be active in HD. However, the administration of single drugs was invariably associated with tumor relapse. In 1964, investigators at the National Cancer Institute began utilizing combinations of chemotherapeutic medications in the treatment of HD. The rationale behind combination chemotherapy is to combine agents known to be effective in the disease that have different mechanisms of action and nonoverlapping toxicities, thereby allowing for the administration of full doses of each drug. This theoretically should decrease the chance of drug resistance and should improve clinical response.

Chemotherapy with Mustargen (nitrogen mustard), Oncovin (vincristine), procarbazine, and prednisone (MOPP) is the prototypic drug combination used to treat HD. The MOPP regimen has become the gold standard to which all other drug programs are compared. Patients with advanced HD or those who relapse following radiation therapy treated with this chemotherapeutic regimen have a complete remission rate of 80 percent. Almost 65 percent of those in complete remission will remain free of disease, resulting in a 50 percent cure rate for all patients who are treated with MOPP. This program is given in 28-day cycles, although all of the medication is administered during the first 14 days of each cycle. This enables the normal tissues of the patient, particularly the bone marrow, to recover from adverse effects before additional therapy is given. Careful attention to dose intensity and drug scheduling is critical if excellent results from chemotherapy are to be obtained. The total duration of therapy is also crucial. Patients who enter complete remission after two or three courses receive a minimum of 6 months of treatment. If patients enter a complete remission after the fourth course, two additional cycles are required. However, there are no data to support the administration of therapy beyond this point.

MOPP chemotherapy is associated with significant toxicity. Nitrogen mustard, an alkylating agent, is associated with significant nausea and emesis, and myelosuppression. The administration of this medication frequently results in a chemical phlebitis, and extensive soft tissue necrosis may develop if it extravasates into the tissues. Vincristine is a vinca alkaloid that acts as a mitotic inhibitor, thereby preventing cell division. This agent is associated with neurotoxicity, characterized by paresthesias, loss of deep tendon reflexes, paralytic ileus, and, rarely, release of antidiuretic hormone. Procarbazine inhibits DNA replication by an unknown mechanism. Unique toxicities associated with this drug include neurotoxicity, which may be ameliorated by the administration of pyridoxine, hypersensitivity pneumonitis, and a disulfiram (Antabuse)-like reaction to alcohol. Lastly, procarbazine is a weak monoamine oxidase inhibitor, and patients must be advised to avoid tricyclic antidepressants, sympathomimetics, and foods that are high in tyrosine (such as aged cheeses, red wine, and bananas). Prednisone, like other corticosteroids, may produce hyperglycemia, exacerbations of hypertension, insomnia, psychosis, and, rarely, aseptic necrosis of the bone.

MOPP chemotherapy is also associated with a significant risk of sterility, with 100 percent of males developing azospermia and testicular atrophy. The effect on ovarian function is less predictable and appears to be age-related. The majority of women less than 25 years of age remains fertile following MOPP therapy, whereas amenorrhea is permanent in more than 50 to 80 percent of women aged 30 or older.

An increased incidence of second malignancies has occurred in patients treated with MOPP chemotherapy with or without radiation. The most frequently encountered is acute nonlymphocytic leukemia (ANLL), which occurs at an estimated frequency of 5 to 10 percent. Patients who received both chemotherapy and radiotherapy are particularly at risk. The peak period of risk occurs between 4 and 7 years following therapy. This secondary acute leukemia is usually characterized by preceding myelodysplasia; abnormalities of chromosome 5 or 7, or both; and refractoriness to antileukemic therapy. NHL may also occur with an increased incidence following successful treatment of HD.

Non–cross-resistant drug combinations provide an alternative for the treatment of HD. Of these, doxorubicin (Adriamycin)-containing regimens have proved most effective. ABVD, a four-drug program consisting of Adriamycin, bleomycin, vinblastine, and dacarbazine (DTIC), has been studied extensively. Potential advantages to this regimen include less neurotoxicity and an apparent significant reduction in the incidence of gonadal dysfunction and secondary leukemia when compared with MOPP therapy. However, significant pulmonary problems due to bleomycin and cardiac toxicity related to Adriamycin may occur, especially in patients previously treated with thoracic irradiation. Other side effects include bone marrow suppression, skin injury from extravasation of doxorubicin, and flulike symptoms related to dacarbazine.

Patients who relapse after MOPP chemotherapy usually respond to retreatment with this regimen if the period of remission lasted longer than 1 year; however, the long-term durability of second MOPP remissions is uncertain. Patients in whom recurrent disease develops within a year of treatment with MOPP, or who fail to respond to MOPP therapy, can be treated with ABVD. Up to 60 percent of these patients treated with "salvage" ABVD may enter a complete remission; 10 to 30 percent of these patients may be cured.

In previously untreated patients with advanced-stage HD, ABVD appears at least equivalent to MOPP with respect to complete remission rate, disease-free survival, and overall survival. The combination of MOPP cycles alternating monthly with ABVD may be superior to MOPP chemotherapy alone. It is unclear whether the alternating combinations are superior to ABVD given alone.

Bone marrow transplantation, either allogeneic or autologous, has been used successfully to produce long-term remissions in some patients with HD disease that has proved refractory to therapy.

Non–Hodgkin's Lymphoma

The therapeutic strategy in non–Hodgkin's disease is guided primarily by the histologic subtype, symptoms, extent of disease, and general medical condition of the patient. For practical purposes, the approach to treatment is generally dictated by whether the patient has a low-grade lymphoma or a disease characterized by a more aggressive natural history, such as that found among the intermediate- or high-grade NHL.

Low-grade lymphomas characteristically have a long natural history, with median survivals of greater than 5 to 7 years. These lymphomas are often responsive to chemotherapy, with complete remission achieved in 50 to 60 percent of cases. However, despite these initial favorable responses, low-grade NHL exhibits a continuous tendency to relapse with time, and cannot be considered curable with present state-of-the-art chemotherapy. As a result, there is little pressure to institute therapy. Indeed, investigators at Stanford University gave no initial treatment to a series of asymptomatic patients with Stages III and IV low-grade NHL. During the period of follow-up study, spontaneous regression of disease occurred in 20 percent of patients and was often durable, lasting more than one year. Ultimately, patients required therapy because of progressive symptoms, bulky adenopathy, or compromise of a vital organ. In this study, treatment was not needed until an average of more than 3 years of observation.

Chemotherapy can be given as a single oral alkylating agent, such as chlorambucil or cyclophosphamide, or can be administered as a combination of several drugs (cyclophosphamide, vincristine, and prednisone, for example). In several well-controlled studies, single-agent therapy was associated with equivalent patient survival to that achieved with combination chemotherapy. However, combination chemotherapy produces responses more quickly than single-agent treatment, thereby making this approach preferable when there is involvement at critical sites. Radiation therapy may be curative in the rare patient with truly localized Stage I or II low-grade NHL and may also palliate patients with more advanced, bulky, or painful disease. Approximately 30 to 40 percent of patients with low-grade NHL will demonstrate transformation to more aggressive histologies. These patients have a poor prognosis and require intensive chemotherapy with regimens appropriate for de novo high-grade lymphomas.

Intermediate- and high-grade non–Hodgkin's lymphomas are characterized by rapid disease progression. However, they are often very responsive to intensive chemotherapy. Frequently used regimens include CHOP (cyclophosphamide, Adriamycin, Oncovin, and prednisone), m-BACOD (methotrexate, bleomycin, Adriamycin, cyclophosphamide, Oncovin, and dexamethasone [Decadron]), MACOP-B (methotrexate, Adriamycin, cyclophosphamide, Oncovin, prednisone, and bleomycin), ProMACE-MOPP (prednisone, methotrexate, Adriamycin, cyclophosphamide, etoposide [VP-16], Mustargen, Oncovin, procarbazine, and prednisone), or COP-BLAM (cyclophosphamide, Oncovin, prednisone, bleomycin, Adriamycin, and procarbazine). These programs produce similar results, with complete remission rates on the order of 60 to 80 percent with approximately one half of these patients presumably cured. Recent studies indicate that the simpler and better tolerated CHOP regimen produces as high of a percentage of durable remissions as do the more complex drug combinations. Selected patients with Stages I and II large cell lymphoma can be treated with a short course of intensive combination chemotherapy, with doxorubicin-containing regimens such as CHOP (cyclophosphamide, hydroxydaunorubicin [Adriamycin], Oncovin, and prednisone), followed by involved-field radiation therapy.

Unfavorable prognostic factors in patients with diffuse large cell lymphoma include bulky masses (> 10 cm in diameter), poor performance status, involvement of more than two extranodal sites, and "B" symptoms (fever, night sweats, or weight loss). Additionally, marked elevation of the serum lactic dehydrogenase level, male sex, and advanced stage are associated with a worse outcome.

Patients with either Hodgkin's disease or aggressive non–Hodgkin's lymphoma who fail to enter a complete remission or who relapse after initial therapy may be candidates for investigational treatment with either allogeneic or autologous bone marrow transplantation. Patients whose lymphomas retain sensitivity to chemotherapy tend to fare better with this approach and have had encouraging results. Other experimental therapies for patients with lymphoma include biologic response modifiers such as α-interferon or interleukin-2, and monoclonal antibodies coupled to radioisotopes or toxins.

Chronic Lymphocytic Leukemia

Chronic lymphocytic leukemia (CLL) is a lymphoproliferative disorder characterized by the accumulation of abnormal but mature-appearing lymphocytes in the peripheral blood (Plate 80) and bone marrow, with frequent involvement of the lymph nodes, spleen, and liver. CLL is the most common leukemia of adults, accounting for approximately 30 percent of all cases in the United States. Generally, patients with CLL are elderly, with a median age at diagnosis of 60 years. In most published series men are affected nearly twice as often as women. The etiology of CLL is presently not well defined, but genetic as well as immunologic factors may play a role. Radiation exposure does not appear to increase the risk of CLL. Patients with CLL seem to have an increased incidence of second malignancies, including skin cancer, sarcomas, and lung cancer.

Chronic lymphocytic leukemia is a neoplastic disorder of lymphocytes, with greater than 95 percent of cases involving B cells and fewer than 5 percent of patients having a monoclonal disease of T lymphocytes. Monoclonality has been demonstrated by a variety of techniques, including the presence of a single surface immunoglobulin light chain (either κ or λ) in the case of B cell CLL and unique immunoglobulin gene or T cell receptor gene rearrangements in B and T CLL, respectively. B cell CLL can be characterized by using a panel of monoclonal markers directed against cell surface antigens. Surface immunoglobulin is most commonly of the IgM variety, but is present in lower density on CLL cells than in normal peripheral blood B cells. Cytoplasmic μ-heavy chain is detectable in high quantities. Additional surface markers typically found include the murine erythrocyte receptor (90% of CLL are positive), B cell surface antigens B1 (CD20), B2 (CD21), and T1 (CD5) (present on normal T cells and CLL B cells, but only rarely on normal B cells), and receptors for the Fc fragment of IgG and for complement. Certain cytogenetic abnormalities have been reported in CLL, with trisomy 12 or 14q+ being the most frequent findings. More complex karyotypic abnormalities have been associated with a worse prognosis. Immunologic derangements include decreased T helper and increased T suppressor activity, as well as inversion in the normal ratio of T helper to suppressor cells. Consequences of this and other immunologic dysfunction lead to many of the clinical features of CLL.

The clinical diagnosis of CLL requires a sustained lymphocytosis of more than 15,000 per milliliter in the absence of other causes. Benign etiologies associated with lymphocytosis include viral infections such as infectious mononucleosis, other infectious conditions such as typhoid fever, autoimmune disorders, and endocrine abnormalities. These states, however, are usually associated with polyclonal proliferation of T lymphocytes. Most often the diagnosis of CLL is suggested by the peripheral blood film, with the demonstration of increased numbers of mature-appearing small lymphocytes (Plate 80). Frequent "smudge" cells, formed by damage to these fragile lymphocytes, may be seen. Although a bone marrow examination is not required for the diagnosis of CLL, it almost invariably shows infiltration with small lymphocytes. The diagnosis can be further confirmed by finding the characteristic cell markers for CLL in peripheral blood or bone marrow lymphocytes. Lymph node biopsies, if obtained, generally reveal diffuse effacement of the architecture by well-differentiated (small) lymphocytes.

Many patients with CLL are asymptomatic and are diagnosed incidentally by a complete blood count. Symptoms, when present, usually relate to tissue infiltration, cytopenias, or immunosuppression, and include fatigue, weight loss, recurrent infections, easy bruisability, or early satiety secondary to splenomegaly. Physical examination should carefully document the presence or absence of lymphadenopathy, splenomegaly, or hepatic enlargement.

Laboratory data reveal anemia or thrombocytopenia, or both, in 25 percent of patients. The mechanism of these hematologic abnormalities is often multifactorial and may include bone marrow infiltration, hypersplenism, and immune destruction. Indeed, 20 percent of patients develop a positive Coombs test and nearly half of these patients have evidence of hemolysis. Immune thrombocytopenic purpura occurs in 5 to 10 percent of cases and, rarely, pure red cell aplasia has been noted. Other immunologic abnormalities include hypogammaglobulinemia in 50 percent of patients and a monoclonal paraprotein spike in 5 to 10 percent, both of which may be diagnosed by serum protein electrophoresis.

Patients with CLL are susceptible to infections as a consequence of hypogammaglobulinemia, defects in cellular immune responses, and neutropenia. Important pathogens include encapsulated bacteria, herpes zoster, and opportunistic organisms. Patients with CLL in whom a fever develops should be evaluated carefully for the presence of a potential infection, as fever is not otherwise routinely encountered in this disorder. It is prudent to avoid vaccination with live organisms, as disseminated vaccinia may develop.

Currently, two staging systems are in use. The Rai classification is a five-stage scheme, as follows: Stage 0 is lymphocytosis only (median survival is 150 months), Stages I is lymphocytosis with enlarged lymph nodes (median survival is 101 months), Stage II is lymphocytosis with splenomegaly (median survival is 71 months), Stage III is lymphocytosis and anemia, and Stage IV is lymphocytosis with thrombocytopenia. The cytopenias seen in Stages III and IV disease must not be on the basis of immune destruction. The median survival of patients with Stages III and IV disease is poor, on the order of 19 months. Patients presenting with early-stage disease typically progress with time through the other stages.

The second classification is referred to as the Binet or International staging system and proposes that patients be divided into three groups, based on the presence of lymphocytosis in the peripheral blood and potential involvement of five additional sites (cervical, axillary, inguinal, liver, or spleen). In Stage A, fewer than three sites are involved (median survival > 10 years); in Stage B, three or more areas are involved (median survival of 7 years); and in Stage C, anemia with a hemoglobin of less than 10 gm/dL or thrombocytopenia with a platelet count of less than 100,000 per milliliter is present (median survival of 2 years or less).

Patients with CLL may not require therapy early in the course of their disease, despite elevated white blood counts. Indications for therapeutic intervention include progressive constitutional symptoms, increasing cytopenias, autoimmune hemolytic anemia, significant splenomegaly, or bulky lymphadenopathy that may obstruct vital organs (with resulting hydronephrosis, for example) or cause cosmetic disfigurement. Infectious complications require prompt antibiotic therapy. Studies utilizing intravenous immunoglobulin suggest that this may be beneficial in reducing the incidence of bacterial infections in selected patients with CLL who have hypogammaglobulinemia. This therapy is costly and time consuming, and should be reserved for patients with frequent, repeated infections.

Alkylating agents remain the cornerstone of therapy for CLL. Chlorambucil is the drug that is most often employed, although cyclophosphamide is equally effective. Chlorambucil can be given on a daily basis or can be administered, with equal efficacy, by pulses every 3 to 4 weeks. The addition of a corticosteroid such as prednisone may increase the response to alkylating agents alone, and is also effective in treating immune-mediated cytopenias. Radiation therapy may play a role in the treatment of localized adenopathy. Indications for splenectomy include significant hypersplenism and immune cytopenias unresponsive to steroid therapy. However, this procedure may be associated with substantial morbidity and mortality in patients with advanced CLL.

Most patients with CLL ultimately succumb to infection, bleeding, or unrelated medical illnesses. However, CLL may also demonstrate progression to more aggressive disorders in a small percentage of cases. High-grade, diffuse, large cell non–Hodgkin's lymphoma develops in 5 to 10 percent of patients. This transformation is referred to as Richter's syndrome, frequently involves the gastrointestinal tract or other extranodal sites, and may present with fever or other constitutional symptoms. The disease is usually resistant to chemotherapy and carries a worse prognosis than large cell lymphoma that arises de novo. Less commonly, transformation to prolymphocytic leukemia may occur. This is associated with the appearance of immature lymphocytes with prominent nucleoli, progressive cytopenias, and splenomegaly.

Hairy Cell Leukemia

Hairy cell leukemia, also known as leukemic reticuloendotheliosis, is an uncommon variant of CLL or NHL. Approximately 600 new cases of hairy cell leukemia are reported a year, accounting for only 2 percent of all adult leukemias. This disorder is characterized by splenomegaly, pancytopenia, and circulating mononuclear cells with cytoplasmic projections simulating "hairs." These leukemic cells contain tartrate-resistant acid phosphatase (TRAP), a feature useful in confirming the diagnosis of hairy cell leukemia. In the overwhelming majority of cases, the neoplastic cell is derived from a B lymphocyte. However, rare cases of T cell hairy cell leukemia have been described in association with a unique retrovirus referred to as human T cell leukemia virus type II (HTLV-II).

The median age at which hairy cell leukemia is diagnosed is 50 to 60 years, and men are affected nearly four times as frequently as women. More than one third of patients present with fatigue, weakness, or infection. Other symptoms include left upper quadrant abdominal discomfort and bleeding. Physical findings are notable for splenomegaly in over 90 percent of patients and hepatomegaly in approximately 40 percent. Significant peripheral lymphadenopathy is unusual. Pancytopenia is present in the majority of patients, with median granulocyte counts of 500 to 600/μL. Careful review of the peripheral blood smear will demonstrate diagnostic hairy cells (Plate 81), and 10 to 20 percent of patients may be frankly leukemic, that is, have large numbers of circulating hairy cells. Bone marrow aspirates are frequently "dry" because of increased reticulin deposition. Biopsies are usually hypercellular, with infiltration by widely spaced mononuclear cells. Splenic pathology is also characteristic, with diffuse involvement of the red pulp and sinuses. The differential diagnosis of hairy cell leukemia includes classic CLL, NHL, LGL lymphocytosis, and aplastic anemia.

Patients with hairy cell leukemia are at risk for a number of complications. Infections with either pyogenic bacteria or opportunistic organisms, such as toxoplasmosis, mycobacteria, *Legionella*, or fungus, produce the majority of deaths from this disorder. Other less commonly encountered problems include bleeding secondary to thrombocytopenia or platelet dysfunction, systemic vasculitis, paraproteinemia, amyloidosis, and bone disease.

Some patients with hairy cell leukemia will require no specific therapy, although the majority will eventually need treatment because of infection, progressive pancytopenia, or marked splenomegaly. In the past splenectomy was the primary treatment utilized, and results in hematologic improvement in more than 75 percent of patients. However, as many as half of these patients will subsequently require additional treatment. Recent advances in the therapy of hairy cell leukemia have come from clinical research using α-interferon. Low dosages of α-interferon will normalize the peripheral blood counts in more than 90 percent of patients, but will rarely result in the complete eradication of bone marrow disease. Toxicity related to interferon administration includes fever, malaise, and fatigue. Chemotherapy with new agents such as deoxycoformycin (Pentostatin), an adenosine deaminase inhibitor, or 2-chlorodeoxyadenosine has been found to be highly efficacious in this disorder, and may be associated with the induction of true complete remissions. These drugs may be useful in patients who progress despite treatment with α-interferon. Eventually they may prove to be the agents of choice for primary treatment. However, more research will be required to determine the optimal sequence of these interventions. With the advent of these newer therapeutic modalities, treatment with chlorambucil, androgens, corticosteroids, or leukapheresis can no longer be recommended.

Infectious Mononucleosis

Infectious mononucleosis is a transmissible, self-limited disease caused by the Epstein-Barr virus (EBV), a ubiquitous human virus belonging to the herpes family of DNA viruses. Epstein-Barr virus infects B lymphocytes as well as epithelial cells, especially of the oropharynx, and is transmitted primarily by contact with saliva from an infected individual. Like other herpeslike viruses, infection with EBV is long-lasting, although generally latent. Frequent reactivation is common, resulting in an increase in the risk of transmission. In industrialized areas of the world, initial exposure to EBV occurs before adolescence and is associated with mild or subclinical disease. However, if initial exposure to the virus is delayed, primary infection in this older-aged group is characterized by the development of infectious mononucleosis. The peak incidence of this disease is in individuals between 15 and 25 years old.

Epstein-Barr virus has also been etiologically linked to Burkitt's lymphoma and other lymphoproliferative diseases, especially among immunosuppressed patients including patients with AIDS and those who have had organ transplants. Epstein-Barr virus infection in patients with the rare X-linked lymphoproliferative syndrome (XLP) results in severe, often fatal, mononucleosis and also predisposes to the subsequent development of lymphoma. Epstein-Barr virus is also associated with the occurrence of aggressive, poorly differentiated nasopharyngeal carcinoma. Most recently, it has been implicated in some cases of aplastic anemia and some cases of Hodgkin's disease.

Infectious mononucleosis is characterized by the triad of fever, lymphadenopathy, and pharyngitis. The fever may be remittent and may be accompanied by drenching night sweats. The lymphadenopathy is especially prominent in the posterior cervical chain, and rarely persists for more than a few weeks. The pharyngitis is most often exudative and may be so severe as to result in respiratory compromise. Other symptoms include headache, dysphagia, jaundice, and malaise. Additional physical findings include splenomegaly in 50 percent of patients, palatal petechiae, and hepatomegaly.

Complications related to infectious mononucleosis are numerous, but occur only rarely. Although chemical hepatitis is characteristic, progressive hepatic failure is most unusual. Acute meningitis, encephalitis, and cranial nerve palsies may all ensue. Cardiac involvement includes pericarditis, myocarditis, and rarely ischemia related to coronary artery abnormalities. Thrombocytopenia is common and, on occasion, may be severe. In the latter instances it is indistinguishable from autoimmune thrombocytopenic purpura. Hemolytic anemia may result from the development of IgM autoantibody to the i antigen on red blood cells. Splenic rupture may also occur.

The diagnosis rests on finding the clinical triad as described above in association with characteristic laboratory abnormalities. Atypical lymphocytosis (Plates 49–51) is present in more than 75 percent of patients, and is related to T cell activation in response to B cell infection with the virus. (These cells are described in the chapter on leukocytes.) Macroglobulins with heterophil antibody activity develop in the majority of patients with infectious mononucleosis. This heterophil antibody will agglutinate sheep red blood cells and can be absorbed completely from the serum by preincubation with beef red cells, but not with guinea pig kidney tissue. These heterophil antibodies are found in the serum of 90 to 95 percent of patients with infectious mononucleosis. More recently, this procedure has been simplified and is commercially available as the Monospot test. The Monospot test is associated with a 3 percent false negative and 3 percent false positive rate. Antibodies to EBV-specific antigens develop in a predictable fashion and may be helpful in the diagnosis of atypical cases.

Heterophil-negative mononucleosis may be due to an acute infection with cytomegalovirus (CMV). This syndrome is clinically similar to EBV-related illness, although pharyngitis and lymphadenopathy are less common. CMV mononucleosis may follow the transfusion of CMV-positive blood to a patient previously unexposed to this virus. The diagnosis can be made by the demonstration of a fourfold rise in the CMV antibody titer.

The treatment of infectious mononucleosis is primarily supportive. Patients should be advised to avoid contact sports because of the presence of splenomegaly and the small but finite risk of splenic rupture. Fever and pharyngitis may be controlled with acetaminophen. Administration of antibiotics is not helpful, and in the case of ampicillin, a characteristic maculopapular rash will develop in virtually all patients with infectious mononucleosis treated with this drug. Corticosteroids may be of benefit in cases involving respiratory compromise, but do not otherwise hasten recovery. Steroids are also useful in the treatment of autoimmune cytopenias. Fatal mononucleosis is extremely rare and patients generally recover without sequelae.

Case Development Problems: Malignant Lymphoma

Patient History No. 1

A 25-year-old woman complains of fever, night sweats, and unexplained itching. On physical examination, a mass of lymph nodes is found on the left side of her neck. They are firm and appear matted together. A complete blood count and peripheral blood smear are normal. Chest x-ray shows left hilar adenopathy.

1. What further information would you require in order to complete the evaluation of this patient?

   Obviously the diagnosis of a malignant lymphoma, such as Hodgkin's disease, should be considered. Biopsy of the lymph node mass should be done soon after such simple procedures as physical examination to determine the size of the liver, spleen, and other lymph nodes, and blood chemistry evaluation including liver function tests, uric acid levels, and serum calcium levels. If the diagnosis of malignant lymphoma, Hodgkin's type, is made by biopsy, then bone marrow biopsy and abdominal and chest CT scans should be considered. Skin tests for tuberculosis and for common antigens to determine whether anergy is present are sometimes helpful.

Lymph node biopsy shows Hodgkin's disease, nodular sclerosis type. The spleen is not palpated in the left upper quadrant. Alkaline phosphatase and transaminase levels (liver function tests) are normal. A bone marrow biopsy and CT scans are negative.

2. What is the clinical stage of this patient?

   Stage IIB, because of two areas of lymphomatous nodes on one side of the diaphragm. The B indicates that she has systemic symptoms, fever, and night sweats. Pruritus is not considered a B symptom.

3. How would you now proceed?

A laparotomy or at least an abdominal exploration with laparoscopy and percutaneous biopsy of suspicious sites should be performed. Abdominal exploration is needed to detect liver involvement by Hodgkin's disease. A splenectomy with all its benefits and possible complications and placement of the ovaries outside the radiation field should also be performed. The abdominal exploration may also locate disease outside the fields treated by routine radiotherapy.

A laparotomy is undertaken. The spleen is removed and found to be involved by Hodgkin's disease. The liver shows small infiltrates with mononuclear cells but no Reed-Sternberg cells. A few granulomas are also found in the liver and spleen. The retroperitoneal lymph nodes are negative for Hodgkin's disease as determined by biopsy.

4. What is the pathologic stage of this patient?

Nonspecific infiltrates and granuloma are not enough to make the diagnosis of Hodgkin's disease of the liver. However, with splenic involvement, there is a good possibility that the liver is also involved, although this was not proved by biopsy. Small foci of Hodgkin's disease can easily be missed by the biopsy procedures used at the time of laparotomy. Despite these possibilities, the patient is staged as PS (pathologic stage) III_sB and not Stage IV.

5. How would you treat this patient?

As a patient with Stage IIIB Hodgkin's disease, she should be treated with combination chemotherapy.

The patient receives six cycles of MOPP therapy and mantle radiotherapy, and all clinically detectable disease disappears. The spleen becomes normal in size, and liver function tests normalize. The patient is in complete remission for 2 years but then suffers a relapse, with growth of lymph nodes in the abdominal area.

6. What therapy can now be offered to this patient?

MOPP chemotherapy can be reintroduced or alternated with ABVD combination chemotherapy. The prognosis is now guarded.

Patient History No. 2

An asymptomatic man, age 60, presents with enlarged lymph nodes throughout his body. Those about his neck, axillae, and groin are particularly enlarged. A lymph node biopsy reveals a malignant lymphoma characterized by sheets of immature lymphocytes replacing normal lymph node architecture. Nodules of lymphocytes are present, but no Reed-Sternberg cells. Cell marker analysis reveals IgM on the surface of the lymphocytes, and many of these cells react with a B1 monoclonal antibody and are CALLA negative. On examination, the patient's spleen is enlarged. Anemia, leukopenia, and thrombocytopenia are discovered. Examination of the peripheral blood smear shows no abnormalities, except a few atypical lymphocytes. The Coombs test is negative.

1. What is the diagnosis? Do the cell markers confirm or contradict the histopathologic diagnosis, and why? How would you further evaluate this patient?

   The patient has non–Hodgkin's lymphoma of the nodular, lymphocytic, poorly differentiated type. The presence of immunoglobulin on the lymphocyte surface indicates that they are B cells. Nodular lymphomas often react with B1 antibody. In contrast to acute lymphocytic leukemia (ALL), nodular lymphomas are usually CALLA negative.

   A bone marrow biopsy is necessary, since many patients with non–Hodgkin's lymphoma of this type will have marrow involvement. An abdominal ultrasound or CT scan will help determine whether the retroperitoneal area is involved. The consequences of malignant lymphoma should be investigated by measurement of serum uric acid levels and renal and liver function tests.

2. Before performing the bone marrow biopsy, what do you give as the clinical stage? (All chemical tests and x-rays are normal.)

   Since the patient has lymph node disease on both sides of the diaphragm, and the spleen is involved, the patient is staged as III$_s$A.

   Bone marrow examination reveals scattered, large nodules of lymphocytes infiltrating the bone marrow.

3. What is the stage now?

   Bone marrow involvement advances the stage to IV. This is commonly the case in low-grade non–Hodgkin's lymphoma and is one reason why radical radiotherapy for cure is seldom considered.

4. What is the likely cause for pancytopenia in this patient?

   The pancytopenia is probably due to two factors: (1) the replacement of the bone marrow by lymphoma and (2) hypersplenism due to infiltration of the spleen by lymphomatous tissue.

5. How would you consider treating this patient?

One possibility is to treat with combination chemotherapy, cyclophosphamide and prednisone. Prednisone would be particularly useful, since he suffers from hypersplenism. If cytotoxic agents alone are used, bone marrow production is often suppressed, and pancytopenia worsens before any beneficial effect of cytotoxic agents becomes evident.

6. What histopathologic feature in the lymph node biopsy will determine the prognosis and the likelihood of response to therapy?

The presence of a nodular lymphoma is associated with a particularly good prognosis.

The patient is treated with chemotherapy, and all evidence of disease disappears. One year later, however, rapidly enlarging nodes are found in his neck.

7. What procedures would you consider now?

Rapidly enlarging nodes in a patient with nodular poorly differentiated lymphocytic lymphoma suggest that the disease has relapsed or possibly has been transformed into a more malignant form of lymphoma, that is, diffuse large cell lymphoma. A repeat biopsy should be done to confirm or deny this possibility.

Diffuse large cell lymphoma is found in the lymph nodes, and the disease progresses rapidly, with more lymph nodes appearing weekly in all areas; the neck nodes are particularly large.

8. What therapy would you consider?

Although the prognosis is not good, treatment with one of several multiple-drug chemotherapy combinations remains his best hope for long-term survival.

At this time atypical lymphocytes with large clefted nuclei and nucleoli are found in the patient's peripheral blood. The total white count rises to 40×10^9 per liter and is made up of 90 percent of these atypical lymphocytes.

9. What is the likely diagnosis, and how does it affect prognosis or therapy?

Most likely the patient's lymphoma has developed a leukemic phase. Prognosis is even worse and treatment more difficult in the development of this leukemic phase.

Selected Readings

Lymphoma—General Considerations

Bertness, V. et al. T-cell receptor gene rearrangements as clinical markers of human T-cell lymphomas. *N. Engl. J. Med.* 313 : 534, 1985.

Blayney, D. W. et al. The human T-cell leukemia/lymphoma virus, lymphoma, lytic bone lesions, and hypercalcemia. *Ann. Intern. Med.* 98 : 144, 1983.

Cohen, P. J., and Jaffe, E. S. Current methods used in the diagnosis and classification of malignant lymphomas. In V. T. Devita, S. Hellman, and S. A. Rosenberg, *Updates of Cancer: principles and practice of oncology* 8 : 1, 1987.

Croce, C. M. et al. Molecular basis of human B-cell neoplasia. *Blood* 65 : 1, 1985.

Foon, K. A., and Todd, R. F. Immunologic classification of leukemia and lymphoma. *Blood* 68 : 1, 1986.

Kirsch, I. R., and Broder, S. The molecular pathology of lymphomas. *J. Clin. Oncol.* 4 : 271, 1986.

Koduru, P. R. K. et al. Cytogenetic and histologic correlations in malignant lymphoma. *Blood* 69 : 97, 1987.

Penn, I. The incidence of malignancies in transplant recipients. *Transplant Proc.* 7 : 323, 1975.

Safai, B., and Good, R. A. Lymphoproliferative disorders of the T-cell series: A review. *Medicine* 59 : 335, 1980.

Waldmann, T. A. et al. Molecular genetic analysis of human lymphoid neoplasms: Immunoglobulin genes and the c-myc oncogene. *Ann. Intern. Med.* 102 : 497, 1985.

Hodgkin's Disease

Blayney, D. W. et al. Decreasing risk of leukemia with prolonged follow-up after chemotherapy and radiotherapy for Hodgkin's disease. *N. Engl. J. Med.* 316 : 710, 1987.

Carbone, P. C. et al. Report of the committee on Hodgkin's disease staging. *Cancer Res.* 31 : 1860, 1971.

Carmel, R. J., and Kaplan, H. S. Mantle irradiation in Hodgkin's disease. An analysis of technique, tumor irradiation, and complications. *Cancer* 37 : 2812, 1976.

Canellos, G. P. Bone marrow transplantation as salvage therapy in advanced Hodgkin's disease: Allogeneic or autologous? *J. Clin. Oncol.* 3 : 1451, 1985.

Canellos, G. P., Come, S. E., and Skarin, A. T. Chemotherapy in the treatment of Hodgkin's disease. *Semin. Hematol.* 20 : 1, 1983.

Connors, J. M., and Klimo, P. MOPP/ABVD hybrid chemotherapy for advanced Hodgkin's disease. *Semin. Hematol.* 24 : 35, 1987.

DeVita, V. T. et al. Curability of advanced Hodgkin's disease with chemotherapy: Long-term follow-up of MOPP-treated patients at the National Cancer Institute. *Ann. Intern. Med.* 92 : 587, 1980.

Gutensohn, N., and Cole, P. Childhood social environment and Hodgkin's disease. *N. Engl. J. Med.* 304 : 135, 1981.

Kadin, M. E. Common activated helper T-cell origin for lymphomatoid papulosis, mycosis fungoides, and some types of Hodgkin's disease. *Lancet* 2 : 864, 1985.

Kaplan, H. S. Tumoricidal dose of radiation therapy for Hodgkin's disease. *Cancer Res.* 26 : 1221, 1966.

Kaplan, H. S. *Hodgkin's Disease* (2nd ed.). Cambridge, MA: Harvard University, 1980.

Lukes, R. J. et al. Reed-Sternberg–like cells in infectious mononucleosis. *Lancet* 2 : 1000, 1969.

Santoro, A., Bonfante, V., and Bonadonna, G. Salvage chemotherapy with ABVD in MOPP-resistant Hodgkin's disease. *Ann. Intern. Med.* 96 : 139, 1982.

Taylor, M. S., Kaplan, H. S., and Nelson, T. S. Staging laparotomy with splenectomy for Hodgkin's disease: The Stanford experience. *World J. Surg.* 9 : 449, 1985.

Tucker, M. A., Coleman, C. N., and Cox, R. S. Risk of second cancers after treatment for Hodgkin's disease. *N. Engl. J. Med.* 318 : 76, 1988.

Non–Hodgkin's Lymphoma

Broder, S, and Bunn, P. A. Cutaneous T-cell lymphomas. *Semin. Oncol.* 7 : 310, 1980.

Broder, S. et al. T-cell lymphoproliferative syndrome associated with human T-cell leukemia/lymphoma virus. *Ann. Intern. Med.* 100 : 543, 1984.

Cohen, L. F. et al. Acute tumor lysis syndrome: A review of 37 patients with Burkitt's lymphoma. *Am. J. Med.* 68 : 486, 1980.

Come, S. E., and Chabner B. A. Staging in non-Hodgkin's lymphoma: approach, results and relationship to histopathology. *Clin. Haematol.* 8 : 645, 1979.

Croce, C. M. et al. Molecular basis of human B cell neoplasia. *Blood* 65 : 1, 1985.

Grogan, T. M., Warnke, R. A., and Kaplan, H. S. A comparative study of Burkitt's and non-Burkitt's "undifferentiated" malignant lymphoma: Immunologic, cytochemical, ultrastructural, cytologic, histopathologic, clinical and cell culture features. *Cancer* 49 : 1817, 1982.

Horning, S. J., and Rosenberg, S. A. The natural history of initially untreated low-grade non-Hodgkin's lymphomas. *N. Engl. J. Med.* 311 : 1471, 1984.

Hubbard, S. M. et al. Histologic progression in non-Hodgkin's lymphoma. *Blood* 59 : 258, 1982.

Kaminski, M. S. et al. Factors predicting survival in adults with stage I and II large cell lymphomas treated with primary radiation therapy. *Ann. Intern. Med.* 104 : 747, 1986.

Knobler, R. M., and Edelson, R. L. Cutaneous T-cell lymphoma. *Med. Clin. North Am.* 70 : 109, 1986.

Lieberman, P. H. et al. Evaluation of malignant lymphomas using three classifications and the working formulation. *Am. J. Med.* 81 : 365, 1986.

Nathwani, B. N. et al. Lymphoblastic lymphoma: A clinicopathologic study of 95 patients. *Cancer* 48 : 2347, 1981.

Pangalis, G. A., Nathwani, B. N., and Rappaport, H. Malignant lymphoma, well differentiated lymphocytic. Its relationship with chronic lymphocytic leukemia and macroglobulinemia of Waldenström. *Cancer* 39 : 999, 1977.

Philip, T. et al. High-dose therapy and autologous bone marrow transplantation after failure of conventional chemotherapy in adults with intermediate or high grade non-Hodgkin's lymphoma. *N. Engl. J. Med.* 316 : 1493, 1987.

Rosenberg, S. A. Karnofsky Memorial Lecture. The low-grade non-Hodgkin's lymphomas: Challenges and opportunities. *J. Clin. Oncol.* 3 : 299, 1985.

Rosenfelt, F., and Rosenberg, S. A. Diffuse histiocytic lymphoma presenting with gastointestinal tract lesions. *Cancer* 45 : 2188, 1980.

Safai, B., and Good, R. A. Lymphoproliferative disorders of the T-cell series: A review. *Medicine* 59 : 335, 1980.

Skarin, A. T. et al. Diffuse aggressive lymphomas: A curable subset of non-Hodgkin's lymphomas. *Semin. Oncol.* 13 (Suppl. 5) : 10, 1986.

Slater, D. E. et al. Lymphoblastic lymphoma in adults. *J. Clin. Oncol.* 4 : 57, 1986.

Takvorian, T. et al. Prolonged disease-free survival after autologous bone marrow transplantation in patients with non–Hodgkin's lymphoma with a poor prognosis. *N. Engl. J. Med.* 316 : 1499, 1987.

Vokes, E. E. et al. Long-term survival of patients with localized diffuse histiocytic lymphoma. *J. Clin. Oncol.* 3 : 1309, 1985.

Ziegler, J. L. Burkitt's lymphoma. *N. Engl. J. Med.* 307 : 735, 1981.

Acquired Immunodeficiency Syndrome (AIDS)

Castella, A. et al. The bone marrow in AIDS. A histologic, hematologic, and microbiologic study. *Am. J. Clin. Pathol.* 84 : 425, 1985.

Donahue, R. E. et al. In-vitro suppression of hematopoiesis after human immunodeficiency virus infection. *Nature* 326 : 200, 1987.

Gartner, S. et al. The role of mononuclear phagocytes in HTLV-III/LAV infection. *Science* 233 : 215, 1986.

Gill, P. S. et al. AIDS-related lymphoma: Results of prospective treatment trials. *J. Clin. Oncol.* 5 : 1322, 1987.

Ioachim, H. L., Cooper, M. C., and Hellman, G. C. Lymphomas in men at high risk for acquired immune deficiency syndrome (AIDS): A study of 21 cases. *Cancer* 56 : 2831, 1985.

Prior, E. et al. Hodgkin's disease in homosexual men: An AIDS-related phenomenon? *Am. J. Med.* 81 : 1085, 1986.

Schneider, D. R., and Picker, L. J. Myelodysplasia in the acquired immune deficiency syndrome. *Am. J. Clin. Pathol.* 84 : 144, 1985.

Spivak, J. L., Bender, B. S., and Quinn, T. C. Hematologic abnormalities in the acquired immune deficiency syndrome. *Am. J. Med.* 77 : 224, 1984.

Steinberg, H. N., Crumpacker, C. S., and Chatis, P. A. In vitro suppression of normal human bone marrow progenitor cells by human immunodeficiency virus. *J. Virol* 65 : 1765, 1991.

Walsh, C., et al. Thrombocytopenia in homosexual patients. Prognosis, response to therapy, and prevalence of antibody to the retrovirus associated with the acquired immunodeficiency syndrome. *Ann. Intern. Med.* 103 : 542, 1985.

Zon, L. I., and Groopman, J E. Hematologic manifestations of the human immune deficiency virus (HIV). *Semin. Hematol.* 25 : 208, 1988.

Chronic Lymphocytic Leukemia and Hairy Cell Leukemia

Aisenberg, A. C. et al. T-cell chronic leukemia. Report of a case studied with monoclonal antibody. *Am. J. Med.* 72 : 695, 1982.

Bearman, R. M., Pangalis, G. A., and Rappaport, H. Prolymphocytic leukemia: Clinical, histopathological, and cytochemical observations. *Cancer* 42 : 2360, 1978.

Binet, J.-L. et al. Chronic lymphocytic leukemia: Proposals for a revised prognostic staging system. *Br. J. Haematol.* 48 : 365, 1981.

Bouroncle, B. A., Wiseman, D. B., and Doan, C. A. Leukemic reticuloendotheliosis. *Blood* 13 : 609, 1958.

Champlin, R. et al. Chronic leukemias: Oncogenes, chromosomes, and advances in therapy. *Ann. Intern. Med.* 104 : 671, 1986.

Chapel, H. M., and Bunch C. Mechanisms of infection in chronic lymphocytic leukemia. *Semin. Hematol.* 24 : 291, 1987.

Cooperative group for the study of immunoglobulin in chronic lymphocytic leukemia. Intravenous immunoglobulin for the prevention of infection in chronic lymphocytic leukemia: A randomized, controlled clinical trial. *N. Engl. J. Med.* 319 : 902, 1988.

Delsol, G. et al. Richter's syndrome: Evidence for the clonal origin of the two proliferations. *Am. J. Clin. Pathol.* 76 : 308, 1981.

Flandrin, G. et al. Hairy cell leukemia: Clinical presentation and follow-up of 211 patients. *Semin. Oncol.* 11 (Suppl. 2) : 458, 1984.

Foon, K. A., and Gale, R. P. Staging and therapy of chronic lymphocytic leukemia. *Semin. Hematol.* 24 : 264, 1987.

Foon, K. A. et al. Recombinant leukocyte α-interferon therapy for advanced hairy cell leukemia: Therapeutic and immunologic results. *Am. J. Med.* 80 : 351, 1986.

Foon, K. A. et al. Response to 2-deoxycoformycin after failure of interferon-alpha in nonsplenectomized patients with hairy cell leukemia. *Blood* 68 : 297, 1986.

Foucar, K., and Rydell, R. E. Richter's syndrome in chronic lymphocytic leukemia. *Cancer* 46 : 118, 1980.

Freedman, A. S., and Nadler, L. M. B cell development in chronic lymphocytic leukemia. *Semin. Hematol.* 24 : 230, 1987.

Gale, R. P., and Foon, K. A. Chronic lymphocytic leukemia: Recent advances in biology and treatment. *Ann. Intern. Med.* 103 : 101, 1985.

Ghani, A. M., Krause, J. R., and Brody, J. P. Prolymphocytic transformation of chronic lymphocytic leukemia: A report of three cases and review of the literature. *Cancer* 57 : 75, 1986.

Golde, D. W. et al. Hairy-cell leukemia: Biology and treatment. *Semin. Hematol.* 23 : 3, 1986.

Golomb, H. M., and Hadad, L. J. Infectious complications in 127 patients with hairy cell leukemia. *Am. J. Hematol.* 16 : 393, 1984.

Han, T. et al. Prognostic importance of cytogenetic abnormalities in patients with chronic lymphocytic leukemia. *N. Engl. J. Med.* 310 : 288, 1984.

Jansen, J. et al. Paraproteinaemia plus osteolytic lesions in typical hairy-cell leukaemia. *Br. J. Haematol.* 54 : 531, 1983.

Knutila, S. et al. Trisomy 12 in B cells of patients with B-cell chronic lymphocytic leukemia. *N. Engl. J. Med.* 314 : 865, 1986.

Rai, K. R., and Montserrat, E. Prognostic factors in chronic lymphocytic leukemia. *Semin. Hematol.* 24 : 252, 1987.

Rai, K. R. et al. Clinical staging of chronic lymphocytic leukemia. *Blood* 46 : 219, 1975.

Ratain, M. J. et al. Treatment of hairy cell leukemia with recombinant alpha-2-interferon. *Blood* 65 : 644, 1985.

Scott, O. S. et al. Prolymphocytoid variants of chronic lymphocytic leukemia. *Leuk. Res.* 11 : 135, 1987.

Spiers, A. S. D. et al. Remissions in hairy-cell leukemia with Pentostatin (2-deoxycoformycin). *N. Engl. J. Med.* 319 : 825, 1987.

Westbrook, C. A., and Golde, D. W. Clinical problems in hairy cell leukemia: Diagnosis and management. *Semin. Oncol.* 11 (Suppl. 2) : 514, 1984.

Westbrook, C. A., and Golde, D. W. Autoimmune disease in hairy-cell leukemia: Clinical syndromes and treatment. *Br. J. Haematol.* 61 : 349, 1985.

Miscellaneous Disorders

Azevedo, S. J., and Yunis, A. A. Angioimmunoblastic lymphadenopathy. *Am. J. Hematol.* 20 : 301, 1985.

Bluming, A. Z., Cohen, H. G., and Saxon, A. Angioimmunoblastic lymphadenopathy with dysproteinemia: A pathologic link between physiologic lymphoid proliferation and malignant lymphoma. *Am. J. Med.* 67 : 421, 1979.

Ducatman, B. S., et al. Malignant histiocytosis: A clinical, histologic, and immunohistochemical study of 20 cases. *Hum. Pathol.* 15 : 368, 1984.

Esseltine, D. W., De Leeuw, N. K., and Berry, G. R. Malignant histiocytosis. *Cancer* 52 : 1904, 1983.

Fauci, A. S. et al. Lymphomatoid granulomatosis: Prospective clinical and therapeutic experience over 10 years. *N. Engl. J. Med.* 306 : 68, 1982.

Katzenstein, A.-L. A., Carrington, C. B., and Liebow, A. A. Lymphomatoid granulomatosis: A clinico-pathologic study of 152 cases. *Cancer* 43 : 360, 1979.

Leibow, A. A., Carrington, C. R. B., and Friedman, P. J. Lymphomatoid granulomatosis. *Hum. Pathol.* 3 : 457, 1972.

Lukes, R. J., and Tindle, B. H. Immunoblastic lymphadenopathy: A hyperimmune entity resembling Hodgkin's disease. *N. Engl. J. Med.* 292 : 1, 1975.

Patton, W. F., and Lynch, J. P. Lymphomatoid granulomatosis: Clinicopathologic study of four cases and literature review. *Medicine* 61 : 1, 1982.

Scott, R. B., and Robb-Smith, A. H. Histiocytic medullary reticulosis. *Lancet* 2 : 194, 1939.

Simon, J. H. et al. Malignant histiocytosis: Complete remission in two pediatric patients. *Cancer* 59 : 1566, 1987.

Steinberg, A. D. et al. Angioimmunoblastic lymphadenopathy with dysproteinemia. *Ann. Intern. Med.* 108 : 575, 1988.

Weiss, L. M. et al. Clonal T-cell populations in angioimmunoblastic lymphadenopathy and angioimmunoblastic lymphadenopathy-like lymphoma. *Am. J. Pathol.* 122 : 392, 1986.

Infectious Mononucleosis

Andiman, W. et al. Use of cloned probes to detect Epstein-Barr viral DNA in tissues of patients with neoplastic and lymphoproliferative disease. *J. Infect. Dis.* 148 : 967, 1983.

Cheeseman, S. H. Infectious mononucleosis. *Semin. Hematol.* 25 : 261, 1988.

Hanto, D. W. et al. Epstein-Barr virus induced B-cell lymphoma after renal transplantation. Acyclovir therapy and transition from polyclonal to monoclonal B-cell proliferation. *N. Engl. J. Med.* 306 : 913, 1982.

Purtilo, D. T. et al. Epstein-Barr virus infections in the X-linked recessive lymphoproliferative syndrome. *Lancet* 1 : 798, 1978.

Sullivan, J. L. Epstein-Barr virus and lymphoproliferative disorders. *Semin. Hematol.* 25 : 269, 1988.

Thorley-Lawson, D. A. Basic virological aspects of Epstein-Barr virus infection. *Semin. Hematol.* 25 : 247, 1988.

14 Dysproteinemias

Joseph Paul Eder, Jr.
Lowell E. Schnipper

The plasma cell dyscrasias (PCD) are a family of disorders that result from abnormal proliferation of immunoglobulin-producing cells. The biologic basis of immunoglobulin synthesis and the nature of these diseases have been the subjects of intensive study by clinicians, biochemists, and molecular biologists. In 1845, William MacIntyre and Henry Bence Jones described a urinary substance in a patient with recurring bone pain that precipitated on heating and redissolved on boiling. Otto Kahler was a neurologist and internist whose descriptions of the clinical disorder, myeloma, have linked his name inseparably to this disease in Central Europe. Nobel Laureate Arne Tiselius developed methods of electrophoresis and chromatography that allowed the separation and purification of biochemical substances. Jan Waldenström, a clinician, and K. O. Pederson, a biochemist, joined together to describe two closely related diseases, macroglobulinemia and multiple myeloma. Edelman was awarded a Nobel Prize for determining the structure of immunoglobulins derived from patients with myeloma, and Tonegawa received a Nobel Prize for the first description of the genetic mechanisms that determine immunoglobulin diversity.

Multiple myeloma, the most common malignant PCD, has complex and variable clinical manifestations that are due to the pathophysiologic consequences of overproduction of a single immunoglobulin resulting from uncontrolled proliferation of a clone of terminally differentiated plasma cells in the bone marrow. Less commonly, other PCDs occur that differ from multiple myeloma in clinical manifestations and the type of monoclonal protein that is produced. Since these diseases are so closely intertwined with immunoglobulin synthesis, a complete description of PCDs requires an understanding of immunoglobulin structure and function and the techniques employed in their analysis.

Immunoglobulins

Structure

General features of the major classes of immunoglobulin are shown in Table 14-1. Immunoglobulin (Ig) molecules are symmetrical

Table 14-1. Characteristics of serum immunoglobulins

	IgG	IgA	IgM	IgD	IgE
Molecular weight (daltons)	160,000	170,000	850,000	180,000	196,000
Sedimentation constant (S)	6.6	6.85[a]	19.0	7.0	8.0
Quantity per dL serum in grams	1.2	0.2	0.1	0.003	0.00003
Half-life (days)[b]	20–30	6–7	5–10	3	2

[a]Secretory IgA with transport piece 11.4S; molecular weight 390,000.
[b]Bence Jones protein has half-life of 24 hours.

polypeptides composed of two H (heavy) chains and two L (light) chains. Each half is composed of one H and one L chain and each half is identical to the other. The H chains determine the class specificity of the immunoglobulin molecules; five antigenic types of H chain and the corresponding Ig have been described (see Table 14-1), and these are designated by the Greek letters γ (IgG), α (IgA), μ (IgM), δ (IgD), and ε (IgE). Each can be identified by its reactivity against a known antibody raised against the specific class of Ig molecules to which it belongs. Subclasses based on further immunologic reactivity have been identified. There are four IgG subclasses (IgG$_1$, IgG$_2$, IgG$_3$, IgG$_4$), and two subclasses each for IgA and IgM. L chains are designated as either κ or λ (Igκ and Igλ). Ig molecules are composed of C (constant) and V (variable) regions. The C regions do not differ within a class (or subclass), but the V regions do, and the diversity of these variable regions is responsible for antibody specificity.

Enzymatic cleavage of an IgG molecule with papain produces two unequal fragments. One of the products contains both L chains and half the H chains and is designated the Fab (fragment–antibody-binding) fragment. The other is the Fc (fragment-crystallizable) fragment, which contains the remaining H chain. The Fab fragment binds to a specific antigen and the Fc fragment binds to recognition sites on reticuloendothelial and B cells. IgM differs from IgG in that it is a pentamer composed of five immunoglobulin molecules, and IgA circulates in monomeric and dimeric forms. Both polymeric forms are bound together by a single J (joining) protein. In the course of secretion into body fluids (e.g., tears, saliva, intestinal juice), IgA molecules are modified by epithelial cells through the addition of a secretory component.

Regulation of Immunoglobulin Diversity

At least two different gene segments contribute to each C and V region of heavy and light chains. Those encoding the H chain are located on chromosome 14, κ-chain genes are on chromosome 2, and λ-genes are on 22.

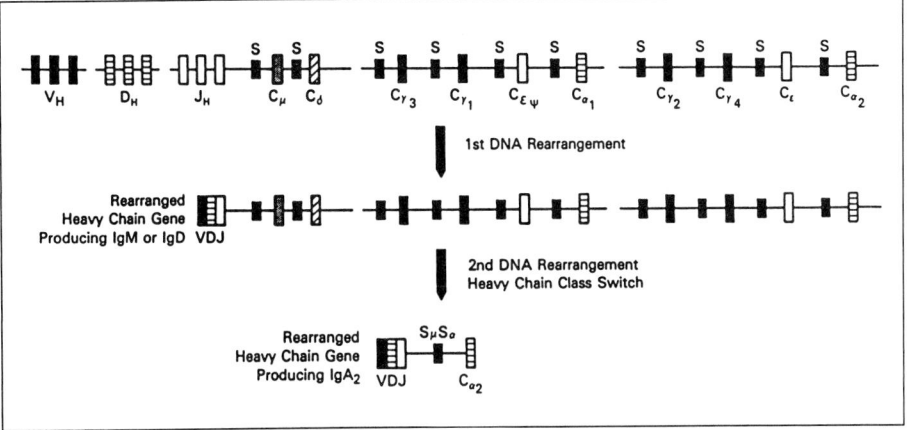

Fig. 14-1. Schematic presentation of the human heavy chain gene locus. The first DNA rearrangement assembles a variable (V_H), diversity $D_{(H)}$, and joining (J_H) region to complete the variable portion of the molecule. Subsequently, a second DNA rearrangement between homologous switch sites (S) can occur, resulting in a heavy chain class switch that moves a more distal constant region next to the assembled VDJ. (From T. T. DeVita, Jr., S. Hellman, and S. A. Rosenberg (eds.), *Important Advances in Oncology 1987.* Philadelphia: Lippincott, 1987. Reproduced with permission.)

The first step in Ig production is H-chain rearrangement, which marks the cell's commitment to the B cell lineage (Fig. 14-1). One of 20 or more diversity (D) genes is transposed next to one of six joining (J) region genes on both chromosomes 14. If a DJ rearrangement is successfully completed, one of the 50 variable (V) region genes on only one of the chromosomes is translocated to form a continuous VDJ_H complex, which can encode the entire variable region of the H chain. Splicing of transcripts is another mechanism that contributes to differential Ig gene expression. In this process RNA transcribed from introns (noncoding regions) is removed, leaving only the RNA from coding regions (exons) to be transported to the ribosomes for translation. Following removal of introns between the VDJ_H complex and the constant region of the μ heavy chain, the μ heavy chain can be translated.

The next step in Ig gene rearrangement occurs on chromosome 2, which encodes the variable region of the κ-chain (Fig. 14-2). DNA fragments from the distinct V and J segments undergo a rearrangement to encode the κ light chain variable region. If a productive VJ rearrangement does not occur, there will be an attempt to undergo a rearrangement on chromosome 22, the locus of the λ-chain. Successful generation of a κ- or λ-chain allows it to bind to the heavy chain to make a complete IgM monomer. This molecule is then transported to the cell surface, where its expression marks the early

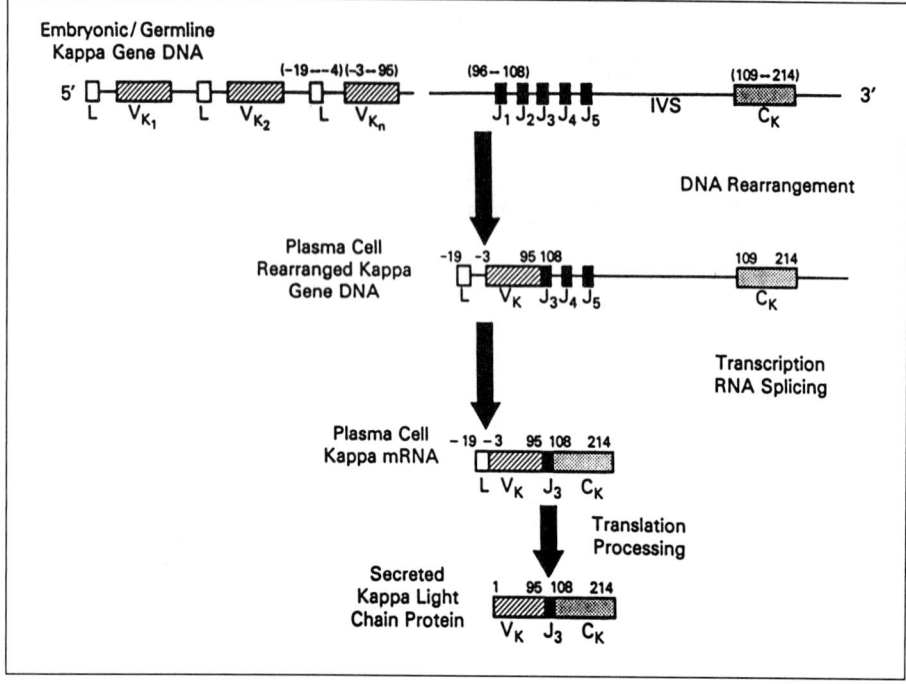

Fig. 14-2. Schematic presentation of the human κ-gene locus. Multiple germline variable (V_K) regions exist with accompanying leader (*L*) sequences. Five alternative joining (J_K) segments each encode amino acids 96–108. There is but one constant (C_K) region per allele. During B cell development, a DNA rearrangement joins a selected V_K and J_K segment. This rearranged allele is transcribed, and the remaining intervening sequences (*IVS*) are removed by RNA splicing. mRNA, messenger RNA. (From V. T. DeVita, Jr., S. Hellman, and S. A. Rosenberg (eds.), *Important Advances in Oncology 1987.* Philadelphia: Lippincott, 1987. Reproduced with permission.)

stage of B cell development. B lymphocytes in an individual cell clone can switch from producing IgM to IgG or IgA with identical variable region binding specificity. When antigen-stimulated B cells lose surface area and begin to accumulate IgG, they become intermediate and then mature B cells, the final step before terminal differentiation to a plasma cell.

In PCDs the production of Ig continues despite the absence of antigenic stimulation, presumably due to uncontrolled lymphocyte or plasma cell proliferation. The generation of normal Igs is often lower than normal in PCDs, leading to functional hypogammaglobulinemia and susceptibility to infection, even though the *total* immunoglobulin level may be very high because of the presence of an abnormal protein derived from the neoplastic cells.

Analysis of Serum Proteins

ELECTROPHORESIS

The electrophoresis of normal serum through a colloid suspension such as cellulose acetate or agarose produces distinct protein bands. Albumin migrates farthest toward the anode while Ig bands remain near the cathode. The major bands seen are albumin, the α_1 fraction (60–70% of which is α_1-antitrypsin), the α_2 fraction, the β fraction (including transferrin, β-lipoprotein, and the C_3 component of complement), and the γ-globulin fraction (predominantly IgG). The other subclasses of Ig usually migrate in the γ-globulin region, but occasionally move farther toward the anode into the β and α_2 regions.

IMMUNOELECTROPHORESIS

Immunoelectrophoresis uses differences in both electrophoretic mobility and antigenic characteristics to identify Ig classes and subclasses. After electrophoresis in a gel, purified anti-Ig serum is placed in wells adjacent to the protein bands, permitting the proteins to diffuse toward the antibody along a concentration gradient until precipitin lines form. These precipitin lines are characterized by shape, size, location, and the specific antisera used. The presence of a monoclonal immunoglobulin—a homogeneous protein produced by a single clone of Ig-producing cells—is detected on immunoelectrophoresis by thickening and shortening of the normal precipitin line. The characterization of the protein is determined by discerning its reaction against specific anti-λ or κ-chain sera, and antibodies against the various heavy-chain classes, IgG, IgA, IgM, and so forth.

The quantity of each serum Ig can be determined by radial immunodiffusion. In this technique anti-Ig is mixed with agar and placed in a Petri dish. Known concentrations of Ig are put in separate wells to generate a standard curve. Precipitin lines form in a circle around each well as the material diffuses into the antibody-impregnated agar; the higher the Ig concentration in the well, the larger will be the diameter of the precipitin circle. The concentration of Ig in unknown samples loaded into other wells is estimated by comparing the diameters of the precipitin arcs formed to a standard curve derived as described above. Using a different Petri dish for each Ig type, the concentration of the five classes can be determined. Concentrations of Ig can also be assayed by nephelometry. In this technique antibodies against each of the Ig classes are added to a solution of the test serum, and the resulting turbidity produced by precipitation of these antibodies with the corresponding Ig type is quantitated spectrophotometrically.

Immunoglobulins in Multiple Myeloma

The Ig abnormalities of multiple myeloma and the other PCDs include suppression of normal Ig synthesis, increased normal Ig catabolism, and the presence in the serum or urine, or both, of monoclonal protein(s), which may be complete Ig or components of Ig, such as free L chains. They appear as "M" (myeloma or monoclonal) spikes, homogeneous peaks observed after densitometric scanning of the serum electrophoretogram. Immunoelectrophoresis that determines the L chain subtype can help decide whether an electrophoretic peak is due to a monoclonal protein. The normal κ : λ ratio in a polyclonal Ig pool is 60 : 40. If only one light chain type is present, the Ig is monoclonal. Approximately 80 to 90 percent of patients with myeloma have a serum M spike. About 75 percent of patients have free L chains in the urine (Bence Jones proteinuria); these are best detected by electrophoresis of the urine. About 10 percent of patients have light chain production only and 1 to 2 percent have a nonsecretory variant in which no abnormal protein is produced. In most patients with fully expressed multiple myeloma, normal serum Ig levels are depressed due to the production of cytokines, which inhibit B cell growth and function.

Somewhat over 50 percent of M proteins are IgG and 21 percent are IgA. Immunoglobulin M disorders account for about 12 percent of PCDs. IgM myeloma is rare and the clinical picture associated with an IgM paraprotein is usually that of Waldenström's macroglobulinemia. Immunoglobulin D myeloma accounts for 2 percent of cases and IgE for fewer than 0.01 percent of patients with multiple myeloma.

Multiple Myeloma

Multiple myeloma (MM) is a malignant neoplasm that is characterized by unregulated proliferation of a monoclonal population of plasma cells, the clinical consequences of which result from an increasing tumor cell mass in bones, bone marrow, and extraosseous sites; the production of vast excesses of monoclonal immunoglobulin; and the underproduction of normal immunoglobulins.

Incidence

Multiple myeloma is a rare disease that accounts for 1 percent of the hematologic malignancies in the United States. Its incidence is correlated with increasing age, and 98 percent of cases occur after age 40. When compared with whites in the United States, African-Americans have a twofold higher incidence of MM. This observation may relate to the higher average immunoglobulin levels in blacks, representing a larger pool of B cells at risk for undergoing malignant transformation.

Predisposing Factors

Genetic factors may be important since first-degree relatives of patients have an increased incidence of both MM and asymptomatic M spikes. Since environmental factors have not been excluded, this area requires further study. As was demonstrated in Japanese atomic bomb survivors, exposure to high doses of ionizing irradiation (≥ 100 cGy) increases the risk of MM after a 20-year latency period.

Diagnosis

The differential diagnosis of MM includes an abundance of benign and malignant disorders. Monoclonal Igs (presumably benign in nature) are frequent in the elderly, with an M-component being observed on the serum protein electrophoresis in 5 percent of healthy individuals over the age of 70. They have been described in patients with autoimmune diseases, and a monoclonal IgM peak is detected in approximately 5 percent of patients with B cell lymphoma and chronic lymphocytic leukemia.

The main criteria for the diagnosis of MM are 30 percent or greater infiltration of the bone marrow by plasma cells (Plate 52) and a monoclonal M spike consisting of at least 3.5 gm/dL IgG, 2.0 gm/dL IgA, or excretion of 1.0 gm per 24 hours or more of κ or λ light chains in the urine (so-called Bence Jones proteinuria). These are general guidelines, and some patients with MM have smaller numbers of plasma cells or lower concentrations of M protein. Many patients have significant depression of normal Ig levels and lytic bone lesions, although the absence of either of these does not preclude the diagnosis. The presence of multiple myeloma is often confirmed by observing clear progression of disease in a previously asymptomatic patient with a monoclonal protein.

The presence of progressive, symptomatic disease is crucial in distinguishing between MM and MGUS (monoclonal gammopathy of unknown significance, previously called benign monoclonal gammopathy). MGUS patients have no symptoms, no bone lesions, marrow plasmacytosis of 10 percent or less, serum M-components usually 3.5 gm/dL or less for IgG and 2.0 gm/dL or less for IgA, and rarely demonstrate substantial Bence Jones proteinuria. The conversion of MGUS to MM occurs at a rate of 2 percent per year, indicating that in many patients malignant disease will never develop. It is appropriate to evaluate patients with MGUS at 1- to 2-month intervals for the first year, after which biannual follow-up study will suffice if the M-component has remained stable.

As is the case for most cancers, total body tumor burden in MM is an important prognostic indicator for survival and response to therapy. Most commonly used is the Durie-Salmon staging system (Table 14-2), which correlates total body plasma cell mass with the clinical features in MM. The median survival is approximately 4 years for Stage I patients, 2.7 years for Stage II, and 2 years for Stage III. Within each staging group, the higher the fraction of plasma cells undergoing DNA synthesis (labeling index), the shorter will be the survival. Subclassification by degree of azotemia is important since Stage A patients (BUN <30 mg%) have about a 3-year survival and B patients (BUN >30 mg%) slightly less than 1 year. β_2-Microglobulin is another important prognostic indicator in MM. This protein is the light chain of the HLA antigen and, when corrected for renal function, serum levels correlate strongly with tumor burden and prognosis in MM.

Clinical Manifestations

Multiple myeloma is a malignant neoplasm that results from monoclonal proliferation of plasma cells. The clinical manifestations of the disease are best understood by considering them to result from an expanding plasma cell mass in the bone marrow, on the one hand, and factors produced by these cells, for example, monoclonal immunoglobulin, Bence Jones protein (i.e., free light chains), and osteoclast activating factor, on the other.

Table 14-2. Simplified myeloma staging system

Stage	Criteria
I	All of following:
	1. Hemoglobin > 10 gm/dL
	2. Serum calcium normal
	3. Normal bones or solitary bone plasmacytoma
	4. M-component:
	a. IgG < 5 gm/dL
	b. IgA < 3 gm/dL
	c. Urine light chains < 4 gm/24 hr
II	Neither stage I nor III
III	One of following:
	1. Hemoglobin < 8.5 gm/dL
	2. Serum calcium > 12 gm/dL
	3. Advanced lytic bone lesions
	4. M-component:
	a. IgG > 7 gm/dL
	b. IgA > 5 gm/dL
	c. Urine light chains > 12 gm/24 hr
Subclassification	
A. Serum creatinine < 2.0 mg/dL	
B. Serum creatinine > 2.0 mg/dL	

Adapted from M. M. Wintrobe (ed.), *Clinical Hematology* (8th ed.). Philadelphia: Lea & Febiger, 1981.

OSSEOUS DISEASE

The vast majority of patients with MM presents with or eventually develops skeletal manifestations that result from diffuse or focal areas of osteolysis in anatomic relation to expanding masses of plasma cells in the bone marrow. Clinically, they present with localized areas of bone pain or swelling, or both, in conjunction with marked bone tenderness. Back pain is particularly common, and may be associated with intractable discomfort that represents a pathologic fracture. Compression fractures of the vertebrae are often seen and are a cause of the patient losing several inches in height. Some early bone lesions that are demonstrable by x-ray are asymptomatic.

On x-ray the most classic observation is the appearance of skeletal lucencies with clearly demarcated borders, so-called punched-out lesions. There is little osteoblastic activity or periosteal reaction, unlike the situation in most other neoplasms that have metastases to bone. In some patients, bone x-rays demonstrate diffuse osteoporosis, but if microradiography were done it would reveal extensive bone destruction. Bone scintigraphy (i.e., bone scanning) is less sensitive than routine x-rays in demonstrating bone involvement by MM, presumably due to the minimal osteoblastic activity and hypovascularity associated with this disease. In the setting of MM and bone pain in which routine radiography of the skeleton is normal, high-resolution computerized tomography (CT) or magnetic resonance imaging (MRI) often permits visualization of lesions that are present early in the course of illness.

Solitary osseous myeloma (SOM) is a variant of the skeletal disease associated with MM. This entity comprises 3 to 5 percent of all patients with plasma cell neoplasia and often presents as pain and tenderness at the site of the bone lesion. There is radiologic evidence of a single area of bone destruction and there may be accompanying neurologic signs due to nerve root compression, radiculopathy, or spinal cord compression. Many of these patients do not have a demonstrable M-component (75%), and among those who do, it is usually less than 1.5 gm/dL. The detectable paraprotein often disappears after radiation therapy. Unfortunately, in many of these patients typical MM develops within 10 years; this risk is greater in those patients in whom the M protein fails to disappear after radiation treatment.

A frequent accompaniment of myelomatous bone involvement is hypercalcemia. Both the bone lysis and the elevations in serum calcium have a humoral basis. Myeloma cells secrete what previously was called "osteoclast activating factor" (OAF). OAF now seems to comprise several cytokines, of which interleukin-1 and tumor necrosis factor are examples; both of these can produce bone lysis. Serum calcium is elevated in 30 percent of patients with MM at presentation, and rises above normal in another 30 percent throughout the course of the illness, roughly correlating with a large tumor burden. Hypercalcemia is often precipitated by the enforced bed rest resulting from painful bone lesions, and can be exacerbated by dehydration. Consequently, both are to be avoided if possible.

HEMATOLOGIC CONSEQUENCES OF MM

At the inception of the illness, the most frequent finding is a normocytic, normochromic anemia. Rouleaux formation is discernible in the peripheral blood smears of patients with high levels of immunoglobulins (Plate 82). Sometimes one can observe with the naked eye a blue background on the slide, due to elevated serum protein concentrations. The reticulocyte count is typically low, and the erythroid suppression may worsen as a function of disease progression or chemotherapy, or both. Leukopenia and thrombocytopenia are frequent, especially as the myeloma cell burden expands in the marrow space, or as the patient is exposed to radiation or chemotherapy. Although serious bleeding is usually due to thrombocytopenia and can often be avoided by platelet transfusions, bleeding will occasionally occur because of interactions between the M-component and clotting factors, or defective platelet function secondary to coating of platelets by immunoglobulin.

Severe neutropenia is an important contributor to the development of bacterial infection, a predisposition that is enhanced by the functional hypogammaglobulinemia that is so often present. The mechanisms underlying the impairment in humoral immunity are probably twofold: an increased rate of normal immunoglobulin catabolism and the production by plasma cells of factors that stimulate macrophages to produce inhibitors of B cell proliferation. These factors appear to include a variety of cytokines including tumor necrosis factor.

RENAL MANIFESTATIONS OF MM
Myeloma Nephropathy
Dense tubular casts are a hallmark of "myeloma kidney," which is typically associated with the urinary excretion of free light chains (Bence Jones proteins). These casts contain immunoglobulin and mucoprotein, and are associated with atrophy of the tubular epithelium. The tubular basement membrane may be ruptured, with interstitial inflammation and fibrosis. Light chains have a direct toxic effect on the tubules; highly cationic protein residues in the variable region are implicated, accounting for the diverse pattern of this complication. Renal failure can be precipitated in patients with MM by acute dehydration, which may occur with preparation for an x-ray study employing iodinated dyes, fever secondary to infection, or hypercalcemia. Dehydration facilitates precipitation of light

chains in tubules, which sometimes is compounded by coprecipitation with calcium. Although light chain nephropathy is an ominous development, acute renal failure arising in the setting of dehydration is sometimes partially reversible by restoration of renal perfusion.

Glomerular Lesions

In some patients with MM, cumulative deposition of the paraprotein in the mesangium develops, resulting in glomerulosclerosis. The morphology is characterized by coarse granular deposits that stain with antibodies to immunoglobulin and κ- or λ-chains and are located at the inner aspect of the glomerular basement membrane. The mechanism by which glomerular damage is produced is not understood.

Renal Amyloidosis

Other glomerular lesions found in some patients with MM are renal amyloid deposits. This material can be found in tubular basement membranes, renal vessels, the interstitium, and, particularly, glomeruli. The glomerular lesions can be associated with nephrotic syndrome in which mixed serum proteins including large amounts of albumin are excreted in the urine. Amyloidosis, which occurs in less than 10 percent of patients with MM, is associated with light-chain production, the light chains in these patients forming the nidus for amyloid deposition in the kidneys and other tissues.

Hypercalcemic Nephropathy

Renal failure in MM often occurs in a setting of hypercalcemia, which causes a failure of renal concentrating ability. This cause of renal insufficiency, unlike the others mentioned, is usually reversible with saline diuresis, loop diuretics, and, most important, control of the underlying cause of the hypercalcemia, that is, the MM.

Other, unusual causes of renal impairment in MM include uric acid stones or nephropathy and direct invasion of the kidney by malignant plasma cells.

The institution of hemodialysis in MM patients with irreversible, profound renal failure is justified if the prospects for systemic control of the MM are good. This management approach has ameliorated the dire consequences otherwise imposed by renal failure, although this complication remains a poor prognostic omen in patients with MM.

NEUROLOGIC COMPLICATIONS

Spinal cord compression is almost always secondary to osseous involvement of vertebrae or ribs in association with an epidural mass. Back or radicular pain is a frequent prelude to this dreaded complication. The importance of prompt diagnosis cannot be overstated, since the neurologic deficits can often progress to complete paraplegia within hours or days. Suspicion of cord compression based on new neurologic signs should stimulate the prompt initiation of CT or MRI scans or myelography to confirm the diagnosis and delineate the upper and lower extent of the lesion(s).

The usual emergent therapy for spinal cord compression is high-dose dexamethasone followed by radiation therapy once the anatomic extent of the lesion is appreciated. Laminectomy is indicated in the circumstance of relapsing cord compression, when further radiation is contraindicated.

Treatment

Multiple myeloma is an incurable disease with a variable survival of about 1 to 15 years, with a median of about 3 years. Initially, some patients may be asymptomatic and in stable condition and do not require treatment for variable periods of time. When symptoms occur, many patients derive considerable relief from chemotherapy, radiotherapy, and supportive care. Relief of bony pain and the prevention of severe fractures and spinal cord compression are the first objectives. Lytic bone disease is treated with chemotherapy or sometimes radiotherapy. Over time, the disease becomes less responsive to therapy, and disease progression in addition to infectious or renal complications results in death.

Objective response to chemotherapy is generally easy to measure because the protein products of the tumor mass are readily quantitated. There must be a significant ($\geq 75\%$) reduction in the serum M-component and/or 90 percent or greater reduction in BJ protein-uria in addition to improvement of anemia, hypoalbuminemia, and hypercalcemia, if present, for an optimal response. Using these strict criteria, about 50 percent of patients treated with chemotherapy will have an objective response. Bone lesions usually do not heal but stabilize with effective therapy.

Alkylating agents (AA), including melphalan, cyclophosphamide, and carmustine, are widely used in MM. These drugs are active against nonproliferating and proliferating cells, and are cytotoxic by cross-linking DNA strands via alkyl bridges. In addition, depurination of alkylated bases or tautomerization of nucleotide bases and subsequent mismatched base pairing may occur. These highly reactive species also bind to cytoplasmic, nuclear, and membrane proteins. In addition to their cytotoxic effects, AAs are mutagenic and late myelodysplasia or leukemia is a real concern.

Vincristine is a periwinkle alkaloid that inhibits mitotic tubule assembly but also affects nonproliferating cells. It is not myelosuppressive or mutagenic, and can be used in combination with AAs. Peripheral neuropathy is the major toxicity.

Doxorubicin is an anthracycline alkaloid that is cytotoxic to cells by several mechanisms, including free radical formation and DNA intercalation and unwinding that result in impaired transcription and DNA cleavage. It is myelosuppressive, a severe vesicant (causing local skin necrosis if extravasated), and causes a cardiomyopathy at high cumulative doses.

Prednisone is a synthetic glucocorticoid that is very valuable in the treatment of MM. It blocks the activation of osteoclasts by cytokines and thus decreases bone resorption and hypercalcemia. It causes catabolism of the MM protein and reduces serum and urinary M-components. Prednisone is cytolytic to plasma cells and does not cause myelosuppression.

Melphalan and prednisone (M+P), used together every 4 to 6 weeks, give a response rate of 50 to 60 percent. The addition of other drugs to melphalan and prednisone is of less certain value, but may be helpful in patients with large or rapidly growing tumor burdens in whom a more rapid response is desirable. It may take 3 to 4 months to achieve a measurable response, particularly with conservative therapy such as M+P, and this can be maintained for months to years, often including a long interval without therapy once a maximal therapeutic response has been achieved.

Therapy with M+P is continued for 1 to 2 years and then stopped if serum and urine M-components have been stable for 6 months and no signs of active disease are present. The ideal duration of treatment is unknown and no survival benefit accrues in patients continued on M+P indefinitely. All patients will eventually relapse after chemotherapy is stopped. Some studies suggest that α_2-interferon given to patients in remission or with stable disease prolongs remission duration and may have an overall survival benefit. When disease progression recurs, M+P therapy is reinstituted and is often effective again for variable periods of time. (Pulsed high dose dexamethasone is an alternative therapy.)

Approximately 40 percent of patients at the initiation of therapy and virtually all who initially respond will ultimately manifest resistance to chemotherapy. A useful salvage regimen of vincristine, doxorubicin, and dexamethasone (VAD) will produce responses in 40 to 70 percent of such patients, sometimes for up to 9 months. Resistance to vincristine and doxorubicin is associated with overexpression of a membrane glycoprotein (p170), the multidrug resistance factor, which actively pumps these drugs out of the cell, preventing cytotoxic concentrations from being achieved. Experimental findings suggest that such drug resistance may be overcome by the addition of the calcium channel blocker, verapamil, or cyclosporin.

Special Complications of MM

THE HYPERVISCOSITY SYNDROME (HVS)

HVS is caused by elevated levels of serum proteins that have a high intrinsic viscosity, and is usually manifest at serum viscosity levels greater than 4 centipoises (Cp). It is unusual in MM and is most common in the setting of Waldenström's macroglobulinemia, which is characterized by marked overproduction of monoclonal IgM protein. In MM it is associated with overproduction of IgG_1 and IgG_3 proteins, since the relevant heavy chains within these categories have a propensity to aggregate. For similar reasons HVS is also observed in IgA myeloma, particularly when the M-component exceeds 5 gm%. The clinical picture of HVS is characterized by fatigue, headache, sluggish mentation, and visual disturbances. These can be compounded by vascular effects of sludging such as myocardial ischemia and purpura. It is important to be alert for the signs of HVS since plasmapheresis can be lifesaving.

CRYOGLOBULINEMIA

Cryoglobulinemia is caused by the precipitation of immunoglobulins on cooling. This is seen in fewer than 10 percent of patients with MM. Eighty percent of patients have cutaneous manifestations, such as purpura, Raynaud's phenomenon, digital necrosis, livedo reticularis, or urticaria. Arthralgias, nephritis, and neurologic complications may occur particularly in "essential mixed cryoglobulinemia" (described below). Type I cryoglobulinemia is due to the intrinsic cryoprecipitable nature of certain monoclonal IgM, IgG, or IgA proteins and may occur in macroglobulinemia, MM, lymphomas, or MGUS. Type II is due to a monoclonal Ig, usually IgM, with rheumatoid factor activity; thus, the cryoglobulin consists of immune complexes of the monoclonal protein and polyclonal immunoglobulins. This disorder is seen in patients with diseases similar to those causing type I cryoglobulinemia and in some patients with autoimmune diseases, hepatitis, and other conditions. Type III cryoglobulinemia is due to polyclonal Igs, one of which, usually an IgM protein, has rheumatoid factor activity. This disorder is also due to immune complexes, and may occur in patients with chronic inflammatory disease, infection, or autoimmune diseases. "Essential mixed cryoglobulinemia" is found in patients with type II or III cryoproteins who have no discernible underlying disease. However, recent studies have implicated the hepatitis C virus in many patients with this syndrome.

BLEEDING DISORDERS

Bleeding disorders are less common in IgG MM than in IgA MM or macroglobulinemia. Immunoglobulin coating of platelets reduces their adhesiveness and makes platelet factor III unavailable. The Fab fragment of the M protein may bind to fibrinogen and prevent polymerization of monomeric fibrin. Amyloid deposits may bind factor X and inhibit clotting. Cryoglobulins and hyperviscosity can impair adequate hemostasis by interfering with small blood vessel perfusion and hence endothelial integrity.

INFECTIONS

Frequent infections with encapsulated gram positive organisms such as *Streptococcus pneumoniae* and *Haemophilus influenzae* occur frequently in MM because of the decrease in normal immunoglobulins. Gram negative rod infections occur with progressive refractory disease, especially when complicated by azotemia. Patients with MM have an impaired primary antibody response and decreased levels of normal Ig. Plasma cells themselves secrete factors or induce macrophages to secrete factors, such as tumor necrosis factor, that suppress B cell proliferation and Ig production. Patients have increased suppressor T cells, which bind the M-component's Fc receptor epitope, thereby further decreasing B cell function. There is relative sparing of cell-mediated immunity. Neutropenia, due to marrow infiltration or the effects of chemotherapy, or both, also predisposes these patients to infection.

ACUTE NONLYMPHOCYTIC LEUKEMIA

Acute nonlymphocytic leukemia may occur in up to 30 percent of patients with MM at 15 years. The sequential presentation of MM and acute leukemia suggests that progression to leukemia may be part of the natural history of MM. It has been hypothesized that this reflects the origin of MM from primordial pluripotential stem cells, although this is primarily speculation. Alkylating agents and radiotherapy are leukemogenic and probably contribute to the high frequency of this complication with time.

Natural History of MM

After an initial high mortality, MM patients die at a constant but inexorable rate. Death during the chronic phase while normal bone marrow reserves are present can occur because of progressive myeloma with renal failure or infection, or both. In the terminal phase, patients develop pancytopenia due to infiltration of the bone marrow by a rapidly expanding plasma cell burden, compounded by profound hypogammaglobulinemia, and usually succumb to infection, uremia, or second tumors, particularly leukemia. Since patients with MM are older (median age is about 60), ischemic vascular disease and other degenerative diseases also cause substantial mortality.

Waldenström's Macroglobulinemia

Waldenström's macroglobulinemia is a neoplasm characterized by monoclonal proliferation of lymphocytoid plasma cells ("plymphocytes") (Plate 53) in association with increased serum levels of a monoclonal IgM. It differs from MM in that patients have hepatosplenomegaly and lymphadenopathy but no lytic bone lesions; that is, they have a clinical picture similar to that of an indolent lymphoma. Hyperviscosity due to the large pentameric molecule is a major complication in many of these patients. In some patients with IgM, renal lesions develop, due to glomerular deposition of IgM; light chain excretion is an infrequent occurrence. A stable asymptomatic chronic phase may last for years. Symptoms, when they develop, can sometimes be controlled by reducing the tumor burden using chemotherapy similar to that employed in MM. Plasmapheresis is reserved for emergent management of the hyperviscosity syndrome, since it is a reliable means of rapidly reducing plasma levels of IgM, which is largely intravascular in distribution.

Heavy Chain Disease

The heavy chain diseases (HCDs) are chronic lymphoproliferative diseases characterized by production of an abnormal H chain that has an intact Fc receptor with a deleted amino terminal end. No L chains are produced. The large H chain fragments do not appear in the urine unless they are less than 60,000 daltons. Though uncommon, the three types of HCD are associated with characteristic clinical syndromes.

α-Chain Disease

Unlike MM, the peak of incidence of α-chain disease is the second and third decade. This is an enteric disease that is most common in tropical climates and the Mediterranean littoral, where viral, bacterial, and parasitic diseases are frequent. There is chronic diarrhea due to severe small intestinal malabsorption, with steatorrhea, dehydration, and electrolyte losses. Fever, abdominal pain with frequent abdominal masses, and weight loss are other presenting features. Lymphoplasmacytic infiltration of the small bowel wall, with villous atrophy and effacement of mesenteric and retroperitoneal lymph nodes due to infiltration with lymphoplasmacytic cells are observed. Serum electrophoresis shows hypoalbuminemia and hypogammaglobulinemia with a monoclonal band. On immunoelectrophoresis this band reacts with anti-IgA, but not anti-κ or anti-λ chains.

Complete regression of the disease has been noted in some cases, although α-chain disease is usually progressive and fatal. Curiously, while some regressions are due to chemotherapy, others have been associated with antibiotic therapy.

γ-*Chain Disease*

γ-Chain disease occurs mainly in older patients, who present with nonspecific findings, such as fever, weight loss, anemia, lymphadenopathy, and hepatosplenomegaly. Palatal lymphadenopathy with pancytopenia and hypogammaglobulinemia with a paraprotein band on serum electrophoresis are often found. This band, on immunoelectrophoresis, reacts with anti-IgG but not with anti-κ or anti-λ chain reagents. Infection or Hodgkin's disease may be suspected initially. The course is variable with some patients surviving up to 5 years but no therapy is of established value.

μ-*Chain Disease*

μ-Chain disease is an extremely rare variant of chronic lymphocytic leukemia (CLL). Patients are older, rarely have lymphadenopathy, and have vacuolated plasma cells in the marrow, and most excrete monoclonal μ-chains in the urine since the μ heavy chain fragment is relatively small. Sometimes a small M spike is seen on serum electrophoresis. Immunoelectrophoresis is again necessary to establish the diagnosis. The treatment is that of CLL.

Case Development Problem: Dysproteinemias

As part of an evaluation for anemia in a 60-year-old man, a serum protein electrophoresis pattern is obtained that shows a tall, thin spike at the most cathodal end of the pattern. Normal immunoglobulins appear to be depressed. On immunoelectrophoresis a thickening and distortion of the IgG precipitin band is seen. The immunoelectrophoretic pattern when anti-κ and anti-λ typing serum is used shows only λ chains. Radial diffusion immunoassay reveals five times the normal amount of IgG and decreased quantities of IgM and IgA.

1. Using these data, characterize the abnormal protein spike.

   This patient has a monoclonal IgG immunoglobulin with λ-L chains and γ-mobility on electrophoresis.

2. What studies would you do to determine whether the patient has malignant lymphoma, multiple myeloma, or Waldenström's macroglobulinemia?

Bone marrow or lymph node examination would be most helpful. A finding of infiltrates of lymphocytes would favor malignant lymphoma, although most monoclonal proteins associated with lymphoma are IgM rather than IgG; "plymphocytes" would suggest macroglobulinemia, although this diagnosis is quite improbable with an IgG rather than an IgM paraprotein; and plasmacytosis, particularly with abnormal or multinucleated forms, would suggest multiple myeloma. A skeletal survey is helpful, because the typical osteolytic lesions of myeloma are infrequently or rarely seen in malignant lymphoma or Waldenström's macroglobulinemia. Lymphadenopathy and hepatosplenomegaly favor lymphoma or Waldenström's macroglobulinemia.

3. List factors that may lead to renal insufficiency in patients with multiple myeloma.

   a. Direct infiltration of kidney with myelomatous tumor (rare)
   b. Hypercalcemia
   c. Hyperuricemia with uric acid nephropathy, uric acid stones, and obstructive uropathy
   d. Toxicity and precipitation of Bence Jones protein in renal tubules ("myeloma kidney")
   e. Development of amyloidosis
   f. Susceptibility to chronic, recurrent renal infections due to immune system dysfunction
   g. Glomerular abnormalities due to inspissation of immunoglobulin

4. Your patient develops bleeding from the nose and gums. What mechanisms could cause this abnormal bleeding tendency?

   a. Interference with the last stages of clotting, due to the presence of the abnormal immunoglobulin
   b. Thrombocytopenia due to infiltration of the bone marrow or chemotherapy
   c. Coating of platelets with immunoglobulin, thereby interfering with function

The patient's skeletal survey shows diffuse osteopenia with discrete lytic lesions in the pelvis and calvarium. His bone marrow shows sheets of atypical plasma cells.

5. What is the most likely diagnosis, and how would you treat this patient?

The most likely diagnosis is multiple myeloma. Treatment should be chemotherapy with an alkylating agent, such as melphalan, and prednisone, as well as treatment of dehydration, hypercalcemia, hyperuricemia, and renal failure, if present.

Before treatment is instituted, the patient is noted to have Raynaud's phenomenon, with blanching and pain in his finger tips following exposure to cold.

6. What is the probable mechanism for this phenomenon?

A cryoglobulin that precipitates from the plasma at low temperature, thereby plugging small capillaries and causing tissue anoxia. In this instance the M protein has cryoprecipitable properties.

Topics for Discussion: Dysproteinemias

Immunologic and structural characterization of immunoglobulins
Hyperviscosity syndrome
Cryoproteins—structure, function, and abnormalities
The immune system in plasma cell dyscrasias
Leukemic phase of multiple myeloma
Heavy chain diseases
Myeloma kidney
Primary amyloidosis
Leukemia and other malignancies as a consequence of chemotherapy and radiotherapy

Selected Readings

Buzaid, A. C., and Drurie, B. G. M. Management of refractory myeloma: A review. *J. Clin. Oncol.* 6 : 889, 1988.

Drurie, B. G. M., and Salmon, S. E. The current status and future prospects of treatment for multiple myeloma. *Clin. Haematol.* 11 : 181, 1982.

Farhangi, M. (ed.). Plasma cell myeloma and the myeloma proteins. *Semin. Oncol.* XIII, 1986.

Johnson, W. J. et al. Treatment of renal failure associated with multiple myeloma. *Arch. Intern. Med.* 150 : 863, 1990.

Kyle, R. A. Diagnosis and management of multiple myeloma and related disorders. *Prog. Hematol.* 14 : 257, 1986.

15 Hemostasis and Thrombosis
Kenneth A. Bauer

Normal Hemostasis

Hemostasis is initiated by vascular injury and culminates in the formation of a firm platelet-fibrin barrier that prevents the escape of blood from the damaged vessel. Vascular damage exposes subendothelial structures to flowing blood, and blood platelets adhere and aggregate on the injured site. Simultaneously, coagulation proteins are sequentially activated to generate thrombin. Thrombin cleaves plasma fibrinogen into fibrin monomers, and these polymerize to form a fibrin mesh over the adherent, aggregated platelets. Blood loss is thereby minimized. Platelet contractile activity then draws the attached fibrin polymers more tightly over the injured vascular surface and away from the luminal blood flow. These hemostatic processes are optimally effective in constricted blood vessels. Plasmin, the active fibrinolytic enzyme generated on fibrin polymers, subsequently hydrolyzes the fibrin to soluble fragments. Properly constructed and metabolically intact vascular wall components, adequate numbers of functional platelets, and sufficient quantities of coagulation proteins are all necessary for normal hemostasis.

Blood Vessels

Endothelial cells line blood vessel walls and synthesize von Willebrand factor (vWF) multimers (Fig. 15-1). These multimers are composed of 230,000-dalton monomers covalently linked by disulfide bonds into structures with molecular weights in the millions of daltons. *vWF multimers* are secreted into the circulation or onto the collagen-containing subendothelium. Following endothelial cell damage and subendothelial exposure, platelets bind to vWF multimers and collagen to initiate hemostasis.

Endothelial cells also synthesize and secrete prostaglandin I_2 (PGI_2 or prostacyclin), a vasodilator that prevents excessive platelet accumulation and occlusive platelet thrombi on subendothelial surfaces after minor vascular injury. PGI_2 stimulates platelet membrane adenylate cyclase and increases platelet cyclic adenosine

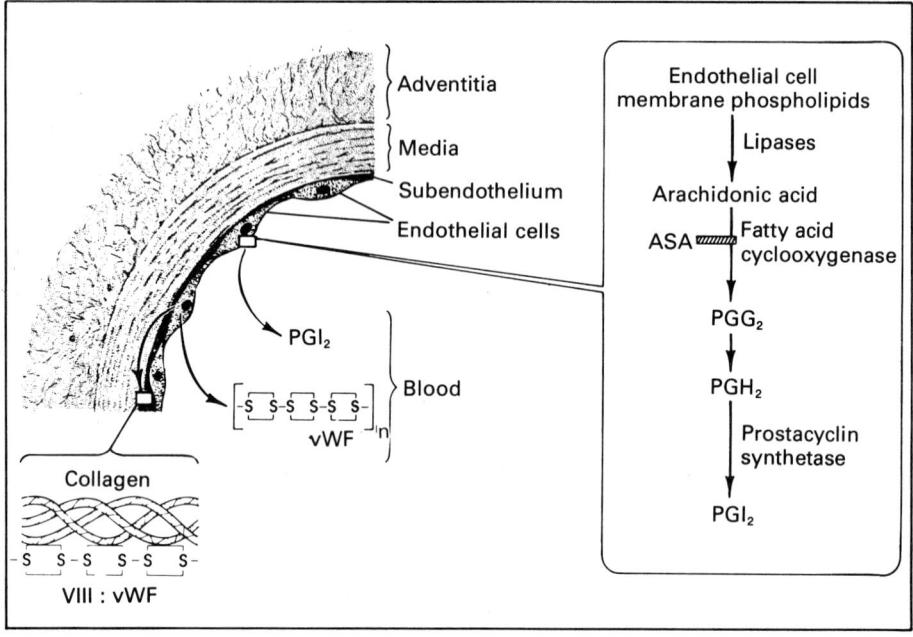

Fig. 15-1. Normal endothelial cell synthesis of prostacyclin (prostaglandin I_2; PGI_2) and von Willebrand factor (vWF) multimers; −S−S−, disulfide bonds between monomeric subunits of vWF multimers, ASA, acetylsalicylic acid (aspirin); PGG_2 and PGH_2, prostaglandins G_2 and H_2 (hydroperoxycyclic and hydroxycyclic endoperoxides, respectively).

monophosphate (cAMP) levels. Increased platelet cAMP levels impair platelet-to-platelet cohesion (aggregation) and suppress platelet release of adenosine diphosphate (ADP) and other granule contents. cAMP-stimulated protein kinase–mediated phosphorylation of platelet membrane or cytoplasmic proteins may be responsible for these inhibitory effects.

Prostaglandin I_2 is synthesized from the arachidonic acid that membrane lipases liberate from endothelial cell membrane phospholipids. Endothelial cell fatty acid cyclooxygenase converts arachidonic acid to short-lived cyclic hydroperoxy (PGG_2) and hydroxy (PGH_2) intermediates, and then via prostacyclin synthetase to PGI_2 (see Fig. 15-1). Prostaglandin I_2 can also be synthesized directly from any PGG_2 and PGH_2 that diffuse into endothelial cells from nearby aggregating platelets.

Platelets

Normal blood contains 150,000 to 350,000 platelets per μL (cu mm). These disk-shaped cells with a diameter of 2 to 3 μg are derived from marrow megakaryocytes. Platelet survival in the blood is normally about 10 days.

Megakaryocytes surround bone marrow sinuses and extend long cytoplasmic projections into the lumina. Megakaryocytes constrict their membranes at varying points and divide these cytoplasmic projections into large fragments and smaller portions (platelets). Both the large fragments and the platelets leave the marrow in sinusoidal blood and enter the systemic circulation. The circulating fragments break down in blood vessels of the lung to produce additional platelets.

In contrast to megakaryocytes, platelets have no nucleus (DNA) and cannot synthesize protein. Plasma coagulation factors are adsorbed onto their surface membranes and several are present in platelet granules. Platelet cytoplasm contains glycogen, mitochondria, enzymes of the glycolytic and hexose monophosphate pathways, microtubules, actin, myosin, and three different types of granules. These are lysosomes, dense granules, and α-granules. Platelet *lysosomes* contain hydrolytic enzymes. *Dense granules* contain adenosine triphosphate and diphosphate (ATP and ADP), calcium, and serotonin. Platelet α-granules contain: β-thromboglobulin, a glycopeptide of unknown function; platelet factor 4, a positively charged glycopeptide capable of binding negatively charged molecules (including heparin); platelet-derived growth factor (PDGF), a glycopeptide that promotes replication of smooth muscle cells and fibroblasts; and several proteins also present in plasma (factor V, vWF, fibrinogen, fibronectin).

When subendothelial structures are exposed to flowing blood, platelets adhere to collagen, bind vWF multimers via specific membrane receptors, change shape from disks to spiny spheres, and release their granule contents (see Fig. 15-2). ADP, a potent platelet-aggregating agent released from dense granules, alters the surface of platelets passing by in the flowing blood. The altered platelet membranes bind fibrinogen from surrounding plasma via the glycoprotein IIb–IIIa complex, and aggregate onto the platelets already adherent to subendothelial vWF and collagen (see Fig. 15-2).

Thrombin, generated by the activation of the coagulation cascade, amplifies platelet aggregation and release responses. Platelet adherence to collagen, as well as thrombin-induced aggregation, causes a change in platelet membrane structure. Collagen and thrombin activate platelet membrane lipases, which then hydrolyze arachidonic acid from ester bonds in platelet membrane phospholipids (see Fig. 15-2A). In a process similar to endothelial cell synthesis of PGI_2, platelet fatty acid cyclooxygenase rapidly converts arachidonic acid to the cyclic endoperoxides PGG_2 and PGH_2. Instead of prostacyclin synthetase, however, platelets contain the enzyme thromboxane synthetase that produces thromboxane A_2 from PGH_2. *Thromboxane* A_2, a short-lived prostaglandin derivative, potentiates the release of platelet granule contents. Any thromboxane A_2 that

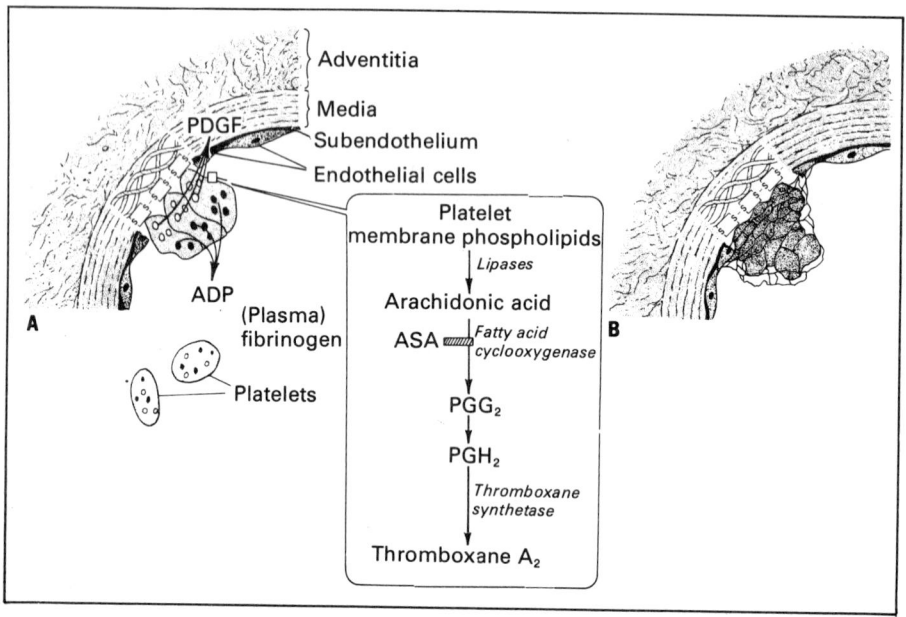

Fig. 15-2. *A.* Normal platelet adhesion and release mechanism. *B.* Platelet aggregation and fibrin polymer formation. ADP, adenosine diphosphate (from dense granules); PDGF, platelet-derived growth factor (from α-granules); ASA, acetylsalicylic acid (aspirin). PGG$_2$, and PGH$_2$, prostaglandins G$_2$ and H$_2$.

leaks from activated platelets also induces other platelets to aggregate, and stimulates local vasoconstriction. It is hydrolyzed rapidly and nonenzymatically into an inactive end product, thromboxane B$_2$.

Coagulation Cascade

By international agreement and common usage, the coagulation proteins are designated by Roman numerals: factor I (fibrinogen), factor II (prothrombin), factor V, and factors VII through XIII. Numerals III, IV, and VI are not used. The numerical order does not reflect reaction sequence. Roman numerals are not used for pre-kallikrein and high molecular weight kininogen. The activated form of a coagulation factor is indicated by the appropriate Roman numeral followed by the suffix "a." For example, factor II (pro-thrombin) is cleaved to the active enzyme, thrombin (IIa). Salient characteristics of the coagulation factors, which are discussed further in the section on coagulation disorders, are shown in Table 15-1.

Although there may be other sites of synthesis, *hepatic cells* probably synthesize and secrete most of the proteins involved in coagulation, including factor VIII. Endothelial cells and megakaryocytes

Table 15-1. Characteristics of coagulation factors

	Storage at 4°C	Half-life in vivo ($t^{1/2}$)	Replacement therapy
VIII complex:			
VIII	Labile	8–12 hrs	Cryoprecipitate or factor VIII concentrate
vWF multimers (largest plasma forms)	Stable	~1 hr	Cryoprecipitate or new forms of VIII concentrate
Vitamin K–dependent factors:			Plasma (usually fresh frozen) or II, VII, IX, X, concentrate
IX		24 hrs	
X		48 hrs	
II (prothrombin)		60 hrs	
VII		4–7 hrs	
Protein C		14 hrs	
Protein S		48 hrs	
Fibrinogen	Stable	3–5days	Plasma (usually fresh frozen) or cryoprecipitate
XI	Stable	40–80 hrs	Plasma (usually fresh frozen)
V	Labile	12–36 hrs	Plasma (fresh frozen)
XIII	Stable	4–14 days	Plasma (usually fresh frozen)

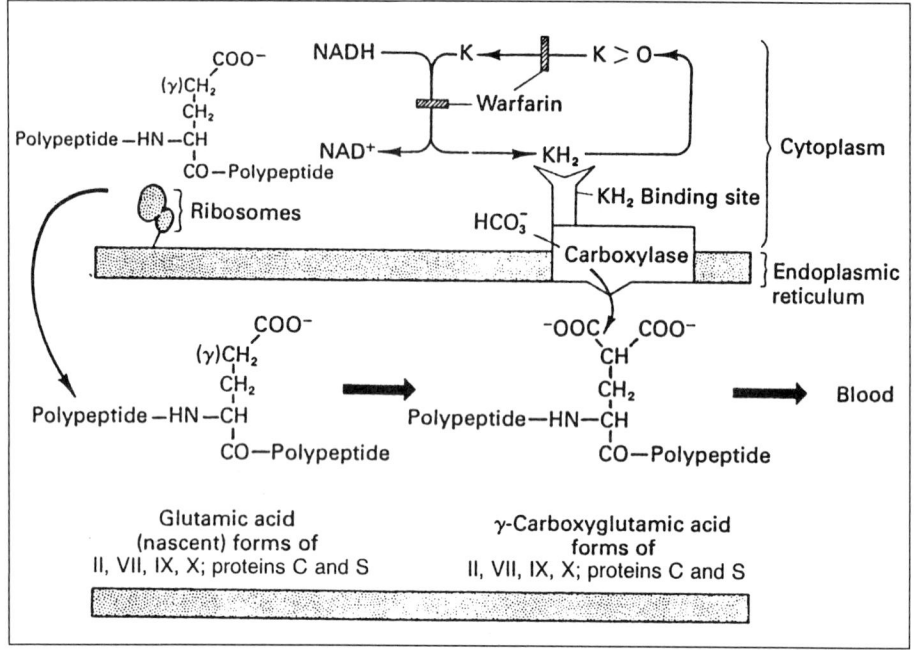

Fig. 15-3. Hepatic cell synthesis of vitamin K–dependent coagulation factors (II, VII, IX, and X). K, vitamin K; KH_2, reduced vitamin K; K > 0, vitamin K epoxide; NADH and NAD^+, reduced and oxidized forms of nicotinamide adenine dinucleotide, respectively.

synthesize and secrete vWF multimers. vWF multimers form ionic bonds with factor VIII molecules and transport this protein in the circulation.

Hepatic synthesis of factors II (prothrombin), VII, IX, and X, is *vitamin K*–dependent (Fig. 15-3). Vitamin K is a quinone with several different phytyl side chains, and the different derivatives are designated K_1, K_2, and so forth. Derived from vegetables (K_1) and, to a lesser extent, from synthesis by intestinal bacteria in the lower ileum and colon (K_2), vitamin K is lipid-soluble. It is absorbed in the small intestine in the presence of bile salts and transported to liver cells. Hepatic cells reduce it to a hydroquinone form (KH_2) that is the effective cofactor for a carboxylase enzyme in their endoplasmic reticulum. The KH_2-activated carboxylase catalyzes the addition of carboxyl groups to the γ-carbon of glutamic acid residues in nascent protein forms of factors II, VII, IX, X, protein C, and protein S as each passes from the ribosomes through the endoplasmic reticulum of liver cells.

In the final common pathway of the coagulation cascade, *thrombin* converts soluble, circulating *fibrinogen* into insoluble *fibrin polymers*. Thrombin generation occurs through two different reaction sequences, the intrinsic and extrinsic coagulation pathways (Fig. 15-4).

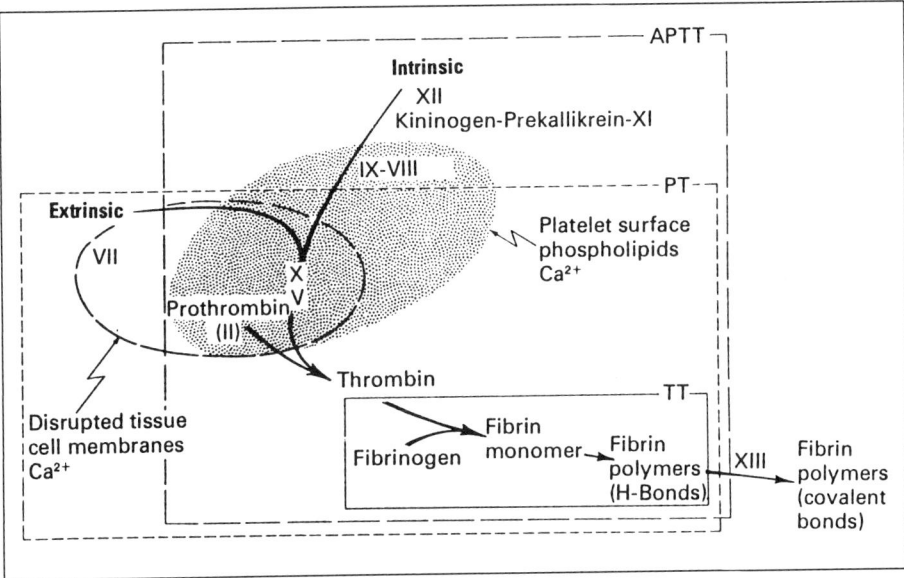

Fig. 15-4. Coagulation mechanisms. *Shaded area* ("platelet surface phospholipids") encloses the intrinsic coagulation reactions that occur on the surface membranes of platelets. *Dashed lines* enclose the extrinsic coagulation reactions that occur on disrupted tissue cell phospholipoprotein membranes intruded into the circulation. APTT, activated partial thromboplastin time; PT, prothrombin time; TT, thrombin time.

Intrinsic Coagulation: Intrinsic Coagulation Pathway

All necessary components for the intrinsic coagulation pathway are present (intrinsic) in the circulating blood. Adsorption of factor *XII* (Hageman factor) and *kininogen* (with bound *prekallikrein* and factor *XI*) to negatively charged subendothelial structures exposed at sites of vascular damage initiates the pathway. Subendothelial adsorption alters and partially activates the factor XII molecule to factor XIIa by exposing an active protease site. Factor XIIa then cleaves nearby kininogen-bound prekallikrein and factor XI molecules to create their active enzyme forms, kallikrein and XIa. In a feedback mechanism, kallikrein cleaves partially activated XIIa molecules adsorbed onto subendothelium to produce a form that is kinetically even more effective in the proteolytic conversion of prekallikrein and factor XI to kallikrein and XIa, respectively.

Calcium is not required for the activation of factor XII, prekallikrein, or factor XI, but is necessary for the proteolytic activation of factor IX by XIa. XIa-mediated activation of IX occurs on the surface of adherent and aggregated platelets where calcium bridges bind the γ-carboxyglutamic acid residues of IX to platelet surface membrane phospholipids. Factor *IX* that has been proteolytically activated to IXa (by XIa) interacts with *VIII* on platelet or endothelial cell surfaces.

Factor VIII, a 260,000-dalton protein, circulates in complexes with vWF multimers. These complexes bind to membrane surfaces by a mechanism yet to be determined, and the VIII molecules are cleaved by thrombin (or factor Xa) to a more active form. Activated VIII then interacts with surface-bound IXa. In association with activated VIII, IXa is optimally effective in cleaving and activating nearby factor *X* molecules. Factor X also binds to membranes by calcium bridges between γ-carboxyglutamic acid residues in X and surface phospholipids. Following the activation of X to Xa, Xa remains platelet-bound and attaches to activated factor *V* molecules (Va). Factor V is either adsorbed from plasma and then cleaved and activated to Va by thrombin, or released in Va form from platelet α-granules. The complex of *Xa-Va* on the platelet surface is formed near *prothrombin* (II) molecules.

The Xa in these platelet-bound *Xa–Va–II complexes* cleaves the prothrombin (II) molecules into two portions. One portion contains all the γ-carboxyglutamic acid residues and may remain bound transiently to the platelets through calcium bridges. The other portion is freed into the blood as *thrombin* (IIa). Thrombin induces local platelet aggregation and can activate factors VIII and V. Thrombin also produces fibrin monomers from plasma *fibrinogen* molecules, and cleaves and activates factor *XIII* to a form (XIIIa) that covalently links *fibrin monomers* into *fibrin polymers*.

Extrinsic Coagulation: Extrinsic Coagulation Pathway

Thrombin and fibrin polymers can also be formed via the extrinsic pathway, initiated by tissue factor, an integral membrane glycoprotein. This protein is normally found on fibroblasts, but can also be expressed by white blood cells, smooth muscle cells, and endothelial cells in some situations. The vitamin K–dependent proenzyme, factor *VII*, binds via γ-carboxyglutamic acid residues and calcium bridges to tissue factor on cell membranes, and is thereby activated to VIIa. VIIa is able to convert factor X to Xa, which is then able to activate prothrombin by mechanisms similar to those described previously.

Normally, the extrinsic and intrinsic pathways are complementary mechanisms and both are essential for the formation of adequate amounts of factor Xa and thrombin in vivo. The factor VII–tissue factor complex, however, is also able to directly convert factor IX to factor IXa and subsequently factor X to factor Xa. This capacity of the extrinsic system to bypass the earliest reactions of the intrinsic cascade may explain the relatively mild hemorrhagic tendency that has been noted in patients with hereditary factor XI deficiency.

The *fibrinogen* molecule (molecular weight 340,000) is composed of two sets of α-, β-, and γ-chains linked by disulfide bonds. Thrombin cleaves the amino terminal portion of the α- and β-chains and releases two small *fibrinopeptides A* (one from each α-chain) and two small *fibrinopeptides B* (one from each γ-chain). The *fibrin monomer* formed binds transiently to unaltered fibrinogen molecules. Continuing fibrinogen cleavage produces more fibrin monomers, and these then become linked by *hydrogen bonds* into fragile *fibrin polymers.* Thrombin-activated factor *XIII* (XIIIa), a calcium-dependent enzyme, catalyzes the formation of *covalent bonds* between the ε-NH$_2$ groups of lysine residues and γ-CONH$_2$ groups of glutamine residues in adjacent γ- and α-chains of the fibrin monomers. The covalent bonds are formed by *transamidation,* and ammonia is released. This final step in blood coagulation forms γ-to-γ *dimers* and α-to-α *polymers,* and creates an insoluble, hemostatically effective fibrin clot. Factor XIIIa also catalyzes the covalent incorporation of the dimeric plasma protein, *fibronectin,* into developing fibrin polymers.

Coagulation Inhibitors

Intrinsic and extrinsic coagulation pathways normally are restricted to the site of injury, thus preventing inappropriate and excessive intravascular thrombosis. The heparan sulfate–antithrombin III and protein C anticoagulant mechanisms function to regulate reactions of the coagulation cascade. Antithrombin III is a plasma protein (molecular weight 56,000), which is the primary physiologic inhibitor of thrombin, but can also neutralize factors IXa, Xa, XIa, and XIIa. In the absence of heparin, antithrombin III is a relatively slow inactivator of these hemostatic enzymes. Heparin is able to bind to antithrombin III, resulting in a conformational change in the inhibitor that leads to a marked acceleration in the rate of enzyme neutralization. Anticoagulantly active heparinlike species (i.e., heparan sulfate) are associated with the vascular endothelium and can locally activate antithrombin III. This is an important mechanism for the inhibition of the various activated factors that are generated in the circulation. Protein C is a vitamin K–dependent glycoprotein (molecular weight 62,000) that circulates in plasma as an inactive zymogen. Thrombin is able to rapidly activate protein C when bound to thrombomodulin, an integral plasma membrane receptor that is present on vascular endothelial cells. Activated protein C inhibits the conversion of prothrombin to thrombin by factor Xa by inactivating factor VIIIa and platelet-bound factor Va. Protein S, another vitamin K–dependent plasma protein, enhances the binding of activated protein C to phospholipid-containing membranes and accelerates the inactivation of the two cofactors. The complement component, C4b-binding protein, forms a complex with protein S, and this molecule normally circulates in both "free" and "bound" (via a noncovalent association) forms in plasma. Only the free form of protein S is functionally active in the protein C anticoagulant pathway.

An additional plasma protein has recently been isolated that inhibits the activity of the factor VIIa–tissue factor complex. This molecule (termed *lipoprotein-associated coagulation inhibitor* or *extrinsic pathway inhibitor*) exists in association with blood lipoproteins and requires the formation of a quaternary complex with factor Xa, factor VIIa, and tissue factor to suppress the activity of the extrinsic pathway.

Fibrinolysis

Once hemostasis has been achieved, vascular repair begins under the stimulus of locally released PDGF, platelet-derived growth factor (PDGF, released from platelet α-granules; see Fig. 15-2A). PDGF is believed to stimulate the replication of vessel wall smooth muscle cells and fibroblasts. Fibrin polymers are then slowly lysed. The active fibrinolytic enzyme is plasmin, produced by partial proteolysis of a fibrin-bound zymogen, plasminogen (Fig. 15-5). *Plasminogen* is adsorbed from plasma via its lysine-binding sites onto the lysine groups in fibrin polymers. Tissue-type plasminogen activator produced by endothelial cells is also able to bind to fibrin, which allows plasminogen to be activated to plasmin at an increased rate. Plasmin remains bound to fibrin and degrades it into fragments ("fibrin degradation products," or "fibrin split products"). The renal glomerular endothelial and tubular cells are especially rich in another type of plasminogen activator (urokinase).

Kallikrein generation by XIIa following initiation of the intrinsic coagulation pathway may convert some fibrin-bound plasminogen to plasmin. Plasmin proteolysis of covalently cross-linked fibrin polymers liberates large, soluble fragments into the circulation. Regions corresponding to portions of the fibrinogen molecule are identifiable in these circulating fragments, including regions designated *D* (90,000 daltons) and *E* (50,000 daltons).

Plasmin Inhibitors

In addition to hydrolyzing fibrin polymers, plasmin has the capacity to cleave fibrinogen, factor V, and factor VIII. Because of the potentially harmful effects of plasmin in the flowing blood, plasmin inhibitors are present in the circulation of normal individuals. α₂-*Antiplasmin* rapidly binds and inactivates plasmin. Some

Fig. 15-5.
Fibrinolysis. Both plasminogen and the hydrolytic enzyme, plasminogen activator (from disrupted endothelial and tissue cells), adsorb onto polymerizing fibrin. Fibrin-bound plasminogen activator cleaves nearby plasminogen molecules to the active enzyme, plasmin, which remains bound to the fibrin polymer and degrades it into soluble fragments ("fibrin degradation products"). ACA, epsilon-aminocaproic acid (a pharmacologic inhibitor of fibrinolysis).

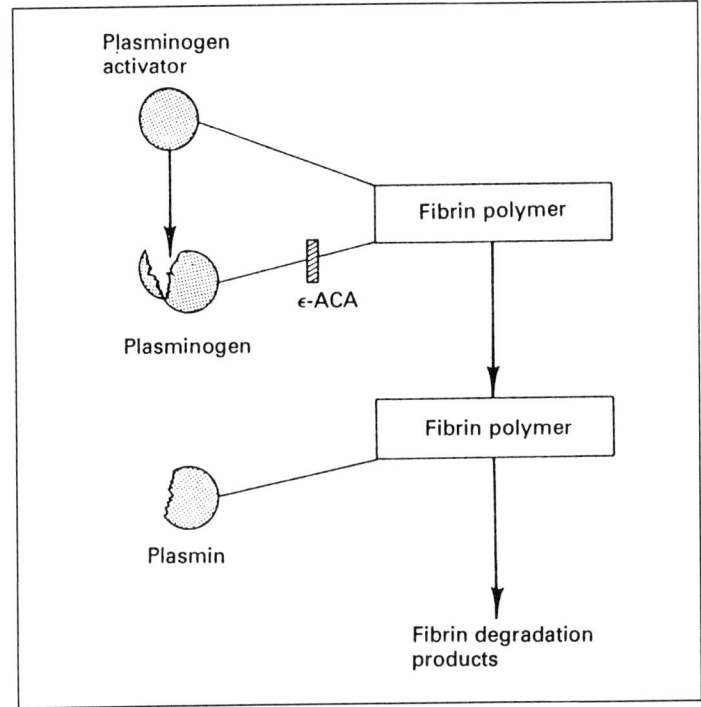

α_2-antiplasmin is even incorporated covalently into fibrin polymers, presumably to ensure that plasmin does not dissociate from fibrin and enter the circulating blood. α_2-*Macroglobulin* binds and inactivates plasmin more slowly than α_2-antiplasmin. A third potential plasmin inhibitor, antithrombin III, inactivates plasmin (as well as XIIa, XIa, IXa, and thrombin) in the presence of heparin.

Human plasma also contains a number of plasminogen activator inhibitors that are important in regulating the activity of the various plasminogen activators.

Evaluation of Hemostasis

History

Any patient who gives a history of "easy bruising" or excessive blood loss should be questioned regarding onset. Symptoms beginning in infancy or childhood suggest a congenital hemostatic defect, while symptoms beginning in later life usually indicate an acquired disorder. Patients with congenital bleeding problems usually have from childhood one or more of the following: ecchymoses or hematomas after minor trauma; excessive bleeding after trauma, surgery, or dental procedures; hemarthroses; or mucosal bleeding from the gums, or into the gastrointestinal or genitourinary tracts. It is important to determine if any previous bleeding has been severe enough to require transfusions, if other family members bleed excessively, or if there is consanguinity in the family.

In patients who have a history of bleeding beginning in later life, a drug-induced defect of platelet function must be considered. This is a common cause of easy bruising and excessive bleeding in association with trauma, menstruation, dental work, or surgical procedures. The patient should be questioned about drugs taken concurrently with any past bleeding episode. It is important to inquire specifically about aspirin (ASA)-containing compounds, nonsteroidal anti-inflammatory agents of the phenylalkanoic acid type (ibuprofen [Motrin], fenoprofen [Nalfon], naproxen [Naprosyn]), and penicillins, because these drugs inhibit platelet function to a modest extent in vivo.

Physical Examination

The skin should be examined for petechiae, purpura, ecchymoses, telangiectatic lesions, angiomas, and jaundice. It should be determined if there is gingival oozing of blood, oropharyngeal petechiae, or gastrointestinal bleeding (black stools). The muscles should be examined for atrophy and hematomas, and the joints tested for range of motion and degeneration. Liver and spleen size should be noted.

In general, either decreased platelet numbers or defective platelet function is associated with bleeding from dermal capillaries (petechiae, purpura, ecchymoses), and from the capillaries of mucosal surfaces (epistaxis, gastrointestinal or genitourinary tract hemorrhage, menorrhagia). Excessive posttraumtic bleeding is usually apparent immediately after injury.

In coagulation disorders, ecchymoses are frequent and often develop into more extensive local collections of blood (hematomas). Bleeding into muscles is also common. Hemarthroses occur in severe coagulation disorders, especially deficiencies of VIII or IX. Platelet adhesion and aggregation after minor trauma are often sufficient to arrest bleeding temporarily, although serious hemorrhage may follow within hours.

Laboratory Tests

In any patient to be evaluated for a bleeding or bruising problem or before a major surgical or invasive diagnostic procedure, a complete bleeding history and a drug history should be obtained. Then, three laboratory screening tests should be ordered: a blood platelet count, a prothrombin time to test the extrinsic coagulation mechanism, and a partial (or activated partial) thromboplastin time to test the intrinsic coagulation pathway (see Fig. 15-4). If any of these tests is abnormal, additional laboratory studies should be done to define the problem precisely.

TESTS OF PLATELET NUMBER AND FUNCTION

To determine the *platelet count,* a blood sample is examined in an electronic particle counter or in a counting chamber under a phase microscope. Examination of the blood film provides a rapid estimate of platelet number. Normally, there are 10 to 20 platelets per oil immersion field.

The *bleeding time* is an in vivo measure of platelet adhesion and aggregation on locally injured vascular subendothelium. A blood pressure cuff is inflated on the upper arm to a pressure of 40 mm Hg and, with guidance from a template (or by using a newer disposable device), a standardized incision about 1 cm long and 1 mm deep is made on the volar surface of the forearm. The wound is blotted gently and the time required for bleeding to cease is recorded (normally ≤9 minutes). A prolonged bleeding time in a patient with a platelet count above 100,000 per microliter usually indicates either *impaired platelet function* or an abnormality of vWF multimers (*von Willebrand's disease*). Aspirin is a common cause of mild platelet dysfunction and a moderately prolonged bleeding time. In a patient with a platelet count *below 100,000 per microliter,* the bleeding time is a superfluous test, as it is usually prolonged at these platelet counts.

Another test of platelet function is *platelet aggregometry,* an in vitro spectrophotometric measurement of platelet cohesion in platelet-rich plasma. Substances that either aggregate platelets directly (*ADP, thrombin, or epinephrine*), induce the release of platelet ADP (collagen or arachidonic acid), or induce the attachment to platelets of large plasma vWF multimers (*ristocetin*) cause the platelets in platelet-rich plasma to clump out of suspension. The resulting increase in the rate and extent of light transmission through the plasma is recorded in graphic patterns. Platelet aggregometry is time-consuming and should not be ordered indiscriminately.

COAGULATION TESTS

The tests described below are all done on citrated platelet-*poor* plasma. The *prothrombin time* (PT) evaluates the generation of thrombin and fibrin polymers via the extrinsic coagulation pathway. *Calcium* and whole tissue cell phospholipoprotein *membranes* ("thromboplastin") are added to citrated platelet-poor plasma and the time required for a fibrin polymer clot to form is determined. A normal PT is 10 to 12 seconds. In the presence of calcium, the added tissue cell membranes form complexes with, and activate, factor VII, and provide surfaces for the attachment and activation of factors X, V, and II (prothrombin). The PT is prolonged whenever plasma levels of one or more of the factors in the extrinsic coagulation pathway (VII, X, V, II, or fibrinogen) fall to levels *below* about 30 percent of normal.

The *partial thromboplastin time (PTT)* measures the time required to generate thrombin and fibrin polymers via the intrinsic coagulation pathway after *calcium* and *phospholipids* are added to citrated platelet-poor plasma. The added phospholipids are substitutes for those on platelet surfaces and are referred to as "partial thromboplastin" to distinguish them from the whole tissue cell phospholipoprotein membranes ("thromboplastin") that initiate the extrinsic coagulation pathway in the PT test. Only whole tissue cell phospholipoprotein membranes activate factor VII.

When blood is placed in a glass tube containing citrate, the coagulation reactions that do not require calcium (the activation of XII → XIIa, prekallikrein → kallikrein, and XI → XIa) occur on the negatively charged surface of the glass tube during the process of transporting and centrifuging the samples and separating the platelet-poor plasma. The contact factors are activated more completely if *additional negatively* charged substances (kaolin or Celite) are added to the platelet-poor plasma before calcium and phospholipid are introduced. Generation of fibrin polymers in this *activated partial thromboplastin time* (APTT) test normally takes about 35 seconds. The APTT becomes prolonged whenever the plasma level of one or more of the coagulation factors other than factor VII drops to levels *below* approximately *30 percent of normal*.

Additional tests to define the precise cause of an abnormal PT or APTT include plasma-mixing studies, specific factor assays, thrombin time, and fibrinogen quantification. For *mixing studies,* one part of normal citrated platelet-poor plasma is combined with one part of patient citrated platelet-poor plasma. An APTT test is then done on the mixture. The APTT should be normal when the level of each of the coagulation factors involved in the intrinsic pathway is at least 30 percent of normal. Normal platelet-poor plasma contains (by definition) 100 percent of each coagulation factor. Therefore, 50 percent of each factor will be present in a 1 : 1 mixture with patient platelet-poor plasma, even if the latter is totally deficient in one or more of the coagulation proteins involved in the intrinsic pathway. Any prolonged patient APTT value that is *corrected completely* by a 1 : 1 mixture of patient and normal plasma indicates that the patient plasma is *deficient* in one or more of the intrinsic coagulation factors. A prolonged patient APTT that is not corrected by this mixture indicates that an inhibitor is present in patient plasma that ultimately interferes with thrombin generation or fibrin polymer production in the normal plasma. This test is referred to as an inhibitor screen and abnormal results can be caused by antibodies directed against coagulation factors. The presence of inhibitors against specific coagulation factors can result in a severe bleeding disorder.

Antibodies to factor VIII are the most common specific factor inhibitors and can be found in patients with hemophilia A, postpartum women, and individuals with systemic lupus erythematosus. The presence of a nonspecific "lupus anticoagulant" is not associated with a bleeding diathesis except when prothrombin deficiency or thrombocytopenia is also present. A confirmatory test for this type of inhibitor is the tissue thromboplastin inhibition test or the Russell's viper venom time. Herparin (which increases the inhibitory effectiveness of antithrombin III) and acquired abnormal forms of fibrinogen can also result in an abnormal inhibitor screen.

Specific *coagulation factor assays* are done using modifications of the PT test for assays of factors VII, X, V, or II (prothrombin). Modifications of the APTT test are used to assay XII, prekallikrein, high molecular weight kininogen, XI, IX, and VIII. Dilutions of citrated platelet-poor patient plasma are added to a citrated platelet-poor substrate plasma that is known to be deficient in the particular factor to be assayed. Dilutions of citrated platelet-poor normal plasma (as a control) are tested separately at the same time. The concentration of the specific coagulation factor being tested in patient plasma is then expressed as a percentage of the activity in normal plasma. One unit of any coagulation factor is the activity of that factor in 1 mL of normal plasma. The characteristics and approximate in vivo survival of coagulation factors, and the appropriate replacement products for deficiency states, are listed in Table 15-1. Factor XII, prekallikrein, and high molecular weight kininogen are not included because deficiencies of these factors do not cause clinical bleeding, although they do prolong the APTT.

The *thrombin time* (TT) measures the clotting time of citrated platelet-poor plasma following the addition of a small amount of thrombin. The test determines the rate of thrombin-induced cleavage of fibrinogen to fibrin monomers, and the subsequent polymerization of fibrin monomers to hydrogen-bonded fibrin polymers. Under usual test conditions this takes about 20 seconds. The thrombin time is prolonged in plasma that contains *fibrinogen* in concentrations less than 100 mg/dL or greater than 400 mg/dL, or in the presence of an abnormal form of fibrinogen (*dysfibrinogenemia*), *heparin*, fibrin degradation products, or high concentrations of *monoclonal immunoglobulins* that interfere with fibrin monomer polymerization (as in myeloma or macroglobulinemia).

Fibrinogen is measured by a modification of the TT test using citrated platelet-poor plasma and several (usually three) concentrations of added thrombin. The fibrinogen value is calculated from the thrombin clotting times of the patient plasma relative to normal control plasma samples containing known concentrations of fibrinogen. Alternatively, the protein content of a fibrin polymer clot produced in patient and normal control plasma is compared as a measure of "clottable" fibrinogen. The normal fibrinogen level is 200 to 400 mg/dL plasma.

Disorders of Hemostasis

Excessive bleeding may occur as a result of an abnormality of blood vessels, platelets, or coagulation factors.

Vascular Disorders

VON WILLEBRAND'S DISEASE

Von Willebrand's disease is a hereditary autosomal dominant disorder that usually results from decreased endothelial cell release or synthesis of vWF multimers (*classic vWD type I*), or both (Table 15-2). Less commonly, either defective endothelial cell polymerization of vWF subunits (*vWD type IIA*) or endothelial cell synthesis of abnormal vWF multimers (*vWD type IIB*) causes the disease. Decreased quantities of vWF multimers, or the presence of inadequately polymerized or abnormal vWF forms, reduce platelet adherence to the subendothelium at sites of vascular injury. The clinical consequences are excessive posttraumatic bleeding, menorrhagia, and spontaneous bleeding from the nasal mucosa, gums, and gastrointestinal and genitourinary tracts. Decreased platelet–subendothelial adherence prolongs the bleeding time. Platelet counts are normal in vWD types I and IIA, but occasionally are moderately decreased in vWD type IIB.

In patients with vWD type I, either one-dimensional electroimmunoassay or radioimmunoassay demonstrates reduced plasma levels of vWF. *Electroimmunoassay* is a technique in which plasma proteins migrate under the influence of an electric field into agarose-containing antibodies, in this case to vWF. The quantity of vWF antigen present in plasma is determined from the height of the precipitated antigen–antibody peak.

The plasma of patients with vWD type IIA contains incompletely polymerized vWF forms. Demonstration by two-dimensional ("crossed") immunoelectrophoresis or sodium dodecyl sulfate-agarose gel electrophoresis that plasma vWF has excessively rapid mobility confirms the defect. In two-dimensional immunoelectrophoresis, plasma proteins are first separated by electrophoresis in agarose. Then, in a second dimension 90 degrees from the first, vWF forms are induced by an electric field to enter agarose-containing antibodies to vWF. The relative mobility of the vWF precipitin arc in the second dimension is determined by comparing the migration of vWF in patient plasma with that in normal plasma.

The positively charged glycopeptide antibiotic, ristocetin, partially neutralizes platelet negative surface charges and enables the largest

Table 15-2. von Willebrand's disease

Excessive bleeding
Prolonged bleeding time with normal platelet count
Low factor VIII level
Heterozygous autosomal defect

von Willebrand's disease (vWD) type I (classic vWD)

Pathogenesis	Diminished endothelial cell secretion of normally constructed vWF multimers (or, in some patients, diminished vWF synthesis)
Laboratory	Decreased plasma vWF Ag, RCoF, VIII coagulant, all vWF multimer forms present in plasma (in reduced quantity)
Treatment	1-deamino-8-D-arginine vasopressin (DDAVP); cryoprecipitate; new types of VIII concentrate

vWD type IIA

Pathogenesis	Defective endothelial cell polymerization of vWF subunits
Laboratory	Modestly decreased plasma vWF Ag and VIII, with very low RCoF; reduced quantity of largest plasma vWF multimers
Treatment	Cryoprecipitate

vWD type IIB

Pathogenesis	Endothelial cell construction of abnormal vWF multimers (from abnormal vWF subunits?)
Laboratory	Modestly decreased plasma vWF Ag and largest vWF multimers; plasma vWF binds to platelets in vitro at low ristocetin concentrations
Treatment	Cryoprecipitate

vWD type III (homozygous or doubly heterozygous vWD)

Pathogenesis	Markedly decreased synthesis of vWF multimers
Laboratory	Very low plasma vWF Ag, RCoF, VIII, all vWF miltimer forms
Treatment	Cryoprecipitate

"Pseudo" (platelet-type) vWD

Pathogenesis	Abnormal platelet surface with decreased affinity for subendothelium, but increased affinity for plasma vWF multimers; intermittent in vivo platelet aggregation and thrombocytopenia
Laboratory	Modestly decreased vWF Ag, RCoF, VIII; reduced quantity of largest plasma vWF multimers
Treatment	Normal platelets

vWF multimer forms present in normal plasma to attach to platelets and induce platelet aggregation. This *ristocetin cofactor activity* (RCoF) is reduced in the plasma of patients with vWD type I or IIA. In patients with vWD type I or IIA, diminished ristocetin cofactor activity correlates with defective platelet adherence to subendothelium.

In patients with vWD type IIB, vWF multimers are abnormally constructed. The largest of these abnormal vWF forms disappear rapidly from plasma, leaving only the relatively small vWF multimers in the circulation. Paradoxically, the abnormal, relatively small vWF multimers in patient plasma attach to patient (or normal) platelets and induce aggregation in vitro in the presence of a very low concentration of ristocetin.

Bleeding problems in vWD are most severe in rare patients who are homozygous or doubly heterozygous for the autosomal gene defect that causes type I vWD (type III). The bleeding time is very long, and plasma levels of vWF antigen, ristocetin cofactor activity, and VIII are extremely low in these patients. In contrast, as mentioned previously, most vWD patients are heterozygous either for the type I, IIA, or IIB gene defect, and their bleeding histories and abnormalities of factor VIII complex components are less severe.

Factor *VIII* is reduced in the plasma of most patients with vWD of all types. The capacity for synthesis of the VIII molecule by hepatocytes is not diminished as it is in hemophilia A. However, if blood levels of vWF multimers are low (vWD type I), vWF in the plasma is inadequately polymerized (vWD type IIA), or the largest plasma vWF multimers disappear rapidly from plasma (vWD type IIB), then VIII is not transported effectively from hepatic cells into the systemic circulation. Furthermore, those VIII molecules that do enter the circulation unbound to vWF multimers are rapidly removed.

When VIII is found to be selectively decreased in a *female* patient with a lifelong bleeding history and a long bleeding time, vWD is the most likely diagnosis.

Treatment of vWD

Cryoprecipitate fractions of normal plasma are transfused in order to arrest bleeding or to prepare the patient for surgery. Cryoprecipitate contains both the vWF and VIII components of the factor VIII complex, as well as fibrinogen and fibronectin. Following cryoprecipitate infusion, the largest transfused vWF multimers bind to the subendothelial surfaces of injured blood vessels. They augment local platelet adherence, decrease bleeding time, and diminish blood loss. In most patients, the therapeutic effect lasts up to 12 hours. Cryoprecipitate transfusion must then be repeated twice daily to maintain normal hemostasis. The majority of lyophilized factor VIII concentrates contains relatively small quantities of the largest vWF multimer forms found in normal plasma, and is not effective in the treatment of vWD. Some newer concentrates can be used to treat vWD.

In most patients with vWD type I, vWF synthesis within endothelial cells is normal, but release of vWF multimers is impaired. An alternative therapeutic agent in these type I patients is 1-deamino-8-D-arginine vasopressin (DDAVP), an analogue of vasopressin (antidiuretic hormone). Infused DDAVP stimulates the endothelial cells of vWD type I patients to release their stored vWF multimers. DDAVP infusion is not effective in heterozygous vWD types II and III. In type IIB vWD, DDAVP infusion can result in thrombocytopenia.

The liver cells of patients with vWD can synthesize VIII as well as normal liver cells. Consequently, vWF multimers in liver arterial blood following cryoprecipitate transfusion, or after DDAVP infusion in vWD type I patients, carry VIII molecules from liver cells into the blood (bound to the vWF multimers). The increase in circulating VIII levels in a patient with vWD who has been transfused with cryoprecipitate is, therefore, greater than can be accounted for by the quantity of VIII in the infused cryoprecipitate.

"PSEUDO" (PLATELET-TYPE) vWD

A few patients have been described with a mild autosomal (heterozygous) bleeding disorder that mimics vWD type IIB, but is due to a *platelet* abnormality. In this "pseudo," or platelet, type vWD, the platelets have an *increased affinity* for the largest vWF multimer forms in plasma. Patient plasma has, in consequence, a reduced quantity of the largest plasma vWF multimer forms, and mild to moderate thrombocytopenia may occur intermittently.

HEREDITARY HEMORRHAGIC TELANGIECTASIA

An autosomal dominant disorder, hereditary hemorrhagic telangiectasia (HHT) is also known as Osler-Weber-Rendu disease. Most mildly affected patients are probably heterozygous for an abnormal gene. The defect is characterized by vascular telangiectasias formed by abnormal blood vessels. Bleeding from telangiectatic sites is a result of vascular fragility.

Telangiectatic lesions are found on oral and nasal mucosal surfaces, lips, fingers, and ears; in the lungs; and throughout the gastrointestinal tract. The lesions may not become obvious until adulthood. Epistaxis and gastrointestinal hemorrhage are common.

Cauterization of bleeding vessels and application of nasal packs are sometimes effective temporarily. Septal mucosal skin flaps have been useful in some patients with intractable epistaxis. Epistaxis and even GI bleeding can sometimes be controlled by oral estrogen therapy. Anemia caused by chronic iron deficiency and intermittent bleeding is common, and often requires intensive iron therapy.

HENOCH-SCHÖNLEIN PURPURA

Henoch-Schönlein purpura is an acquired vascular defect that usually occurs in children following viral or bacterial infection, or after exposure to drugs or chemicals. It may represent an evanescent formation or deposition of immune complexes within blood vessel walls, with subsequent complement activation. Chemotactic attraction of neutrophils to affected vessels may occur in response to the local generation of C5a (the chemotactic complement peptide fragment). Local release of neutrophil lysosomal proteolytic enzymes may then cause vascular injury. The disorder is characterized by purpura, joint and/or abdominal pain, and glomerulonephritis with hematuria and proteinuria. Purpuric lesions are usually raised and therefore palpable, and are often symmetrically located at sites of increased intracapillary pressure (buttocks, legs, dorsal surface of the arms), vary in size, and may be preceded by urticaria. The platelet count is normal. Purpura usually lasts days to weeks. Episodes may recur, however, and occasionally irreversible renal damage occurs. Therapy with glucocorticoids is possibly beneficial, probably because these agents interfere with the interaction between neutrophils and the chemotactic peptide, C5a.

OTHER CAUSES OF VASCULAR PURPURA

In *mechanical* or *orthostatic purpura,* there is dermal vascular damage in areas subjected to stasis or abrupt increases in intravascular pressure (as during strong muscular contraction or paroxysms of coughing). Chronic stasis and purpura lead to local accumulation of iron–ferritin complexes (hemosiderin) and skin pigmentation.

Elderly individuals, patients with *Cushing's syndrome,* and patients receiving long-term *glucocorticoids* frequently have sharply demarcated ecchymoses on hands and forearms. Decreased synthesis or increased catabolism of dermal collagen and other connective tissue components, and the associated decreased vascular support, are responsible for the skin bleeding in these conditions.

Increased blood viscosity and sludging of cells in the microcirculation (as in *polycythemia vera* and *macroglobulinemia*) can result in the leakage of blood from packed capillaries with endothelial cells stretched apart by the increased intravascular volume or rendered ischemic by sluggish blood flow. The deposition of *amyloid* in dermal blood vessels can also result in increased vascular fragility and purpura.

Vitamin C is necessary for enzymatic posttranslational hydroxylation of proline and lysine in nascent collagen molecules synthesized by fibroblasts and other cells. Deficiency of vitamin C (*scurvy*) results in the deposition of defective collagen in blood vessel walls. Gingival, perifollicular, and subperiosteal hemorrhages are characteristic.

Platelet Disorders

THROMBOCYTOPENIA
Decreased Platelet Production
Acquired thrombocytopenias are common manifestations of many *toxic, nutritional, or neoplastic* disturbances of bone marrow hematopoietic stem cell proliferation and differentiation. In marrows that are hypoplastic because of injury by irradiation, drugs, or chemicals, the numbers of all hematopoietic cells, including megakaryocytes

and their precursors, are reduced. Bone marrow infiltration by metastatic cancer cells, leukemia, Hodgkin's disease, non–Hodgkin's lymphoma, or disseminated tuberculosis (*Mycobacterium tuberculosis* or atypical mycobacteria) may also reduce the number of marrow megakaryocytes. In megaloblastic anemias caused by *folate* or *vitamin* B_{12} deficiency, the defect in thymidine (and DNA) synthesis affects megakaryocytes and causes ineffective thrombopoiesis. In these various conditions the numbers of circulating red cells and leukocytes are usually reduced as well. Rarely, one may see patients with "amegakaryocytic thrombocytopenia," an acquired form of isolated thrombocytopenia due to decreased platelet production in the bone marrow.

Ethanol or its major metabolite, acetaldehyde, suppresses megakaryocyte proliferation. Thrombocytopenia is a common complication of chronic ethanol abuse, even in the absence of folate or other vitamin deficiency. A mild qualitative platelet defect may also be associated with excessive ethanol intake. Both the thrombocytopenia and mild platelet dysfunction improve rapidly after ethanol ingestion is stopped.

Increased Platelet Destruction

Thrombocytopenia caused by increased peripheral destruction of platelets is characterized by shortened platelet survival and increased marrow megakaryocytes (in an effort to compensate for shortened platelet survival). Severity of bleeding is proportional to the degree of thrombocytopenia.

Drug-induced immune thrombocytopenia. Drugs or drug metabolites can induce immune platelet destruction and severe thrombocytopenia (platelets < 20,000/μL) in individuals who produce antibodies to the drug or metabolite. Drugs implicated include *quinidine* and *quinine* (stereoisomers of one another), *sulfonamides* and structurally similar drugs, digitoxin, rifampicin, heroin, and morphine. Either the drug or its metabolite, as hapten, binds noncovalently to albumin and other plasma proteins to form complete antigenic structures. The patient produces antibodies that combine specifically with the protein-bound haptenic drug or metabolite, and the complex of antibody + drug (or metabolite) + plasma protein adsorbs onto platelet surfaces. The antigen–antibody complex adsorbed to platelets fixes and activates complement component C1 whenever IgM, IgG_1, or IgG_3 is involved in the immune complex. If the classic complement pathway on platelet surfaces is activated completely via C1, C4, C2, and C3 through the terminal attack complex (C5–C9), platelets lyse in the circulation. If the classic complement pathway is not activated beyond C3, as is common because of the presence in plasma of a circulating C3 inactivator, platelets are destroyed predominantly within splenic and hepatic macrophages. Macrophages have specific surface receptors for the Fc portion of IgG_1 and IgG_3 molecules, and for the C3b portion of the C3 molecule. Macrophages phagocytose and destroy adherent IgG- or C3-coated platelets.

For immune reactions to occur on platelet surfaces, the drug or drug metabolite must be continuously present. Thrombocytopenia abates within days to weeks following discontinuation and catabolism of the drug and its complete removal from the blood and body tissues. If bleeding persists after the drug is stopped, and hours have passed (during which clearance of the drug or metabolite may have occurred), then a platelet transfusion can be attempted. If the offending antigen (drug or metabolite) has been removed, immune complexes will no longer be present in the circulation to destroy transfused platelets, even though antibodies to the drug or metabolite persist in the blood. Glucocorticoids are sometimes helpful in treating drug-induced immune thrombocytopenia, although this has not been proved with certainty.

Idiopathic thrombocytopenic purpura (ITP). Acute ITP occurs most often in children following viral infections. Although the mechanism of immune damage has not been defined precisely, the attachment to platelet surfaces of complexes composed of virus–viral antibody (with or without complement fixation and activation) is a possible cause. The extent of complement activation presumably determines if platelets are lysed directly in the blood or phagocytosed by splenic and hepatic macrophages. Other possible causes of acute ITP are viral (or other microbial) interference with suppressor T lymphocyte function, or alterations in the patient's own platelet membrane antigens as a consequence of viral attachment to platelet surface structures. Either of these processes could cause transient production of autoantibodies against the patient's own platelet membrane antigens. In acute ITP, thrombocytopenia usually persists for a few weeks and then abates spontaneously. A glucocorticoid or a course of intravenous γ-globulin may be useful in severe cases. Occasionally, the patient fails to recover and chronic ITP develops, requiring protracted therapy with a glucocorticoid and eventual splenectomy. Because of the danger of subsequent pneumococcal (or other bacterial) sepsis, splenectomy should be avoided in children if possible. Polyvalent pneumococcal vaccination should precede splenectomy in both children and adults.

Chronic ITP occurs predominantly in adults. It is a relatively common disorder that may complicate other diseases associated with defective immune responses (systemic lupus erythematosus, B lymphoproliferative disorders). More often, ITP is idiopathic, as its name implies. Onset of thrombocytopenia and hemorrhage is usually less abrupt than in drug-induced immune thrombocytopenia or acute ITP, and the disorder seldom remits spontaneously. Thrombocytopenia results from the development and persistence of IgG antibodies that react with platelet antigens (primarily GPIIb-IIIa) present on all platelets, both the patient's own and those obtained from normal individuals. The IgG antibodies may fix and activate complement components on platelet surfaces, although complement-mediated intravascular platelet lysis is less common than in drug-induced immune thrombocytopenia.

Clinical manifestations include petechiae, bruising, menorrhagia, and bleeding after minor trauma. The diagnosis is made after other possible nonimmune and drug-induced immune causes of thrombocytopenia have been excluded. Demonstration of anti-platelet antibodies may help in diagnosis, but these are present in only about two-thirds of all patients with chronic ITP. In chronic ITP, platelet counts may sometimes be less than 20,000 per microliter. Usually, however, platelets are in the 20,000 to 80,000 per microliter range. Anemia, when present, is often caused by blood loss. Rarely, auto-immune hemolytic anemia may occur concurrently with ITP (Evans syndrome).

Chronic ITP is treated initially with a glucocorticoid (1–2 mg/kg/ day prednisone). Platelet survival and platelet counts usually increase within days to weeks as a result of the effects of glucocorticoids on splenic and hepatic macrophages. In contrast, a longer time is required for glucocorticoid suppression of immunoglobulin synthesis. The therapeutic dosage of glucocorticoids used in chronic ITP produces inadequate defense against infection, abnormal glucose utilization, and excessive protein catabolism (including the proteins in bone). Consequently, splenectomy is usually necessary to interrupt permanently phagocytosis by splenic macrophages of IgG ($\pm$C3b)-coated platelets. In most patients, platelet survival and platelet counts return to normal (or above) after splenectomy, although IgG platelet autoantibodies often persist in the circulation and on patient platelets.

Because of blood flow patterns through the macrophage-packed red pulp, the spleen is the major site of platelet destruction. If platelets are very extensively coated with IgG ($\pm$C3b), phagocytosis also occurs in macrophage-lined liver sinusoids. These patients (~20% of those with chronic ITP) do not respond to glucocorticoids and splenectomy. Such patients and those who are not candidates for splenectomy may benefit from intravenous vincristine infusions, and may achieve long-term remission with 6-mercaptopurine or cyclophosphamide. These agents are immunosuppressive. Intravenous polyvalent IgG concentrate is also effective in treating both chronic and acute ITP by blocking splenic and hepatic macrophage IgG Fc receptors. The benefit is usually only temporary. An attenuated androgen with diminished virilizing capacity, danazol, may also be useful in ITP.

Transfusion of platelet concentrates is either ineffective or of evanescent benefit because normal donor platelets also react with the circulating platelet autoantibodies. Consequently, transfused platelets survive only briefly, and should be reserved for situations in which bleeding is life-threatening.

Neonatal autoimmune thrombocytopenia occurs in infants born to mothers with chronic ITP following transplacental passage of maternal IgG platelet autoantibodies. The mothers usually have been splenectomized and may have normal (or near-normal) platelet counts, but have persistent IgG platelet autoantibodies in their blood. The IgG platelet autoantibodies are passively transferred to the fetus, which develops thrombocytopenia and is at increased risk for intracerebral bleeding during vaginal delivery. Thrombocytopenia in the neonate lasts for weeks (until the maternal IgG is catabolized). Occasionally, the degree of thrombocytopenia is so severe that the neonate requires glucocorticoids, platelet transfusions (for temporary hemostasis), intravenous IgG, or exchange transfusions to accelerate the removal of maternal platelet autoantibodies from the blood. The application of fetal scalp vein sampling for the measurement of platelet counts before birth has been of questionable assistance in determining the optimal mode of delivery for these mothers (low platelet counts being taken as an indication for cesarean section).

Isoimmune neonatal thrombocytopenia. Isoimmune neonatal thrombocytopenia results from isoimmunization of the mother by a fetal platelet antigen inherited from the father but absent on maternal platelets. The fetal platelet antigen is usually either a histocompatibility (HLA) antigen or the common platelet-specific Pl^{A1} antigen (present in about 98% of people). Fetal platelets that leak into the maternal circulation carry the immunizing antigen. Thrombocytopenia in the neonate is caused by subsequent transplacental passage to the fetus of IgG isoantibodies produced by the mother against the specific fetal platelet antigen. The mother's platelets lack the antigen that stimulated production of the isoantibodies and are unaffected. The syndrome is pathogenetically similar to erythroblastosis fetalis, except that fetal platelets (rather than fetal red cells) carry the immunizing antigen and are the targets of the IgG isoantibodies. Transfusions of maternal platelets (which lack the offending antigen, but must be washed free of maternal plasma containing platelet isoantibodies) may be required to control thrombocytopenia and bleeding in the baby.

Posttransfusion purpura. A rare form of isoimmune thrombocytopenia, this develops in Pl^{A1}-negative individuals about 1 week after transfusion of a blood product containing Pl^{A1}-positive platelets (usually whole blood or platelet concentrates). Pl^{A1} isoantibodies are produced and combine with any residual Pl^{A1} antigen that remains in the circulation from the previous transfusion. Circulating immune complexes form and are believed to attach to the patient's own (Pl^{A1}-negative) platelets, where they fix and activate complement and cause platelet destruction. Severe and often fatal bleeding may ensue. Otherwise, the thrombocytopenia subsides spontaneously in several weeks.

Bacterial sepsis. Sepsis may be complicated by mild thrombocytopenia. This may be due to attachment to platelets of bacterial antigen–antibody immune complexes ($\pm$complement). Alternatively, certain microbial antigens may attach to platelets, followed by specific antibodies to the microbe ($\pm$complement). The latter mechanism has been reported to cause the thrombocytopenia that frequently complicates *Plasmodium falciparum* malaria. Disseminated intravascular coagulation (with thrombin-induced platelet aggregation in vivo) often contributes to the thrombocytopenia associated with microbial sepsis.

Increased Platelet Consumption

Thrombotic thrombocytopenic purpura (TTP). TTP is a combination of thrombocytopenia, hemolytic anemia, fever, and fluctuating signs of ischemic vascular occlusion (including neurologic and renal abnormalities). In the clinically similar *hemolytic-uremic syndrome* (HUS), a constellation of thrombocytopenia, hemolytic anemia, and acute renal failure is usually unaccompanied by neurologic signs. TTP and HUS are abrupt in onset and the outcome is sometimes fatal. TTP is associated with widespread vascular occlusive lesions, whereas renal lesions predominate in HUS. The vascular lesions consist of thrombi within arterioles and capillaries, unaccompanied by inflammation. These thrombi contain aggregated platelets with some fibrin, and account for the clinical signs and symptoms of concurrent vascular thrombosis and ischemia either in many organs (TTP) or in the kidney alone (HUS). Fragmentation of erythrocytes occurs as the red cells circulate through partially occluded small blood vessels, causing "microangiopathic" hemolytic anemia and the characteristic schistocytes on peripheral blood films. Both megakaryocytic and erythroid hyperplasia occur in the bone marrow in response to the increased intravascular aggregation of platelets and the mechanical injury and destruction of red cells.

Recent observations suggest that TTP may be caused by several different mechanisms. *Widespread endothelial damage (or stimulation)* may cause the release into the blood of large, endothelial cell–derived vWF multimers. These vWF forms are larger than the vWF multimers that normally circulate. The unusually large vWF multimers may then attach to platelets, resulting in intravascular platelet aggregation, thrombocytopenia, organ ischemia, and mechanical hemolysis.

Therapy of TTP in the past included drugs that interfere with the function of platelets in vivo (aspirin, dipyridamole). Even splenectomy was tried, often in desperation. More satisfactory results have been obtained in the past several years with exchange transfusion (normal plasma infusion combined with plasmapheresis) or the transfusion of normal plasma alone.

Mortality from *HUS* has been reduced by *dialysis* combined with infusions of normal *plasma,* although some degree of renal impairment often persists.

Disseminated intravascular coagulation. This entity is described later in this chapter.

Other Causes of Thrombocytopenia

Thrombocytopenia is sometimes the result of increased platelet sequestration in *splenomegaly.* About one third of the total body platelets are normally found in the spleen at any one time. Splenic enlargement, as in cirrhosis with portal hypertension, results in delayed intrasplenic transit of platelets. Splenomegaly and thrombocytopenia also occur in lymphoma, sarcoidosis, and lipidoses (e.g., Gaucher's disease). If a small number of patient platelets are labeled with a radioisotope (^{51}Cr or ^{111}In) and returned to the patients, their survival in the body is normal. The number of labeled platelets in the circulation at any one time is reduced, however. Patients with splenomegaly usually have only modest thrombocytopenia (50,000–150,000 platelets/μL).

Dilutional thrombocytopenia can complicate the *massive transfusion* of platelet-poor whole blood in a patient with severe hemorrhage. Thrombocytopenia can also result from damage or consumption of platelets during *extracorporeal circulation* (cardiopulmonary bypass, hemodialysis); platelet loss is due to platelet damage and lysis by shear stresses generated in the apparatus, by platelet adhesion to the foreign surfaces, and by platelet aggregation induced by the ADP released from damaged red cells, leukocytes, and other platelets.

INHERITED QUALITATIVE PLATELET DEFECTS

Congenital defects of platelet adhesion, release, or aggregation are associated with a modestly prolonged bleeding time and with mild to moderate spontaneous and posttraumatic bleeding. Although these syndromes are rare, they demonstrate that platelet adhesion, release, and aggregation must all be intact in order for hemostasis to be perfectly normal. The fact that bleeding in each is usually relatively mild indicates that adhesion, release, and aggregation are a complementary set of hemostatic reactions.

In the *Bernard-Soulier* syndrome, extremely large platelets are present in the circulation in reduced numbers. The giant platelets lack several externally exposed membrane glycoproteins including glycoprotein Ib and therefore adhere poorly to vWF multimers. Both spontaneous and posttraumatic bleeding occurs from infancy because of thrombocytopenia and reduced platelet adhesion to subendothelial components. The syndrome has an autosomal recessive inheritance pattern, with defective platelets, thrombocytopenia, and bleeding only manifest in homozygous individuals.

In the rare congenital defects of release, platelets either do not "package" ADP and serotonin properly in dense granules (*"storage pool disease"*) or platelets do not release ADP and serotonin normally following adhesion to sites of injury (*"ADP release defect"*). Both abnormalities result in less than optimal platelet aggregation and accumulation on sites of vascular damage.

In *Glanzmann's thrombasthenia*, platelets bind to vWF multimers and collagen, generate thromboxane A_2 from membrane arachidonic acid, and release ADP and serotonin from dense granules. Thrombasthenic platelets do not aggregate, however, in response to exogenous ADP plus fibrinogen, thrombin, or epinephrine. Externally exposed fibrinogen-binding sites and platelet–platelet cohesion sites are decreased on thrombasthenic platelets. The platelet membrane glycoproteins IIb and IIIa (which are normally held together as a complex by calcium) are either absent or abnormal on thrombasthenic platelets.

Thrombasthenia is inherited as an autosomal recessive disorder. Moderate to severe bleeding occurs only in homozygous individuals. Laboratory findings include normal platelet count; prolonged bleeding time; decreased or absent aggregation of platelets in platelet-rich plasma in response to ADP, thrombin, epinephrine, collagen, or arachidonic acid (the latter two agents induce the release of ADP from thrombasthenic platelets, but the platelets cannot aggregate in response to released ADP and plasma fibrinogen); and defective platelet-mediated fibrin clot retraction, either because of defective attachment of fibrin polymers to thrombasthenic platelets or diminished thrombin-induced aggregation of thrombasthenic platelets within the fibrin polymer clot. Ristocetin-induced attachment of vWF multimers to thrombasthenic platelets, and subsequent aggregation, are normal.

ACQUIRED QUALITATIVE PLATELET DEFECTS

Acquired abnormalities of platelet function are characterized by posttraumatic bleeding and prolonged bleeding times in patients with normal platelet counts. Associated conditions are uremia, macroglobulinemia, myeloproliferative disorders, and the administration of several different drugs. The basis for the hemostatic defect in *uremia* is poorly understood, but may in part be related to an accumulation of derivatives of the hepatic urea cycle (e.g., guanidinosuccinic acid). It has also been reported that platelets in uremic plasma have diminished fatty acid cyclooxygenase activity and, consequently, reduced thromboxane A_2 production. Serious bleeding in uremia is uncommon in patients who are not also concurrently receiving drugs that interfere with platelet function. When bleeding occurs it can be treated by dialysis to remove the uremic metabolites. Infusion of *DDAVP* has been used in uremic patients to induce the secretion of additional quantities of large vWF multimers from endothelial cells. These multimers presumably attach to subendothelial structures, augment platelet–subendothelial adherence, and improve hemostasis. The transfusion of cryoprecipitate containing vWF multimers is effective in the control of bleeding in some uremic patients. Administration of estrogens can also be useful; their effect is more delayed but better sustained than those of the foregoing agents.

Platelet–subendothelial interactions may be impaired in *macroglobulinemia* by the monoclonal IgM adsorbed nonspecifically onto platelet membranes or subendothelial surfaces. Defective megakaryocyte and platelet membrane construction may cause a mild degree of platelet dysfunction in patients with *myeloproliferative disorders.*

Drugs that inhibit platelet function in vivo include acetylsalicylic acid (ASA, *aspirin*) and large doses of certain *penicillin* compounds (carbenicillin, ticarcillin, and penicillin G). Ampicillin in usual dosages, methicillin, and the cephalosporins do not have this effect. ASA acetylates the active site of platelet fatty acid cyclooxygenase and inhibits conversion of platelet membrane arachidonic acid to cyclic endoperoxides (and subsequently to thromboxane A_2) following platelet adherence to subendothelial components and collagen (see Fig. 15-2). Platelet release of ADP and other granule contents is, thereby, reduced, as is the number of platelets induced to cohere to those already adhering to the subendothelium.

ASA and the penicillins interfere irreversibly with platelet function. Consequently, propensity for bleeding and a prolonged bleeding time persist for days after their discontinuation. ASA or large doses of penicillin G, carbenicillin, or ticarcillin can induce or increase bleeding in association with coagulation abnormalities, thrombocytopenia, or ethanol ingestion. Transfusion of platelet concentrates is occasionally necessary to control severe bleeding (after the offending drug is discontinued).

Several other agents interfere with platelet fatty acid cyclooxygenase in vitro, and thus suppress platelet release and aggregation in the aggregometer. These drugs include indomethacin, phenylbutazone, sulfinpyrazone, and the phenylalkanoic acid–type analgesics (Motrin, Nalfon, Naprosyn). With the exception of the alkanoic compounds, however, these agents do not cause bleeding or prolong bleeding times. This is probably because indomethacin, phenylbutazone, and sulfinpyrazone are only transient inhibitors in vivo of platelet fatty acid cyclooxygenase.

THROMBOCYTOSIS

Elevated platelet counts reflect increased megakaryocytic proliferation and platelet production. Platelet counts of 500,000 to 1 million/μL are often associated with iron deficiency, Hodgkin's disease, other neoplastic disorders (e.g., lung cancer), and several other conditions (see Chap. 11). The pathogenesis of this *secondary* or *reactive thrombocytosis* is unknown, although excessive production of a "thrombopoietin" is suspected. This increased thrombopoietic activity may be due to the release of cytokines and growth factors, for example interleukin-1 and interleukin-6. Effective therapy of the underlying disorder results in reduction of platelet counts to the normal range. Thrombotic and hemorrhagic complications are unusual.

Thrombocytosis is also associated frequently with *myeloproliferative disorders,* in which there is excessive hematopoiesis (polycythemia vera, chronic myelogenous leukemia, myelofibrosis–myeloid metaplasia). Platelet counts in the myeloproliferative disorders often are over 1 million/μL, and the platelets frequently have mild functional defects (as determined by bleeding time and aggregometry). The specific platelet defects that have been identified in the myeloproliferative disorders include acquired storage pool–like defects, platelet membrane abnormalities, and alterations in arachidonic acid metabolism. A clear relationship between any of these defects and the bleeding or thrombosis that may occur in patients with these disorders has not been established.

Essential thrombocythemia is a myeloproliferative disease with a predominant neoplastic proliferation of megakaryocytes. Platelet counts can be seen in the millions per microliter. Therapy with myelosuppressive drugs (e.g., hydroxyurea) is directed at reducing megakaryocytic proliferation and platelet production.

Coagulation Disorders

Decreased or defective synthesis of one or more of the coagulation factors can cause bleeding. In disorders other than vWD, the defect is probably within hepatic cells. A single factor is deficient in all inherited coagulopathies except the rare combined deficiency of factor VIII and factor V. In contrast, several coagulation factors are deficient in most acquired disorders.

INHERITED COAGULATION DISORDERS

With the exception of hemophilia A and B, all inherited coagulation defects have autosomal inheritance patterns. vWD and the inherited thrombotic disorders are usually transmitted as autosomal dominant disorders in which there is a single abnormal gene (heterozygosity). Most of the other inherited bleeding disorders are autosomal recessive. Two abnormal genes (homozygosity or double heterozygosity) must be present for there to be abnormal bleeding, and this rarely occurs.

Hemophilia A and B are X-chromosome–linked recessive disorders. Bleeding occurs in males who are hemizygous for the abnormal X chromosome. This usually has been transmitted by a heterozygous, asymptomatic mother. Hemophilia A is a deficiency of factor VIII activity and hemophilia B a deficiency of factor IX activity. Each disorder results from a defect at a different locus on the X chromosome. In most *female carriers,* VIII or IX activity is approximately 50 percent of normal. Levels differ from one female carrier to another because of variable inactivation of the normal and abnormal X chromosomes in somatic cells during embryonic cell replication (Lyon phenomenon).

Probability considerations indicate that a female carrier of hemophilia will transmit the defective X chromosome to half of her sons, who will be hemophiliacs, and to half of her daughters, who will be carriers. A male hemophiliac will transmit his defective X chromosome only to his daughters, all of whom will be carriers. When there is no family history, a spontaneous *mutation* in the X chromosome of the male patient may have occurred during embryogenesis. Alternatively, a mutation may have occurred in one of the mother's X chromosomes before the patient's conception, or in one of the X chromosomes transmitted from a maternal grandparent to the mother (so that the mother is the first in the family to be a carrier).

Hemophiliac bleeding can be *severe* (VIII or IX activity <1% of normal), *moderate* (coagulant activity 1–5% of normal), or *mild* (coagulant activity >5% of normal). In severe hemophilia, "spontaneous" bleeding occurs repeatedly in areas subject to mechanical stress (joints and muscles) or minor trauma (skin). *Hemarthroses,* hematomas, and ecchymoses are frequent. Recurrent hemarthroses can cause destructive joint disease and hematomas can cause tissue damage by restricting blood flow. In moderate and mild hemophilia, bleeding often is a problem only during and after surgery, or in association with trauma.

In both hemophilia A and B, the APTT is prolonged. The PT, fibrinogen level, thrombin time, platelet count, and bleeding time are normal. Specific assays of VIII and IX activity must be done to distinguish hemophilia A from hemophilia B.

Hemophilia A

Synthesis or secretion of the VIII molecule is either mildly, moderately, or severely decreased in most patients. In others, a defective form of the VIII molecule is synthesized and secreted. Hemophilia A patients have normal plasma and subendothelial levels of vWF multimers, with normal bleeding times.

Bleeding episodes in patients with hemophilia A are treated by transfusions of *cryoprecipitate* prepared from normal plasma. Cryoprecipitate contains both of the components of the factor VIII complex (VIII bound electrostatically to large vWF multimers), as well as fibrinogen and fibronectin. Lyophilized *concentrate*, which contains VIII in complexes with usually smaller vWF multimer forms, is available commercially and can be reconstituted quickly for infusion. Until recently, concentrates were contaminated with hepatitis B virus; viruses of the non-A, non-B type (most of which have been found to be hepatitis C); cytomegalovirus; and the agent responsible for the acquired immunodeficiency syndrome (AIDS). Although fresh and fresh frozen plasma contain the factor VIII complex, cryoprecipitate and lyophilized concentrate contain a greater quantity in a smaller volume, and are more effective as replacement therapy.

The attenuated androgen, danazol, has been reported to increase modestly the plasma VIII level in a few patients with hemophilia A (and the plasma IX level in hemophilia B). The precise mechanisms, as well as the place of danazol in the treatment of hemophilia A (and B) patients, remain to be determined.

Factor VIII levels that are 10 to 20 percent of normal are usually adequate to sustain hemostasis after minor trauma. For major injuries, surgery, or bleeding into dangerous sites (e.g., the central nervous system or respiratory tract), VIII levels must be maintained at 50 to 100 percent of normal for several days.

The half-life of transfused factor VIII is 8 to 12 hours, and transfusions must be repeated two or three times a day. Home therapy programs, in which patients with hemophilia A transfuse themselves with cryoprecipitate or lyophilized factor VIII concentrate at the earliest sign of bleeding, have reduced hospital dependence.

In patients with hemophilia A or B, vWD, or other inherited coagulopathies, deposition of fibrin polymers during dental surgery is reduced and there is a risk of hemorrhage, because of the fibrinolytic properties of saliva as well the decreased coagulant activity. Oral administration of ε-aminocaproic acid (EACA) before and for several days after the dental procedure reduces bleeding and decreases transfusion requirements. *EACA* is a lysine analogue that competitively impairs attachment of plasminogen to fibrin polymers, which normally involves lysine-binding sites on plasminogen and lysine groups in fibrin polymers. Because EACA impairs plasminogen–fibrin binding, there is reduced generation of plasmin on the limited quantities of fibrin deposited at the dental surgery site.

The hepatic cells of patients with *mild* hemophilia A produce some functional VIII molecules. In these patients, intravenous infusion of *DDAVP* to raise plasma VIII levels is an alternative to transfusion of cryoprecipitate or lyophilized factor VIII concentrate. DDAVP causes endothelial release of stored vWF multimers. These multimers circulate through the liver of patients with mild hemophilia A and carry additional functional VIII molecules into the bloodstream. DDAVP also increases endothelial cell release of plasminogen activator, and thus enhances the activation of plasminogen to plasmin on fibrin polymers. EACA is given concurrently to prevent augmented local fibrinolysis.

Patients with severe hemophilia A lack or have an abnormal form of VIII protein, and require repeated transfusions of blood products containing the factor VIII complex. In some of these patients (10–20%), *antibodies* (usually of the IgG type) develop against VIII. These antibodies inhibit the coagulant activity of transfused VIII molecules. The plasma of patients with VIII antibodies prolongs the APTT and lowers the VIII activity of *normal* plasma. In mixing studies using dilutions of patient and normal plasma, inhibitor levels can be titrated and expressed in "Bethesda units." (One Bethesda unit of VIII antibody destroys 50% of the VIII activity in one mL of normal plasma during a 2-hour incubation at 37°C.) Inhibitor titers in a hemophiliac often increase anamnestically following infusion of cryoprecipitate or commercial factor VIII concentrate.

Treatment of patients with circulating antibodies to VIII has been generally unsatisfactory because the antibodies rapidly inactivate transfused VIII. Therapeutic approaches have included massive or continuous infusion of cryoprecipitate or lyophilized factor VIII concentrate; plasmapheresis to remove intravascular antibodies to VIII; transfusion of porcine factor VIII concentrate containing VIII molecules that may be less susceptible to inactivation by circulating VIII antibodies; administration of immunosuppressive drugs (e.g., cyclophosphamide [Cytoxan]); administration of intravenous γ-globulin; transfusion of "activated" commercial II, VII, IX, X concentrate that contains IXa, Xa, or a small quantity of activated VII capable of bypassing the coagulation defect induced by VIII antibodies; and extracorporeal removal of IgG antibodies to VIII on affinity columns of immobilized staphylococcal protein A (to which IgG attaches via its Fc portion). The combination of several of these therapeutic modalities has recently been used successfully to treat patients with VIII inhibitor.

Occasionally, a patient who does not have hemophilia A or a history of transfusion produces antibodies to VIII, perhaps because of an acquired defect in a suppressor T lymphocyte population. Predisposing conditions include immunologic disorders (e.g., systemic lupus erythematosus) and the postpartum state. Bleeding is often severe. The antibodies are usually IgG and are sometimes monoclonal (i.e., heavy chain of one subtype with either κ or λ light chain).

Hemophilia B

Congenital deficiency of factor *IX* is characterized by decreased or defective synthesis or secretion of factor IX molecules. The disorder is not corrected by vitamin K. Factor IX deficiency (Christmas disease) and hemophilia A are indistinguishable clinically.

Bleeding episodes in hemophilia B are treated by transfusing either normal fresh frozen *plasma* or a lyophilized *concentrate*, containing functional forms of the vitamin K–dependent coagulation factors (II, VII, IX, X). The risk of hepatitis with the concentrate has been considerable. Factor IX is stable in blood or plasma stored at refrigerator temperature (4°C), as well as in fresh frozen plasma. Transfused IX has a half-life of 24 hours.

Contact Factor Deficiencies

A deficiency of either *XII, prekallikrein, or high molecular weight kininogen* is not associated with bleeding. In factor *XI* deficiency, bleeding is usually mild. Spontaneous bleeding is unusual, but postoperative and posttraumatic hemorrhage may occur. Replacement of XI during a bleeding episode or in preparation for surgery is with fresh frozen plasma. Patients with deficiencies of XII, prekallikrein, kininogen, or XI have a prolonged APTT and normal PT.

The absence of bleeding in even severe deficiencies of XII, prekallikrein, or kininogen—and the relatively mild bleeding in patients with severe XI deficiency—indicate that a mechanism alternative to the contact factor system must exist for activating factor IX in vivo. It has been shown that complexes of relipidated tissue factor and factor VIIa are capable of activating factor IX.

Deficiencies of VII, X, V, II (Prothrombin), or Fibrinogen

A deficiency or defect of *VII* is suspected if the PT is prolonged with a normal APTT. A deficiency or defect in the activity of *X, V, prothrombin,* or *fibrinogen* is suspected if both PT and APTT are prolonged. Confirmation of each defect requires a specific factor assay. Bleeding episodes associated with deficiencies of VII, X, V, or prothrombin are treated with transfusions of fresh frozen plasma. Bleeding as a consequence of fibrinogen deficiency is treated by transfusion of cryoprecipitate, which contains fibrinogen (as well as the factor VIII complex and fibronectin).

Congenital dysfibrinogenemias are a heterogeneous group of disorders characterized by the synthesis of abnormal fibrinogen molecules with different functional characteristics. In some patients, thrombin cleavage of fibrinopeptides from the abnormal fibrinogen is defective. In others, there is abnormal polymerization of the "dys" form of fibrin monomers generated by thrombin cleavage of the dysfibrinogen molecules. Most affected individuals have little or no bleeding. A few have had thrombotic disorders, which may result from the resistance of abnormal fibrin molecules to plasmin digestion.

The thrombin time is prolonged, and levels of fibrinogen antigen (determined by immunoassay) exceed the levels of fibrinogen determined by functional assays (based on thrombin clotting times). APTT and PT are often slightly prolonged. The dysfibrinogen molecules present in patient plasma interfere with the generation and polymerization of fibrin monomers present in normal plasma. Consequently, the prolonged APTT, PT, and thrombin times of patient plasma are not corrected by a 1 : 1 mixture of patient and normal platelet-poor plasma.

Factor XIII Deficiency

In rare patients with deficiences or defects of factor XIII, coagulation mechanisms proceed normally up to the production of hydrogen-bonded fibrin polymers. In the absence of XIIIa-mediated covalent linkage, these hydrogen-bonded polymers depolymerize readily and are extremely susceptible to fibrinolysis by adsorbed plasmin. In vitro the fragile fibrin polymers dissolve in urea or mono-chloroacetic acid, agents that disrupt hydrogen bonds but do not affect normal covalently linked fibrin polymers. Delayed bleeding occurs at trauma sites, and wound healing may be defective. Miscarriage is frequent.

Very small amounts of XIIIa are required for the covalent cross-linking of fibrin monomers into stable polymers. Therefore, XIII deficiency must be severe before fibrin dissolves in urea or mono-chloroacetic acid. Replacement of XIII is with fresh frozen plasma.

Deficiences of Coagulation Inhibitors

Congenital antithrombin III deficiency is an autosomal dominant disorder. Affected patients are usually heterozygous for an abnormal gene. Patients with antithrombin III deficiency have plasma levels that are approximately 50 percent of normal and suffer repeated episodes of venous (and rarely arterial) thrombotic occlusions. Adequate anticoagulation with heparin (which accelerates the interaction of antithrombin III in plasma and on endothelial surfaces with activated forms of XII, XI, IX, X, and thrombin) can usually be achieved with plasma antithrombin III levels of about 50 percent. However, the transfusion of antithrombin III in either concentrates or fresh frozen plasma may occasionally be required. Patients with recurrent thrombotic episodes are anticoagulated chronically with oral warfarin (Coumadin).

Congenital deficiencies of protein C and protein S have also been associated with venous thrombosis. The prevalence of heterozygous protein C deficiency appears to be quite high (1 per 200–300) in the general population. Many of these individuals, however, do not exhibit thrombotic diatheses. The factors responsible for the variable clinical expression of protein C deficiency are not known at present. Warfarin-induced skin necrosis may occur in association with protein C deficiency during the initiation of oral anticoagulation. A homozygous or doubly heterozygous form of protein C deficiency (levels < 5% of normal) can present as neonatal purpura fulminans.

ACQUIRED COAGULATION DISORDERS
Deficiency of Vitamin K–Dependent Coagulation Factors
In the absence of vitamin K, the blood contains nascent, nonfunctional forms of factors II (prothrombin), VII, IX, and X, which lack γ-carboxylated glutamic acids and cannot bind via calcium bridges to phospholipid membranes. Nascent, nonfunctional forms of protein C and protein S also circulate in vitamin K deficiency.

Concomitant deficiency of factors II, VII, IX, and X in vitamin K deficiency causes bleeding. Vitamin K deficiency occurs when intake, endogenous bacterial synthesis, absorption, or hepatic utilization of the vitamin is impaired. If no vitamin K is ingested, deficiency develops within a few weeks—and even more rapidly if the patient is receiving antibiotics that kill vitamin K–producing intestinal bacteria.

Levels of II, VII, IX, and X in newborns are reduced because neonatal body stores of vitamin K are low, intestinal bacterial synthesis of the vitamin is minimal, and the hepatic γ-carboxylating enzyme system is immature. Deficiency of vitamin K and reduced levels of circulating, functional forms of II, VII, IX, and X may be severe enough to cause hemorrhagic disease in premature infants.

In patients with vitamin K deficiency, both the PT and APTT become prolonged when functional levels of II, VII, IX, and X decrease below approximately 30 percent of normal. Excessive bleeding is then a danger. The various preparations of vitamin K available for therapeutic use include water-soluble oral and parenteral forms. Synthesis of functional forms of II, VII, IX, and X results in correction of the coagulopathy within 1 to 2 days after administration of vitamin K. If bleeding is severe or surgery imminent, the coagulation defect can be corrected immediately by the transfusion of fresh frozen plasma.

Liver Disease
Because hepatic cells probably synthesize all the plasma coagulation proteins with the exception of vWF multimers, coagulation abnormalities are common complications of liver disease. In obstructive liver or biliary tract disease, the synthesis of functional vitamin K–dependent coagulation factors is decreased because the absorption of lipid-soluble vitamin K requires bile salts in the gastrointestinal lumen. This defect can be corrected by parenteral vitamin K. In severe hepatocellular disease the synthesis of all the plasma coagulation factors (except vWF) is impaired.

Thrombocytopenia is common in patients with liver disease and portal hypertension and congestive splenomegaly, and may contribute to the likelihood and severity of bleeding. Impaired clearance of activated coagulation factors and fibrin degradation products and diminished synthesis of coagulation inhibitor proteins, including antithrombin III and protein C, may also occur. An acquired dysfibrinogenemia may also be seen in patients with liver disease. Laboratory test abnormalities in liver disease often include prolonged plasma PT and APTT and modestly decreased platelet and plasma fibrinogen levels.

Bleeding episodes are treated with *fresh frozen plasma* containing functional forms of all of the coagulation factors. In thrombocytopenic patients, the infusion of platelet concentrates may also be necessary.

Disseminated Intravascular Coagulation (DIC)

This follows excessive activation of the extrinsic or intrinsic coagulation pathway. Excessive hemostatic system activation can follow extensive cellular destruction. Many surface and organelle membranes from disrupted tissue can enter the circulation. Common clinical problems that predispose patients to DIC include sepsis with phagocytosis of microbes and consequent white cell disruption; necrosis of neoplastic tissue by ischemia, cytoxic drugs, or irradiation; premature separation of the placenta; hypertonic saline-induced abortion; a retained dead fetus; heat stroke with hypovolemia and widespread tissue ischemia; and severe injuries, especially those involving membrane-rich brain tissue.

Excessive activation of the coagulation mechanism also occurs in patients with endothelial abnormalities (e.g., the giant hemangioma of Kasabach-Merritt syndrome) or extensive endothelial damage (as in a dissecting aneurysm).

The most frequent complication of DIC is *bleeding* from sites of injury, surgery, or vascular invasion (e.g., venipuncture or catheter placement). This can result from the presence of severe thrombocytopenia and coagulation factor depletion. Thromboembolic complications may also occur in patients with DIC.

Fibrinolysis inevitably accompanies DIC. It is the result of the liberation of plasminogen activators from endothelial cells, or disrupted tissue cells, or both; plasminogen activators and plasminogen then bind to fibrin polymers. Fibrin polymers are proteolytically degraded, usually within hours of formation. Because of this associated fibrinolysis, occlusive vascular symptoms and signs occur less frequently than bleeding in DIC. In a seriously ill or injured non-ambulatory patient with DIC, however, the risk of venous thromboembolism is enhanced. In some patients, fibrin polymers remain in the microcirculation long enough to damage and hemolyze red cells flowing through the fibrin mesh. This results in the formation of fragmented red cells (schistocytes) on blood films.

The diagnosis of DIC (and associated fibrinolysis) is suspected whenever fibrin degradation products are found in patient plasma and serum samples. Increased levels of fibrin degradation products in patient plasma impair in vitro interaction of fibrinogen molecules with thrombi, impede fibrin monomer polymerization, and prolong the thrombin time. In laboratory assays abnormally increased quantities of fibrin degradation products in serum samples attach to latex particles coated with antibodies made against the D and E regions of fibrinogen, and cause the particles to clump. The thrombin time and the immunoassay of fibrin degradation products are standard laboratory tests for the detection of DIC. The recently introduced test for D-dimer complements that for fibrin degradation products. The D-dimer test is specific for degradation products of cross-linked fibrin, whereas the standard test for fibrin degradation products detects fragments derived from fibrinogen as well. Thus, the D-dimer test is specific for in vivo clot formation.

Patients with DIC and associated fibrinolysis usually have increased serum levels of fibrin degradation products; D-dimer; thrombocytopenia; prolonged thrombin time, PT and APTT; and declining fibrinogen levels. Occasionally, the PT and APTT are normal or only slightly prolonged. Medical or surgical treatment of the underlying disorder is the most effective means of controlling the condition. Until this can be achieved, *fresh frozen plasma* (containing coagulation factors), *platelet concentrates,* and cryoprecipitate (containing fibrinogen, as well as factor VIII complex) are used as necessary for clinical bleeding.

Patients with DIC who are not bleeding and in whom *venous thromboembolism* develops are treated with *heparin*—if anticoagulation is not contraindicated. If heparin cannot be used (as in patients with head injury, recent central nervous system surgery, or open wounds), then a prosthetic filter can be placed in the inferior vena cava to prevent the passage of clot fragments from distal veins to the pulmonary vessels.

Arterial thromboses occur occasionally in patients with DIC. A dramatic example is purpura fulminans in children, a condition of widespread skin infarction and hemorrhage caused by thrombotic occlusion of dermal arterioles and capillaries. Purpura fulminans usually follows an infection, and is treated with heparin.

Excessive Local Fibrinolysis

Following prostate surgery, there is increased local release (and binding to fibrin) of plasminogen activator (urokinase). Local fibrin-bound plasminogen is then converted by this plasminogen activator to plasmin at an excessive rate, causing rapid local lysis of fibrin polymers and ineffective hemostasis.

Excessive local fibrinolysis is likely to be the cause of bleeding in a patient who passes blood devoid of clots from a urethral catheter placed after prostate surgery. On the other hand, if clots are present, defective surgical hemostasis is the more likely cause of excessive postoperative bleeding.

Relatively excessive fibrinolysis follows dental procedures in hemophiliacs, patients with von Willebrand's disease, and patients with other congenital coagulopathies, all of whom have reduced local fibrin formation because of the coagulopathy, superimposed on which is the fibrinolytic property of saliva.

Excessive local fibrinolysis can be treated effectively with oral or intravenous *EACA* (~ 1 gm/hr). EACA must be used with caution if the patient is also at risk for DIC. In the presence of DIC, EACA-induced inhibition of fibrinolysis promotes vascular occlusion and tissue infarction.

In Vitro Clotting Defects Unassociated with Clinical Bleeding

The lupus anticoagulant causes in vitro laboratory abnormalities that are not accompanied by bleeding in vivo.

The *lupus anticoagulant* is a circulating immunoglobulin that reacts with phosphoryl groups in phospholipids. It impairs the interaction of IX, X, V, and II (prothrombin) with the phospholipids that are added in vitro (along with calcium) to initiate the APTT test, but does not impair the interaction of these coagulation factors with phospholipids embedded in platelet membranes either in vivo or in vitro. Clotting times and the consumption of coagulation factors following the addition of calcium to citrated *platelet-rich* plasma are normal, as is in vivo interaction of platelets and clotting factors.

The lupus anticoagulant appears in patients with systemic lupus erythematosus and in other patients treated with *drugs* that induce a lupuslike syndrome (e.g., chlorpromazine and procainamide). However, it may develop in healthy individuals or those with a variety of disease states. The APTT is prolonged and is not corrected by a 1 : 1 mixture of patient and normal platelet-poor plasma. The PT may be slightly prolonged as well in some patients. This laboratory abnormality has been associated with a thrombotic tendency in some individuals, as well as spontaneous abortions on the basis of placental infarction. The mechanisms responsible for these thrombotic diatheses are uncertain at present.

Thrombosis

Venous Thrombosis

In venous thrombosis there is usually no obvious venous endothelial injury. For example, if blood flow is slowed (as in the leg veins of a patient at bed rest) or tissue damage is present (as in the perioperative period or after trauma), then coagulation factor activation can result in local thrombin generation, thrombin-induced platelet aggregation, and fibrin polymer formation within the venous lumen that can overwhelm the inhibitory actions of the natural anticoagulant mechanisms. The thrombus then grows by extension in the vein lumen.

Arterial Thrombosis

Arterial thrombosis is believed to be initiated by vascular injury and the exposure of subendothelial surfaces to flowing blood. This invariably occurs at sites of atherosclerotic lesions. The primary pathophysiologic event is probably the adherence of platelets to exposed subendothelial components including collagen, with subsequent platelet aggregation. Coagulation inhibitors (antithrombin III, protein C) are continuously present in flowing blood and represent an important defense against intravascular thrombin generation and fibrin formation. These two anticoagulant mechanisms are dependent for their normal functioning on cofactors (anticoagulantly active heparan sulfate, thrombomodulin) associated with the vascular endothelium. Once the arterial lumen is occluded, blood flow becomes turbulent proximal to the occlusion and stagnant distally, a hydrostatic situation that favors continued thrombin generation, platelet aggregation, fibrin polymer formation, and thrombus extension both above and below the site of vessel injury.

Anticoagulants

Anticoagulant therapy is used in thrombosis to accelerate the inactivation of coagulation factors (heparin) or to retard the synthesis of functional forms of the vitamin K–dependent coagulation factors (warfarin). The goal is to retard the deposition or extension of fibrin thrombi and to prevent additional thromboses from occurring.

HEPARIN

A naturally occurring, sulfated, negatively charged mucopolysaccharide, heparin is stored in the granules of human basophils and perivascular mast cells. The substance used for anticoagulation is heterogeneous in size and composition. It is prepared from the mast cells of bovine lung or porcine intestinal mucosa.

Heparin binds to *antithrombin III* molecules in plasma, and accelerates the inhibition by antithrombin III of XIIa, XIa, IXa, Xa, thrombin, and plasmin. Heparin in higher concentration also accelerates the inhibitory activity against thrombin of another plasma protein, *heparin cofactor II*. The physiologic role of heparin cofactor II is not yet known.

The half-life of an intravenous dose is approximately 1 hour. The major toxic effect is bleeding from sites of injury or surgery. An effective antidote is the positively charged substance, protamine, which forms an ionic complex with heparin and competitively impairs its binding to antithrombin III.

Intravenous heparin is used for the immediate treatment of thromboembolism. Heparin therapy is monitored with the APTT. To minimize the risk of thrombotic extension or recurrent embolism, APTT values should be at least $1^{1}/_{2}$ to 2 times control values at any time during the continuous infusion of heparin, or immediately before the next dose if heparin is given intermittently. When heparin is given continuously, the adult patient receives 5,000 to 10,000 units of the drug as a bolus, followed by 1,000 to 2,000 units per hour. Alternatively, intermittent heparin can be given to the adult patient in a dosage of 5,000 to 10,000 inhibitor units every 6 hours.

Subcutaneous heparin in lower dosage (5,000 units 2 to 3 times per day) provides *prophylaxis* against thromboembolism in many groups of medical and surgical patients, and does not usually result in a substantial prolongation of the APTT. Antithrombin III activation by subcutaneous heparin does, however, prolong the thrombin time and impede the interaction of activated coagulation factors sufficiently to provide protection against thrombosis.

Heparin-induced thrombocytopenia is relatively common. Some individuals form antibodies to the heparin extracted from animal tissue, and the antibody–heparin complexes probably result in the immune destruction of platelets in the circulation. Discontinuation of heparin reverses these processes within hours and platelets return to normal levels within days. Occasionally, patients with severe heparin-induced thrombocytopenia develop arterial and venous thromboses on the basis of intravascular platelet aggregation in vivo.

WARFARIN

Initial intravenous anticoagulation with heparin in a patient with venous thromboembolism is followed by long-term *oral* anticoagulation with a coumarin compound. *Warfarin,* the agent most commonly used, is started between days 1 and 5 of heparin therapy. Heparin is continued during the next 3 to 5 days that are required for the anticoagulant effect of warfarin to occur. Heparin is then stopped and warfarin administered for 3 to 6 months.

Warfarin is a water-soluble structural analogue of vitamin K that inhibits the posttranslational γ-carboxylation of factors II, VII, IX, and X, and proteins C and S by a carboxylase enzyme in liver cells. During the γ-carboxylation of glutamic acid residues in these proteins, reduced vitamin K (KH_2) is oxidized to vitamin K epoxide ($K>O$). The subsequent reduction steps that convert $K>O$ back to vitamin K, and then KH_2, utilize a reduced nicotinamide adenine dinucleotide (NADH) as cofactor and are inhibited by warfarin (see Fig. 15-3). In the presence of warfarin, levels of KH_2, the effective cofactor for hepatic carboxylase, decline in hepatic cells. Forms of II, VII, IX, and X that are incompletely γ-carboxylated enter the blood. These forms are less capable (or incapable) of binding via calcium bridges to phospholipids in the membranes of platelets or disrupted tissue cell membranes.

Warfarin prolongs both the APTT and PT, but is monitored with the PT. It has been customary to give a dosage of warfarin that maintains PT values at 1½ to 2 times control, in order to minimize the risk of recurrent thrombosis or embolism. Recent studies have demonstrated that less intense warfarin therapy may be equally as effective for the prevention of recurrent thromboembolism, with a lessened risk of bleeding complications. The dose of warfarin required is usually between 2.5 and 15.0 mg per day, and depends in each patient on the rate of warfarin inactivation by hepatic mixed-function oxidase enzymes.

Warfarin is absorbed from the small intestine and transported in the blood bound to albumin, from which it can be displaced by negatively charged *drugs* (sulfonamides, sulfonylureas, indomethacin, phenylbutazone, sulfinpyrazone). The concurrent administration of one of these compounds produces levels of free warfarin in the circulation that are greater than expected. The rate of transport of free warfarin into liver cells is, thereby, increased. In addition, phenylbutazone, diphenylhydantoin, sulfinpyrazone, and the sulfonylureas compete with warfarin for binding sites on hepatic mixed-function oxidase catabolizing enzymes. The inactivation of warfarin, as well as the inactivation of phenylbutazone, diphenylhydantoin, sulfinpyrazone, or sulfonylurea concurrently administered, is impeded. When any of these drugs is given along with warfarin, anticoagulation is likely to be excessive and to lead to ecchymoses, epistaxis, or bleeding from the gastrointestinal or genitourinary tracts.

Excessive warfarin anticoagulation occurs often in patients who take both warfarin and a barbiturate, and then discontinue the barbiturate. *Barbiturates* increase mixed-function oxidase activity in the endoplasmic reticulum of hepatic cells, and thus accelerate the catabolism of warfarin. Therefore, a patient who is receiving a barbiturate requires a higher dosage of warfarin for effective anticoagulation. After the barbiturate is discontinued, the rate of warfarin catabolism decreases. Bleeding from excessive warfarin anticoagulation is likely if the warfarin dosage is not reduced.

If bleeding occurs during warfarin therapy, the drug should be stopped and a water-soluble form of *vitamin K* given orally or subcutaneously. Intramuscular drugs should be avoided, if possible, in a patient with a bleeding disorder because of the danger of hematoma formation. Intravenous water-soluble vitamin K causes hypotensive reactions in some patients, and must be infused slowly. If bleeding is severe, the patient should be transfused with fresh frozen *plasma* or concentrate containing functional forms of factors II, VII, IX, and X. In patients who are to be continued on warfarin subsequently, it is preferable to transfuse plasma and withhold vitamin K, as the latter will impede the reestablishment of effective anticoagulation.

Warfarin crosses the placenta. Because of the danger of anticoagulation in the fetus or neonates, warfarin (or any other coumarin compound) should not be used in pregnant women. If given during the first trimester of pregnancy, warfarin may cause fetal skeletal malformations by impairing the γ-carboxylation of glutamic acid residues required for normal Ca^{2+}-binding by bone protein.

DRUGS THAT INTERFERE WITH PLATELET FUNCTION

Platelet adhesion, release, and aggregation are considered to be important in the pathophysiology of coronary, cerebrovascular, and peripheral arterial thrombosis. Release of the platelet α-granule growth factor (PDGF), which stimulates the replication of subintimal smooth muscle cells and fibroblasts, may be involved in the pathogenesis of atherosclerosis.

Several drugs have been used in an effort to suppress platelet function sufficiently to prevent excessive platelet accumulation. The drugs that have been used most commonly are aspirin and dipyridamole (Persantin).

Aspirin: Acetylsalicylic acid (ASA)

ASA inhibits the fatty acid cyclooxygenase activity both of platelets and endothelial cells (see Figs. 15-1 and 15-2). The synthesis of PGG_2, PGH_2, and thromboxane A_2 is irreversibly inhibited in platelets whose fatty acid cyclooxygenase enzymes are acetylated by ASA (see Fig. 15-2). The synthesis of the antiaggregation compound, PGI_2, by endothelial cells is also suppressed, even by a very low dosage (20 mg/day or ~ $1/15$ of an adult aspirin tablet) of ASA (see Fig. 15-1). However, endothelial cells, unlike platelets, can synthesize new enzyme, allowing for the rapid regeneration of PGI_2.

Dipyridamole

While it is controversial as to whether dipyridamole is effective as an antithrombotic agent, it has been widely used for the prevention of arterial thrombosis in conjunction with aspirin.

FIBRINOLYTIC AGENTS

Fibrinolytic agents are used on the premise that by activating endogenous plasminogen an increased rate or extent of fibrin digestion can be induced at local sites of thrombosis. *Streptokinase,* a bacterial exoenzyme, forms a complex with circulating plasminogen and results in the exposure of the active enzyme site in the zymogen.

Streptokinase-bound plasminogen then cleaves other plasminogen molecules to plasmin. When the amount of plasmin exceeds the inhibitory capacity of plasma α_2-antiplasmin and α-macroglobulin, the free plasmin adsorbs to fibrin polymers and proteolyzes them.

Urokinase is a type of plasminogen activator that can directly activate plasminogen to plasma. It is synthesized by renal tubular epithelial cells and is excreted into the urine, but endothelial cells are also capable of releasing this enzyme. Streptokinase and urokinase are given by intravenous infusion and cannot discriminate between free and fibrin-bound plasminogen. Both agents can therefore produce significant fibrinogenolysis.

Because streptokinase is a bacterial enzyme, and because streptococcal infections are common, *streptokinase antibodies* are often present in a patient before treatment. These antibodies usually increase during the first several days of therapy, rendering further infusion of streptokinase ineffective. Circulating immune complexes, tissue injury, and fever may also complicate therapy. None of these limitations is encountered with the human enzyme urokinase.

Tissue plasminogen activator (TPA) is the major physiologic plasminogen activator and is normally synthesized by vascular endothelial cells. Unlike streptokinase or urokinase, TPA preferentially converts plasminogen to plasmin when the zymogen is adsorbed to fibrin clots. TPA has been produced by recombinant DNA techniques, and is currently used to lyse coronary artery thrombi in patients with acute myocardial infarction. Streptokinase and urokinase have also been successfully employed in this setting.

Bleeding is a significant complication of fibrinolytic therapy. It occurs because free plasmin generated in excess of plasma inhibitory capacity proteolyzes fibrinogen, factor V, factor VIII, and other coagulation proteins. In addition, free plasmin in the circulation binds to, and degrades, fibrin polymers that are important in hemostasis.

Fibrinolytic therapy has been useful in patients with extensive pulmonary emboli and has also been recommended for use soon after venous thrombosis (before fibroblast invasion and collagen formation). At present, it is uncertain whether fibrinolytic therapy in the latter condition prevents venous valvular damage and decreases postthrombophlebitic complications (i.e., venous congestion and edema).

Case Development Problems: Hemostasis and Thrombosis

Patient History No. 1

An 8-year-old girl has a rash on the lower extremities. The mother states that the child had a cold 2 weeks previously, but otherwise had been well without fever, chills, malaise, anorexia, nausea, vomiting, or abdominal pain. The child says that her gums bled recently when she brushed her teeth, and that she has not taken any medications.

Her only physical findings are petechiae on the ankles. Hemoglobin (Hb) is 13.0 gm%, hematocrit (hct) 38 percent, WBC 7,500/μL with a normal differential count 1, and platelet count 5,000μ/L.

1. What is the diagnosis?

In the absence of drug ingestion, the problem is most likely to be acute idiopathic (autoimmune) thrombocytopenic purpura (ITP).

2. What is the natural history of the disease?

ITP in childhood frequently abates spontaneously.

3. What therapy is indicated? What would be the therapeutic approach if the thrombocytopenia were to persist for 3 to 6 months?

Often no therapy is needed. Short-term therapy with prednisone (or another glucocorticoid) or intravenous γ-globulin is appropriate if thrombocytopenia is severe (<20,000/μL), if bleeding occurs, if surgery is required, or if the child suffers trauma. Long persistent thrombocytopenia is rare in acute ITP in childhood but might require splenectomy.

Patient History No. 2

A 70-year-old insulin-dependent diabetic woman is admitted for evaluation of thrombocytopenia and severe metrorrhagia that requires transfusion of 2 units of packed red cells. Two years before she noted easy bruising but no blood count was performed. For the past 4 years, she has been on digoxin, a thiazide diuretic, and KCl elixir for treatment of congestive heart failure following a myocardial infarction. On physical examination many purpuric and ecchymotic lesions are noted on the legs and the flexor surface of the arms. Vital signs are normal. The chest is clear, heart sounds are normal, and the liver and spleen are not enlarged.

Admitting laboratory values are: Hb 11.2 gm%, hct 36 percent, WBC 9,000/μL with normal differential count, reticulocytes 6.1 percent, and platelets 4,000/μL. Bone marrow is hypercellular, with orderly maturation of the erythroid and myeloid series, abundant megakaryocytes, and hemosiderin present.

Prednisone (60 mg/day) is begun and after 4 days the platelet count is 18,000/μL with no petechiae. After 7 days the platelet count is 164,000/μL. She is discharged on 50 mg prednisone every other day and an attempt is made to decrease the dosage further. At 15 mg prednisone every other day, her platelet count drops precipitously. The dosage is increased to 10 mg prednisone twice a day, and her platelets increase to normal. After 6 weeks she complains of epigastric pain. She has gained 30 pounds, her blood pressure is elevated, and her diabetes has become more difficult to control. The prednisone is decreased again; she does well for 3 months, and then returns with petechiae and a platelet count of 3,000/μL. She is hospitalized, given prednisone (100 mg/day), and by the fifth day her platelets are 45,000/μL. Splenectomy is performed without complication. Prednisone is continued and 7 days after surgery the platelet count is 425,000/μL. Over the next several months, each attempt to reduce prednisone dosage results in a recurrence of thrombocytopenia. Immunosuppressive therapy with 6-mercaptopurine is begun and prednisone is discontinued over a period of months. During the next year her platelet counts remain normal on immunosuppressive therapy alone. She is now receiving no therapy and has had no recurrence of thrombocytopenia.

1. What was the reason for her thrombocytopenia?

Chronic ITP.

2. Did she have the usual response to therapy?

The response to high-dose prednisone and relapse with lower doses are common in patients with adult-onset chronic ITP. However, the majority of these patients will respond well to splenectomy and will not require immunosuppressive therapy.

3. Would any of the patient's medications have been suspected of causing the thrombocytopenia?

Digoxin is a rare cause of drug-induced thrombocytopenia. Thiazide diuretics result in thrombocytopenia more frequently; this is usually due to suppression of platelet production via a toxic effect on bone marrow megakaryocytes, and the degree of thrombocytopenia is usually mild. Rarely, a thiazide may produce severe thrombocytopenia due to increased platelet destruction.

4. In any thrombocytopenic patient, what two standing orders should be entered in the chart to prevent iatrogenic bleeding complications?

The patient is to receive no intramuscular injections and no aspirin-containing drugs!

Patient History No. 3

A 6-year-old boy is struck in the thigh by a baseball and an extensive hematoma subsequently develops. He is admitted to a local hospital and the hematoma is drained. Following the operation, the patient bleeds profusely, requiring 4 units of blood. A PT before the operation is normal.

1. What coagulation factors are tested in the prothrombin time? What factors are not measured?

   VII, X, V, II, and fibrinogen (tested); XII, kininogen, prekallikrein, XI, IX, and VIII (not measured).

2. What additional screening tests should have been done before surgery? What further historical information would you request?

   A platelet count, PT and APTT are screening tests to consider before major surgical procedures. A drug history should always be obtained. It should also have been determined if this child had previously bled excessively after injury, surgery, or dental care, and if any relative had a bleeding history.

Additional history revealed that the mother's nephew had bled following dental extraction, although he had taken no medication at the time. The following data were obtained on plasma of the patient and his family members:

APTT	(sec.)
Normal	35
Patient	52
Father	35
Mother	34
Mother's sister	35
Sister's son (patient's cousin)	58

3. What does the pattern of inheritance suggest? Deficiencies of which factors are compatible with this inheritance pattern?

   An X-chromosome–linked recessive disorder, either IX or VIII deficiency.
   The patient was found to have a plasma VIII level of 5 percent, confirming the diagnosis of mild hemophilia A.

4. Would vWF antigen levels likely be normal or reduced in this family?

   Normal.

Patient History No. 4

A 17-year-old young man bruises easily, bleeds excessively after minor cuts, and has epistaxis that has required transfusion on several occasions beginning in childhood. He has intermittent hematuria, and frequent painful swelling of the right knee, ankle, and elbow for which he has received transfusions of fresh frozen plasma.

He lives in a small town and withdrew from school because he was unable to climb stairs to the 10th grade classroom. Although he has obtained several jobs in local stores, he cannot work regularly because of recurrent hemarthroses.

The patient's mother states that she "bruises easily"; however, she had dental surgery without excessive bleeding. The patient's maternal aunt also "bruises easily." The mother has four asymptomatic sisters and a nephew who died in infancy of bleeding after a laceration; three of her seven brothers are "bleeders."

On physical examination the patient appears healthy except for limitation of motion in large joints. His mucus membranes are pink and he has no jaundice, hepatosplenomegaly, or cardiovascular abnormalities. He has a normal CBC, platelet count, and differential count. Liver function tests and urinalysis are normal.

1. The differential diagnosis includes which coagulation abnormalities?

   The history of death from hemorrhage in a male cousin on the maternal side suggests that the defect is likely to be X-chromosomed–linked. A history of "easy bruising" is obtained frequently in clinical practice, and is probably not important in this case since the patient's mother had uneventful dental surgery. Hemarthroses most frequently occur in patients with severe deficiency of either VIII or IX.

2. What coagulation factor assays should be done?

   VIII and IX.

3. What are the psychological and sociologic implications of this disorder?

   The extreme problems of daily living in patients with severe hemophilia A and B are exemplified by the patient's difficulties with education and employment. Moreover, many hemophiliacs who received factor concentrates in the early 1980s have developed antibodies to the virus responsible for AIDS (human immunodeficiency virus–1).

4. Why were liver function tests obtained?

Patients with severe hemophilia A or B have been exposed to hepatitis virus, as well as other infectious agents, in the blood products used for replacement therapy.

Patient History No. 5

A 34-year-old woman gives a history of excessive bleeding after trauma. Her bleeding tendency was first noted in childhood, when she had several episodes of spontaneous epistaxis that required transfusions and local cauterization. Epistaxis occurred less frequently during adolescence. The patient bruises easily and has menorrhagia (7–10 days of bleeding) that has not been corrected by several dilatation and curettage procedures. Vaginal bleeding lasted for 2 to 3 weeks after the birth of each of her four children. Her 5-year-old son has frequent epistaxis. The patient's mother and sister have menorrhagia and a history of excessive postoperative hemorrhage.

Physical examination is normal. Laboratory values include: Hb, 13.3 gm% hct 39 percent, WBC 7,500/μL with normal differential count, and platelets 282,000/μL. Her bleeding time is 16 minutes. She denies taking any medications.

1. What is the most likely diagnosis? Which type of the disease is most prevalent?

von Willebrand's disease; type I (classic) vWD.

2. Predict the results of the following studies:

Assays of VIII, IX, and XI
Ristocetin cofactor activity
vWF antigen level
Platelet aggregation in response to arachidonic acid, collagen, ADP, thrombin, and epinephrine

Factor VIII, ristocetin cofactor activity and vWF antigen levels will be low in patient plasma. Factors IX and XI and platelet aggregation (in response to all agents other than ristocetin) will be normal.

3. How is this disorder transmitted?

As an autosomal dominant trait.

4. What is the appropriate therapy in anticipation of a surgical procedure?

Cryoprecipitate (for all vWD types) or DDAVP (for vWD type I patients).

Patient History No. 6

A 51-year-old woman is admitted with lethargy, dizziness, and bilateral edema of the legs. In the past she underwent abdominal surgery without excessive bleeding. On physical examination she is afebrile with bilateral rales. Cardiac and abdominal evaluation is normal. Blood gases are pO_2, 52 mm Hg; pCO_2, 41 mm Hg; and pH, 7.41. Bilateral lower-lobe perfusion defects are seen on ventilation–perfusion lung scan, consistent with pulmonary emboli. She is placed on heparin, and then warfarin. Her PT at discharge is 21 seconds (control, 11 seconds) on a warfarin dosage of 5 mg by mouth each day.

During a subsequent clinic visit, bruises and ecchymoses are noted. The patient also has a cough and hoarseness. An ecchymotic lesion is present on the uvula and direct laryngoscopy reveals a vocal cord hematoma. PT is 60 seconds (control, 12 seconds). Warfarin is discontinued and she is transfused with II, VII, IX, X concentrate. Posttransfusion PT is 12 seconds. Her hoarseness and cough resolve and she is discharged.

Two months later she is admitted for a recurrence of the initial pulmonary problem. She is given heparin and subsequently discharged on 7.5 mg warfarin daily. One month later she returns with ecchymoses, epistaxis, gingival bleeding, right upper quadrant pain, and anorexia. On physical examination scleral icterus and a subconjunctival hemorrhage are found. The liver is tender, with a span of 17 cm. Hb is 11 gm%, hct 33 percent, platelet count 142,000/μL, and WBC 5,400/μL. Serum bilirubin is 6.1 mg% and alkaline phosphatase, SGOT and SGPT ("liver enzymes") are all markedly elevated. PT and APTT are both greater than 120 seconds. She is given oral vitamin K and transfused with fresh frozen plasma. PT and APTT are corrected partially by plasma; however, they remain about three times control values until her hepatic enzymes return to normal. At discharge her PT is 13 seconds (control, 11 seconds) and APTT is 34 seconds (control, 35 seconds).

1. What was the patient's initial thrombotic problem?

Pulmonary embolism.

2. Was anticoagulation with warfarin adequate when she was discharged from her first hospitalization?

Yes. However, the PT was on the high side of the therapeutic range.

3. Why was she given II, VII, IX, X concentrate?

Bleeding into the airway because of excessive anticoagulation is a medical emergency, requiring immediate replacement of functional forms of II, VII, IX, and X. Her physician elected to use lyophilized II, VII, IX, X concentrate in order to provide considerable quantities of these coagulation factors rapidly. It is usually preferable, however, to administer fresh frozen plasma in this setting.

4. What was her diagnosis on the last admission? What was the probable etiology of this abnormality? Why was anticoagulation excessive at this time?

She acquired hepatitis from the lyophilized II, VII, IX, X concentrate transfused previously. Liver cell synthesis of functional forms of II, VII, IX and X was reduced by the viral infection.

Patient History No. 7

The following vignettes are examples of clinical mishaps. What errors in clinical management were made?

1. A 15-year-old boy is admitted with deep venous thrombosis following tryouts for the school football team several days earlier. By physical examination he has a swollen, tender, erythematous left leg. The only abnormal laboratory values are a protein C level of 40 percent (normal range, 65–135%). The patient is started on intravenous heparin and is given 30 mg warfarin by mouth. One day later he develops skin necrosis on the extremities and a prothrombin time of 30 seconds. What led to this thrombotic complication so soon after the patient received warfarin? (Refer to the half-lives [$t^{1/2}$] in Table 15-1.)

The 30-mg dosage of warfarin was excessive and caused profound reduction in the capacity of liver cells to synthesize functional forms of factor II, VII, IX, and X; protein C; and protein S. Factor VII and protein C have short in vivo half-lives and are the first coagulation factors to be depleted. Warfarin induced acute, severe protein C deficiency in this patient, who already had pre-existing hereditary protein C deficiency, at a time when considerable quantities of functional forms of II, IX, and X still remained in his plasma, resulting in the development of skin necrosis. Heparin therapy did not prevent this complication. There is no reason to use large loading doses of warfarin. The half-lives of prothrombin and factor X are relatively long and it will take 3 to 5 days to lower the functional levels of these factors to concentrations at which antithrombotic protection is afforded.

2. A 58-year-old man is admitted with pulmonary emboli. During the hospitalization he is treated with phenobarbital and 5 mg per day warfarin; PT values are 16 to 18 seconds. He is discharged on

5 mg per day of warfarin and no other drugs. Two weeks later hematuria develops and he is found to have a PT of 52 seconds. The catabolism of warfarin was accelerated by phenobarbital in this patient while he was hospitalized. When he was discharged the phenobarbital was discontinued, the rate of warfarin catabolism decreased subsequently, and a 5 mg/day warfarin dosage proved to be excessive.

3. A 34-year-old woman with epilepsy, controlled by diphenylhydantoin (Dilantin), is admitted with deep venous thrombosis. She is treated initially with heparin and then with warfarin. Her PT values are 16 to 20 seconds on an extremely low warfarin dosage (2.5 mg every other day). Three weeks after discharge she develops a staggering gait, swollen gums, and epistaxis. Her PT is 43 seconds.

Warfarin and Dilantin compete for hepatic mixed-function oxidase enzymes. When the drugs were given concurrently, the catabolic rate of each was decreased. Excessive levels of both drugs were present in the circulation, and caused both Dilantin toxicity and bleeding from warfarin overdose.

Selected Readings

Bloom, A. L. Factor VIII inhibitors revisited. *Br. J. Haematol.* 49 : 319, 1981.

Cimo, P. L. et al. Heparin-induced thrombocytopenia associated with platelet aggregating antibodies and arterial thrombosis. *Am. J. Hematol.* 6 : 125, 1979.

Deykin, D. Warfarin therapy. *N. Engl. J. Med.* 283 : 801, 1970.

Esmon, C. T., and Owen, W. G. Identification of an endothelial cell cofactor for thrombin-catalyzed activation of protein C. *Proc. Natl. Acad. Sci. USA* 78 : 2249, 1981.

Feinstein, D. I. Diagnosis and management of disseminated intravascular coagulation: The role of heparin therapy. *Blood* 60 : 284, 1982.

Gallop, P. M. et al. Carboxylated calcium-binding proteins and vitamin K. *N. Engl. J. Med.* 302 : 1460, 1980.

Gallus, A. S., and Hirsh, J. Treatment of venous thromboembolic disease. *Semin. Thromb. Hemost.* 2 : 291, 1976.

Hoyer, L. W. The factor VIII complex—structure and function. *Blood* 58 : 1, 1981.

Jackson, C. M., and Nemerson, Y. Blood coagulation. *Ann. Rev. Biochem.* 49 : 765, 1980.

Jaffe, E. A. Endothelial cells and the biology of factor VIII. *N. Engl. J. Med.* 296 : 377, 1977.

Karpatkin, S. Autoimmune thrombocytopenic purpura. *Blood* 56 : 329, 1980.

Lijnen, H. R., and Collen, D. Interaction of plasminogen activators and inhibitors with plasminogen and fibrin. *Semin. Thromb. Hemost.* 8 : 2, 1982.

Mammen, E. F. Congenital coagulation disorders. *Semin. Thromb. Hemost.* 9 : 1, 1983.

Moake, J. L. et al. Unusually large plasma factor VIII: von Willebrand factor multimers in chronic relapsing thrombotic thrombocytopenic purpura. *N. Engl. J. Med.* 307 : 1432, 1982.

Moncada S., and Vane, J. V. R. Arachidonic acid metabolites and the interactions between platelets and blood-vessel walls. *N. Engl. J. Med.* 300 : 1142, 1979.

Moss, R. A. Drug-induced immune thrombocytopenia. *Am. J. Hematol.* 9 : 439, 1980.

Rosenberg, R. D. Action and interaction of antithrombin and heparin. *N. Engl. J. Med.* 292 : 146, 1975.

Ruggeri, Z. M. et al. Multimeric composition of factor VIII/von Willebrand factor following administration of DDAVP: Implications for pathophysiology and therapy of von Willebrand's disease subtypes. *Blood* 59 : 1272, 1278, 1982.

Zucker, M. B. The functioning of blood platelets. *Sci. Am.* June 1980, p. 86.

Index